An **OUTCOME INDICATOR** is a specific, observable, and measurable characteristic or change that will represent achievement of the outcome.

From: United Way of America. *Measuring Program Outcomes: A Practical Approach.* Alexandria, VA: United Way of America; 1996.

For more information, contact
CDC Office on Smoking and Health
770-488-5703

For additional copies, e-mail your request to:
tobaccoinfo@cdc.gov

Suggested citation

Starr G, Rogers T, Schooley M, Porter S, Wiesen E, Jamison N. *Key Outcome Indicators for Evaluating Comprehensive Tobacco Control Programs.* Atlanta, GA: Centers for Disease Control and Prevention; 2005.

Naming of surveillance systems, databases, and evaluation tools is for example purposes only and does not constitute endorsement by the Centers for Disease Control and Prevention or the U.S. Department of Health and Human Services.

KEY OUTCOME INDICATORS FOR

Evaluating Comprehensive
Tobacco Control Programs

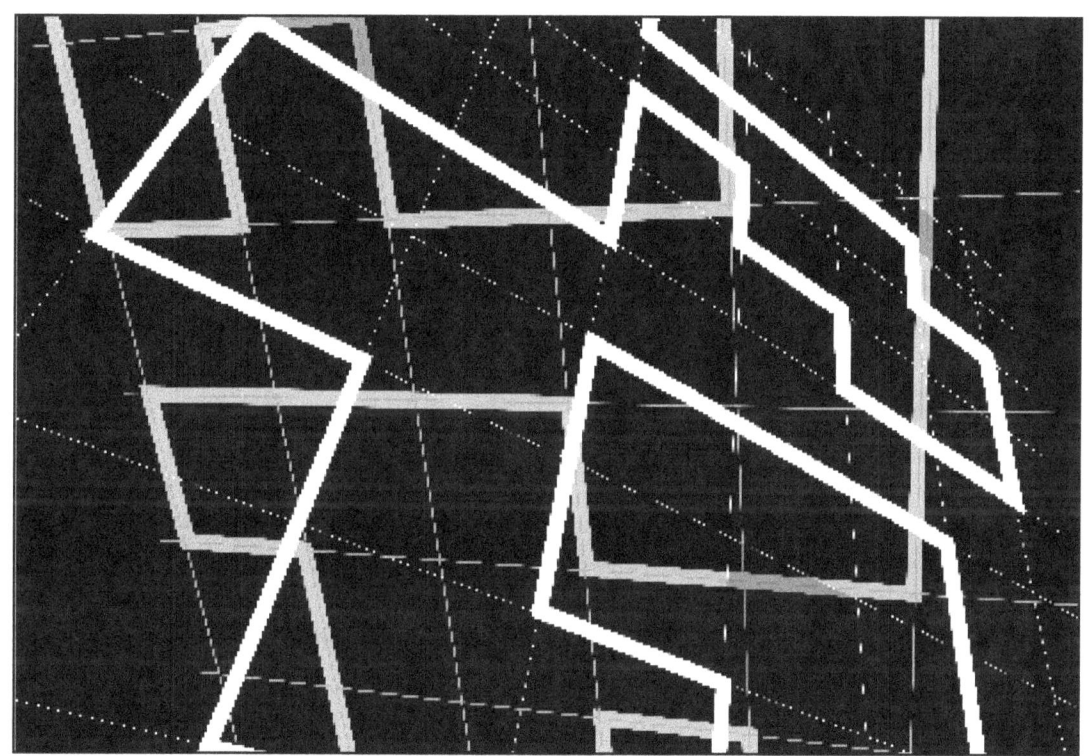

Acknowledgments

We would like to extend special thanks to the following individuals for their assistance in preparing and reviewing this publication.

Expert Panel Members (Appendix C)

Centers for Disease Control and Prevention (in alphabetical order):
Stephen Babb
Patrick Cox
Linda Crossett
Martha Engstrom
Reba Griffith
Corinne Husten
Kat Jackson
Jerelyn Jordan
Brian Judd
Sharon Kohout
Goldie MacDonald
Allison MacNeil
Helen McClintock
Bill Marx
Patrick Nadol
Terry Pechacek
Linda Pederson
Lisa Petersen
Jamilyn Renna
Robert Robinson
Abby Rosenthal
Angela Trosclair

We also give special thanks to:

Pamela Clark
Battelle Centers for Public Health Research and Evaluation

Matthew Farrelly
Research Triangle Institute

Gary Giovino
Roswell Park Cancer Institute

Preface

If the United States were to meet the *Healthy People 2010* goal of reducing smoking prevalence to 12% among adults and 16% among young people aged 14 through 17 years, more than 7 million premature deaths after 2010 could be prevented.[1,2] Studies show that investing in state tobacco control programs and implementing effective tobacco control policies significantly reduces cigarette consumption and improves health outcomes.[3-9] To continue funding state programs, however, legislators, policy makers, and other funders of state programs want to see evidence that the program is effective and that resources are being used wisely.

To produce such evidence, state tobacco control programs must evaluate their programs. Good evaluation is the key to persuading policy makers that your program is producing results that will lead to improved health for the community.

If good evaluation is key to proving that your program is effective, then selecting the right indicators to measure is key to a good evaluation. That's where this book will help.

This publication is a companion to the 2001 publication *Introduction to Program Evaluation for Comprehensive Tobacco Control Programs*, which is based on the Centers for Disease Control and Prevention's (CDC's) *Framework for Program Evaluation*.[10,11] In *Introduction to Program Evaluation for Comprehensive Tobacco Control Programs*, we discuss in detail the six steps of a good evaluation as they apply to tobacco prevention and control programs:

1. Engage stakeholders.
2. Describe the program.
3. Focus the evaluation.
4. Gather credible evidence.
5. Justify your conclusions.
6. Ensure evaluation findings are used and share lessons learned.

This new publication provides information on selecting indicators and linking them to outcomes, the main focus of step 3 (focus the evaluation) and step 4 (gather credible evidence).

In *Introduction to Program Evaluation for Comprehensive Tobacco Control Programs*, we described how to select indicators to measure program outcomes. We also gave examples of indicators and suggested sources of data on those indicators.[10] This publication goes further. Here we discuss in detail 120 evidence-based key indicators that have been scientifically linked to program outcomes. We also document the evidence that shows the value of using these indicators to measure the progress of a state tobacco control program.

To help you make informed choices about which indicators are most suitable for your program, we engaged a panel of experts in the field of tobacco control to rate each indicator on various criteria, including overall quality, resources needed, strength of evaluation evidence, utility, accepted practice, and face validity to policy makers. The ratings will help the reader decide, for example, which indicators can be measured within budget or which indicators are likely to carry the most weight with policy makers. In essence, this publication is a consumer's guide to tobacco control indicators for program managers and evaluators.

In this publication we provide examples of data sources and survey questions that evaluators can use to gather data from their programs' target populations. We were particularly careful about our choice of example data sources and survey questions. Most come from commonly used state and national surveys and surveillance systems, and using them will allow managers and evaluators to compare their findings with data from other states and over time.

Evaluation of key indicators over time will help monitor progress toward expected outcomes and refine program activities as needed. Using well designed evaluation methods will increase your program's and your evaluation's chance of success. We encourage you to read more about the multiple purposes of program evaluation in *Introduction to Program Evaluation for Comprehensive Tobacco Control Programs*.[10]

We also hope that this publication will help to advance national evaluation and surveillance efforts by encouraging managers and evaluators of state tobacco control programs to use standard questions from commonly used state or national surveys or surveillance systems. If states use comparable indicators, questions, and collection methods, we will be better able to assess the national impact of state tobacco control programs.

Technical Assistance

CDC is ready to help state and territorial health departments plan, implement, and evaluate tobacco prevention and control programs. To contact CDC's Office on Smoking and Health, please call (770) 488–5703 or e-mail at tobaccoinfo@cdc.gov.

References

1. U.S. Department of Health and Human Services. *Healthy people 2010*. 2nd edition. With *Understanding and improving health and objectives for improving health*. 2 vols. Washington, DC: Government Printing Office; 2000.

2. U.S. Department of Health and Human Services. *The health consequences of smoking: a report of the Surgeon General*. Atlanta, GA: Centers for Disease Control and Prevention; 2004.

3. Farrelly M, Pechacek T, Chaloupka F. The impact of tobacco control program expenditures on aggregate cigarette sales: 1981–2000. *Journal of Health Economics*. 2003;22(5):843–59.

4. Sargent R, Shepard R, Glantz S. Reduced incidence of admissions for myocardial infarction associated with public smoking ban before and after study. *British Medical Journal.* 2004 Apr 24;328(7446):977–80.

5. Cowling DW, Kwong SL, Schlag R, Lloyd JC, Bal DG. Declines in lung cancer rates: California, 1988–1997. *Morbidity and Mortality Weekly Report.* 2000;49:1066–9.

6. Jemal A, Cokkinides VE, Shafey O, Thun MJ. Lung cancer trends in young adults: an early indicator of progress in tobacco control (United States). *Cancer Causes & Control.* 2003;14(6):579–85.

7. Barnoya J, Glantz S. Association of the California tobacco control program with declines in lung cancer incidence. *Cancer Causes & Control.* 2004;15(7):689–95.

8. Max W, Rice DP, Sung HY, Zhang X, Miller L. The economic burden of smoking in California. *Tobacco Control.* 2004;13(3):264–7.

9. Tauras JA, Chaloupka FJ, Farrelly MC, Giovino GA, Wakefield M, Johnston LD, O'Malley PM, Kloska DD, Pechacek TF. State tobacco control spending and youth smoking. *American Journal of Public Health.* 2005;95:338–44.

10. MacDonald G, Starr G, Schooley M, Yee SL, Klimowski K, Turner K. *Introduction to program evaluation for comprehensive tobacco control programs.* Atlanta, GA: Centers for Disease Control and Prevention; 2001.

11. Centers for Disease Control and Prevention. Framework for program evaluation in public health practice. *Morbidity and Mortality Weekly Report.* 1999;48 (RR-11): 1–40.

Table of Contents

Preface iii
How This Book Is Organized ix

Chapter 1 Introduction 1

Chapter 2 Goal Area 1: Preventing Initiation of Tobacco Use Among Young People 17
    Logic Model: Preventing Initiation of Tobacco Use Among Young People. 19
    Outcome 6: Increased Knowledge of, Improved Anti-tobacco Attitudes Toward, and Increased Support for Policies to Reduce Youth Initiation. 25
    Outcome 7: Increased Anti-tobacco Policies and Programs in Schools. 39
    Outcome 8: Increased Restriction and Enforcement of Restrictions on Tobacco Sales to Minors 61
    Outcome 9: Reduced Tobacco Industry Influences 72
    Outcome 10: Reduced Susceptibility to Experimentation with Tobacco Products 89
    Outcome 11: Decreased Access to Tobacco Products. 98
    Outcome 12: Increased Price of Tobacco Products 108
    Outcome 13: Reduced Initiation of Tobacco Use by Young People 112
    Outcome 14: Reduced Tobacco-use Prevalence Among Young People. 116

Chapter 3 Goal Area 2: Eliminating Nonsmokers' Exposure to Secondhand Smoke 121
    Logic Model: Eliminating Nonsmokers' Exposure to Secondhand Smoke 123
    Outcome 3: Increased Knowledge of, Improved Attitudes Toward, and Increased Support for the Creation and Active Enforcement of Tobacco-free Policies 127
    Outcome 4: Creation of Tobacco-free Policies 147
    Outcome 5: Enforcement of Tobacco-free Public Policies 159
    Outcome 6: Compliance with Tobacco-free Policies 165
    Outcome 7: Reduced Exposure to Secondhand Smoke. 174
    Outcome 8: Reduced Tobacco Consumption 184

Chapter 4 Goal Area 3: Promoting Quitting Among Adults and Young People 191
    Logic Model: Promoting Quitting Among Adults and Young People 193
    Outcome 7: Establishment or Increased Use of Cessation Services. 197
    Outcome 8: Increased Awareness, Knowledge, Intention to Quit, and Support for Policies That Support Cessation 209
    Outcome 9: Increase in the Number of Health Care Providers and Health Care Systems Following Public Health Service (PHS) Guidelines. 223
    Outcome 10: Increased Insurance Coverage for Cessation Services 237
    Outcome 11: Increased Number of Quit Attempts and Quit Attempts Using Proven Cessation Methods 242
    Outcome 12: Increased Price of Tobacco Products 249
    Outcome 13: Increased Cessation Among Adults and Young People 252
    Outcome 14: Reduced Tobacco-use Prevalence and Consumption 259

Chapter 5 ▸ Future Directions 267

Appendices and Glossary 273
    Appendix A: National Tobacco Control Program 275
    Appendix B: Selecting and Rating the Indicators 279
    Appendix C: Expert Panel Members 293
    Appendix D: Data Source Indicator Table 295
    Glossary 301

How This Book Is Organized

The chart below shows the layout of this book.

General Information

Preface

How This Book Is Organized

Chapter 1: Introduction
- Purpose
- Audience
- The National Tobacco Control Program
- Logic Models
- Outcome Components
- Indicators

Using This Book to Plan a State Tobacco Control Program Evaluation

Merging program planning and evaluation planning for state tobacco control programs. Included is a hypothetical example.

First Three Goals of the National Tobacco Control Program

Chapter 2: Goal Area 1
Preventing Initiation of Tobacco Use Among Young People

Chapter 3: Goal Area 2
Eliminating Nonsmokers' Exposure to Secondhand Smoke

Chapter 4: Goal Area 3
Promoting Quitting Among Adults and Young People

Each goal area has three major sections

Logic Model
Depicts causal pathways that link outcome components

Indicators
A list of indicators for each outcome component in the logic model

Outcome Component
- Outcome overview: Empirical support
- Key indicators: Measurable characteristics
- Indicator rating table: Indicator ratings by criterion
- Indicator profiles: Indicator details

Additional Information

Chapter 5: Future Directions
- Develop process indicators
- Identify indicators to measure tobacco-related disparities
- Encourage evaluation research

Appendices
A. National Tobacco Control Program
B. Selecting and Rating the Indicators
C. Expert Panel Members
D. Data Source Indicator Table

Glossary
Definitions of words and terms used in this book

CHAPTER 1
Introduction

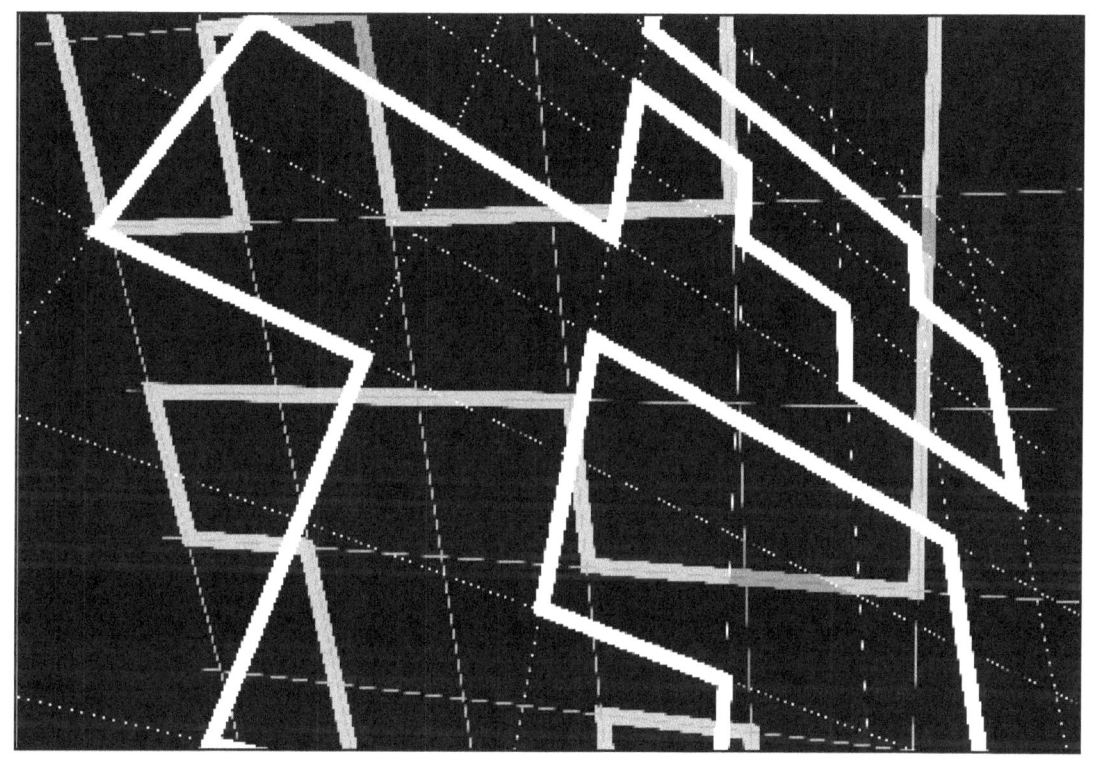

Introduction

Purpose

CDC developed this publication to help state and territorial health departments plan and evaluate state tobacco control programs. This publication is a companion to *Best Practices for Comprehensive Tobacco Control Programs, Introduction to Program Evaluation for Comprehensive Tobacco Control Programs,* and *Surveillance and Evaluation Data Sources for Comprehensive Tobacco Control Programs.*[1-3]

Audience

The primary audiences for this publication are (1) planners, managers, and evaluators of state programs to prevent or control tobacco use and (2) CDC's national partners in the fight against tobacco use.

The National Tobacco Control Program

As part of its mission to reduce the incidence of tobacco-related disease and preventable death, CDC created the National Tobacco Control Program (NTCP) to encourage coordinated, nationwide activities. The goal of the NTCP is to reduce tobacco-related disease, disability, and death. This overarching goal is subdivided into four goal areas:

- Preventing initiation of tobacco use among young people.
- Eliminating nonsmokers' exposure to secondhand smoke.
- Promoting quitting among adults and young people.
- Identifying and eliminating tobacco-related disparities.

For more information on the NTCP, see Appendix A.

Logic Models

As explained in *Introduction to Program Evaluation for Comprehensive Tobacco Control Programs*, logic models depict the presumed causal pathways that connect program inputs, activities, and outputs with short-term, intermediate, and long-term outcomes.[2] An example of a basic logic model is provided in Figure 1.

To help tobacco control programs with planning and evaluation, we updated logic models previously published in the *Introduction to Program Evaluation for Comprehensive Tobacco Control Programs.*

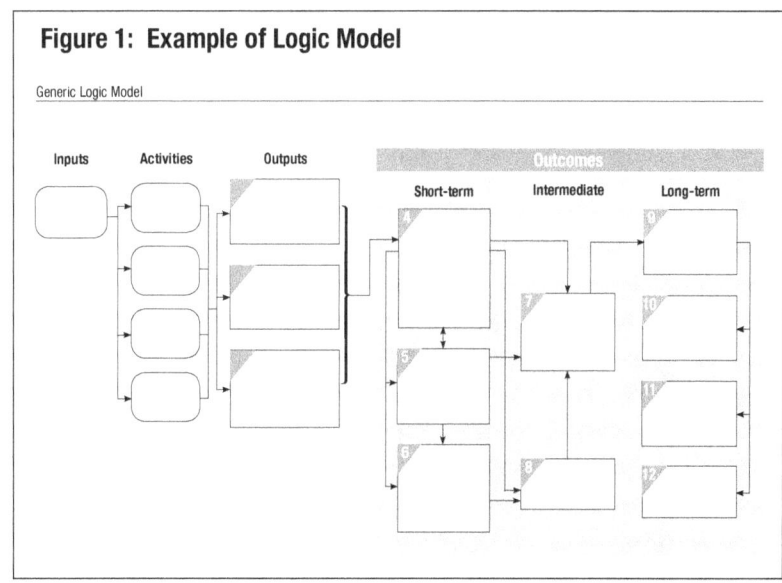

Figure 1: Example of Logic Model

We numbered the outputs (direct results of program activities) and outcomes in each logic model to allow for easy reference in discussing the links between logic model components.

The logic models for the NTCP's goal areas can be used in several ways:
- To see the links between program activities; outputs; and short-term, intermediate, and long-term outcomes.
- To identify relevant short-term, intermediate, and long-term outcomes.
- To assist in selecting indicators to measure outcomes.

Outcome Components

The outcome components in the logic models are categorized as short-term, intermediate, or long-term to indicate a presumed causal sequence.

For each outcome component, we provide an outcome overview in which we summarize the scientific evidence in support of the assumption that implementing the program activities shown in the NTCP logic model for a particular goal area will lead to the short-term or intermediate outcomes shown in the same NTCP logic model. In turn, achieving the short-term and intermediate outcomes will affect the long-term outcomes in the logic model. For example, if a program is working with the example logic model shown in Figure 1 and the program selects outcome component 7 as its intermediate outcome, program activities designed to achieve changes in short-term outcomes 4, 5, and 6 (linked vertically on the logic model) should lead to changes in outcome 7 (linked horizontally with outcomes 4, 5, and 6 on the logic model). Indeed, not only will changes to outcomes 4, 5, and 6 affect outcome 7, but they will also affect intermediate outcome 8 as well as long-term outcomes 9 and 10 and distal outcomes 11 and 12. Distal outcomes are the last two outcomes in each logic model. They are the longest-term outcomes and are the same for the first three NTCP goal areas.

Indicators

Outcome indicators are specific, observable, and measurable characteristics or changes that represent achievement of an outcome.[4]

For example, if your program is trying to increase restrictions on young people's access to tobacco and you measured the proportion of jurisdictions with policies that control the location, number, and density of retail outlets that sell cigarettes, the result would indicate the extent of your progress toward creating restricted access policies in all jurisdictions.

Most indicators we discuss in this publication are useful for measuring progress toward reducing cigarette use. However, we encourage programs to broaden their surveillance and evaluation activities to include measuring all forms of tobacco use, including spit tobacco (smokeless), bidis, small cigars, and loose tobacco (roll your own).

In this publication, indicators are organized by outcome component in the logic models for goal areas 1, 2, and 3 of the NTCP. We list indicators for only the first three NTCP goal areas because the logic models for these goal areas focus on evaluating and measuring the *effects* of a state tobacco prevention and control program. The focus of the logic model for goal area 4 (page 271) is on developing and increasing organizational capacity to plan and implement activities to identify and eliminate tobacco-related disparities. Currently, few well-established, evidence-based indicators are available for measuring a program's success in increasing organizational capacity in this area. See Chapter 5 for more details.

Indicators to measure distal outcomes in each goal area (i.e., reduced tobacco-related morbidity, mortality, and disparities) are not included in this book for two reasons. First, the research base establishing linkage between behavioral outcomes (e.g., reductions in tobacco consumption and tobacco use prevalence) and the distal outcomes is well established. Therefore, tobacco control programs need to demonstrate only an effect on behavioral outcomes and they can assume that these will lead to favorable health effects. Second, we determined that the greatest expressed needs of the states for evaluation assistance would be addressed by identifying short-term and intermediate outcome indicators.

This does not mean that programs should not monitor their effect on the distal outcomes in the NTCP logic models. Although some tobacco-related diseases (e.g., lung cancer) are slow to be affected by tobacco prevention and control programs, many positive health effects are realized relatively quickly (e.g., reductions in the risk of cardiovascular disease and low birthweight in babies).[5] Some long-standing programs (e.g., California Tobacco Control Program) have been able to show an effect on long-term outcomes, but most states have not had comprehensive programs in place long enough to show such effects.[6-8]

We also do not intend to imply that measuring outcomes is sufficient for evaluating a tobacco control program. It is not. Equally important is process evaluation, which focuses on measuring program implementation. (See *Introduction to Program Evaluation for Comprehensive Tobacco Control Programs* for information on process evaluation.)[2] CDC has begun researching indicators for use in process evaluation. See Chapter 5 for a brief discussion of this topic.

Program managers and evaluators who want to evaluate their progress toward NTCP goal area 4 (identifying and eliminating tobacco-related disparities) can do so by using the indicators for the other three goal areas and analyzing the data gathered by race, ethnicity, or tobacco-related disparity. For example, by measuring the level of confirmed awareness of media messages on the dangers of secondhand smoke (indicator 2.3.1) across various racial populations, evaluators can learn whether the messages' reach varied among racial groups.

Indicator Selection and Rating

CDC proposed a set of outcome indicators and engaged a panel of 16 experts in tobacco control practice, evaluation, and research to assess each indicator on the basis of the following criteria: strength of evaluation evidence, utility, face validity to policy makers, conformity with accepted practice, uniqueness, overall quality, and how essential the indicator is for evaluating state tobacco control programs.

The experts also indicated the level of resources needed to collect and analyze data on the indicator. In addition to rating the indicators that CDC proposed, the experts suggested other indicators and sources of data for those indicators.

CDC reviewed the experts' responses, comments, and suggestions and compiled the results into an individual rating across criteria for each indicator. A few indicators, however, have no ratings because they were added at the suggestion of the experts after the rating process was complete. These indicators have the symbol NR after their numbers.

In addition, the experts' ratings showed that the criterion "essential for evaluation" was highly correlated with "overall quality" and is therefore omitted from the indicator rating tables described below. Likewise, the "uniqueness" criterion was used only to narrow the indicator lists (see Appendix B).

For a list of expert panel members, see Appendix C.

Because some reviewers said they were not familiar with all the research on all goal areas, we do not report their ratings on the "strength of evaluation evidence" criterion. Instead, under contract with CDC, the Battelle Centers for Public Health Research and Evaluation rated the strength of scientific evidence that supports using each indicator to measure a downstream outcome of a tobacco control program. This information can be found in the indicator rating tables (described below) for each outcome in the related logic model.

For detailed information on how CDC selected indicators, how the expert panelists and Battelle Centers for Public Health Research and Evaluation went about their tasks, and how the ratings were calculated, see Appendix B. Also in Appendix B is a full explanation of how CDC compiled the indicator ratings.

Indicator Rating Tables

For each outcome component of the logic models, we provide an indicator rating table. In each table is a list of all the indicators associated with the outcome component and the ratings for each indicator by criterion. Using this table makes it easy to compare all the indicators for one outcome. The number and name of each relevant indicator is provided in each table, as are graphic displays of the criteria scores for each indicator.

An example of an indicator rating and an explanation of how to read it is provided in Figure 2.

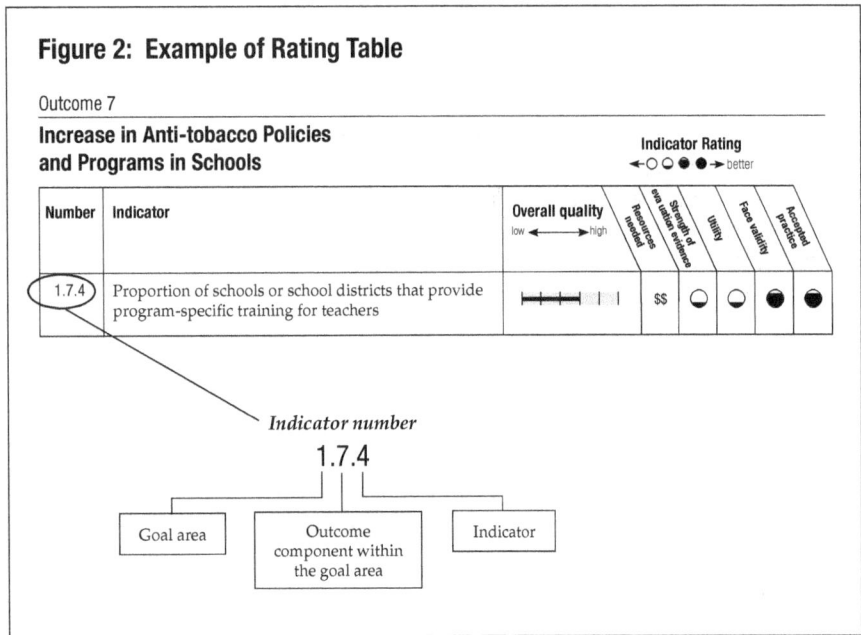

Figure 2: Example of Rating Table

The following are definitions of the criteria on which the ratings are based:

Overall quality. The general worth of the indicator as it relates to evaluating state tobacco control programs.

Resources needed. Dollar signs show the amount of resources (funds, time, and effort) needed to collect and analyze data on the indicator using the most commonly available data source: the more dollar signs (maximum four), the more resources needed. The dollar signs do not represent specific amounts because the actual cost of measuring and analyzing an indicator varies according to the existing capacity of a state health department or organization to evaluate its programs.

Strength of evaluation evidence. The degree to which scientific evidence supports the assumption that implementing interventions to effect change in a given indicator (e.g., proportion of schools or school districts that provide program-specific training for teachers) will lead to measurable downstream outcome (e.g., reduced susceptibility to experimentation with tobacco products).

Utility. The extent to which the indicator is useful for answering evaluation questions for comprehensive state tobacco control programs.

Face validity. The degree to which data on the indicator would appear valid to tobacco program stakeholders, such as policy makers.

Accepted practice. The degree to which using the indicator to measure a tobacco control program's progress is consistent with accepted practice.

In addition, certain symbols are associated with some of the ratings:

An asterisk (*) indicates low reviewer response: if less than 75% of experts rated the indicator or if more than 75% of experts gave a certain criterion an invalid rating (e.g., "don't know"), we considered the indicator to have low reviewer response. A low response suggests a high degree of uncertainty among raters. An example of such an indicator is 2.3.2: Level of receptivity to media messages about secondhand smoke.

A dagger (†) indicates a low level of agreement among reviewers: if less than 75% of the valid ratings were within one point of each other, we considered the rating to have a low level of agreement. An example of an indicator with a low level of agreement is 1.6.3: Proportion of students who would ever wear or use something with a tobacco company name or picture. This low level of agreement represents a relatively high degree of variability in the raters' responses for the criterion.

A diamond (◊) indicates that the "resources needed" rating for this indicator was modified by CDC after the experts provided their ratings for this criterion. An example of such an indicator is 1.9.1: Extent and type of retail tobacco advertising and promotions.

Indicator Profiles

Each indicator listed in this publication is associated with one short-term, intermediate, or long-term outcome component in a specific logic model for each of the NTCP's first three goal areas. Several indicators, however, are associated with more than one NTCP goal area. These indicators may have different indicator ratings, depending on the NTCP goal area and logic model component. In addition, the number of indicators for each logic model component varies considerably; some have only one indicator, while others have many.

For each indicator, we provide an indicator profile. These profiles provide detailed information about each indicator, as follows:

- **Indicator number and name.** Each indicator is uniquely identified by three numbers. The first number represents the goal area, the second number represents the outcome component within the goal area logic model, and the third number represents the indicator. For example, indicator 1.6.3 is number 3 on the list of indicators associated with outcome component 6 in the logic model for NTCP goal area 1.

- **Outcome component.** The title of the outcome component (i.e., logic model box) is provided in the logic model.

- **What to measure.** A description is included of what to measure in order to gather data on the indicator.

- **Why this indicator is useful.** The rationale is provided for using the indicator as a measure of a specific outcome in the logic model.

- **Example data source(s).** Listed are some example surveys and sources of data to measure the indicator as well as the population from which the data could be collected (if not apparent from the title). Most sources we list are well known and widely used state or national surveys or surveillance systems.[3] We also list non-standardized topic-specific data sources (e.g., media tracking, policy tracking, worksite surveys, environmental scans, and other tobacco-related state surveys) that may not be widely used by state tobacco programs but can be useful for evaluation. If similar survey questions are in multiple data sources, we list the data source most commonly available to state tobacco control programs. In addition to measuring the suggested indicator, evaluators may want to collect demographic data such as survey respondents' age, sex, race, ethnicity, and city or county of residence.

- **Population group(s).** The population group(s) include(s) the individuals from which data about this indicator are most commonly collected, if applicable.

- **Example survey question(s).** These are usually survey questions from state or national surveys or surveillance systems. When appropriate, the range of possible responses to the survey questions is also given. If no state or national survey has an appropriate question, we created an example question.

- **Comments.** Here we provide any additional information we have on this indicator. For example, we may suggest other uses for the indicator, the indicator's limitations (if any) as a measure of a program's progress, or sources of information on data collection methods.

- **Reviewers' ratings.** The rating tables include the criterion ratings given to the indicator by the panel of experts and Battelle Centers for Public Health Research and Evaluation ("strength of evaluation evidence" criterion only).

Using This Book to Plan a State Tobacco Control Program Evaluation

State tobacco control program managers need to evaluate their programs to demonstrate their effects, account for their funding, and improve their programs. Effective tobacco control programs require careful planning, implementation, and evaluation. To develop a successful program and a useful evaluation, program staff and program evaluators must work collaboratively on program planning and evaluation planning. A strong evaluation will not salvage a weak program, and a strong program cannot be proven effective without a defensible evaluation.

Managers and evaluators can use this publication to help them select the program's outcomes and the key indicators for evaluating the program's success in achieving the selected outcomes. Programs need to avoid two common pitfalls: (1) choosing interventions without sufficient plans or funds for evaluation; and (2) only selecting indicators primarily for research purposes rather than for program evaluation.[1]

Seven major steps are involved in planning an effective program and program evaluation. The order in which each step is taken can vary depending on the program's circumstances. For example, the first step of a program with limited funds for evaluation might be to examine the indicator rating tables to see which indicators require the fewest resources for data collection and analysis. Alternatively, the first step might be to review Appendix D (Data Source Indicator Table) to determine which indicators are being measured by surveillance and evaluation methods already in place in the state. Another program might be given funds specifically to reduce nonsmokers' exposure to secondhand smoke. Since the funders selected this program's long-term outcome, the planners' first step could be to examine the logic model of goal area 2 (eliminating nonsmokers' exposure to secondhand smoke) to select the short-term and intermediate outcomes they will work toward achieving.

Below are the seven major steps involved in planning and evaluating a state tobacco control program. This book provides assistance for steps 1–4 and step 7.

States are not restricted to addressing one goal area. In fact, we encourage programs to work across several goal areas. However, it is best to go through the steps separately for each selected goal area and then consider program strategies and indicators across goal areas. This approach can help produce efficiencies of scale in both operating programs and in evaluating them.

Step 1. Select the NTCP goal area that suits your program best.

Look at the logic models for each NTCP goal area carefully, keeping in mind that we do not list outcome indicators for goal area 4 in this publication (see page 5 in this chapter and page 269 in Chapter 5 for an explanation). For program planning, it is often helpful to read logic models backward; that is, begin with the long-term outcomes and trace a causal pathway back through intermediate outcomes, to short-term outcomes, to program outputs and program activities. After reviewing the logic models and your state's circumstances (e.g., political situation, resources, and tobacco-related statistics), select the goal area(s) that best fit your state's needs.

Step 2. Select long-term outcomes for your program.

Read the outcome overviews for the long-term outcome components in the selected goal area's logic model. This information will help you understand the rationale and empirical support for the logic model pathway that links specific program activities with specific outcomes. If you need more information, read some of the related articles listed after the references for each outcome overview in the section titled "For Further Reading." Then, on the basis of this information, select one or more long-term outcomes, again keeping in mind your state's circumstances, resources, and needs.

Step 3. Select short-term and intermediate outcomes for your program.

Read the outcome overviews for each short-term and intermediate outcome component that is linked to your selected long-term outcomes. If you need more information, read some of the related articles listed after the references for each outcome overview in the section titled "For Further Reading." Based on what you have read and your program's circumstances, select short-term and intermediate outcomes that will lead to your selected long-term outcomes.

Step 4. Select indicators of progress toward your selected short-term, intermediate, and long-term outcomes.

Examine the indicator rating tables relevant to the long-term, intermediate, and short-term outcomes you have selected. Compare ratings pertaining to the indicators' overall quality, resources needed, strength of evaluation evidence, utility, face validity, and accepted practice. Select candidate indicators and learn more about them by reading each indicator profile. On the basis of your reading and your program's circumstances, select indicators to show progress toward your selected short-term, intermediate, and long-term outcomes.

Step 5. Select or design activities to achieve your selected outcomes.

Program activities should be designed to achieve intended outcomes. To learn more about designing, planning, and implementing evidence-based tobacco control activities, managers and evaluators should refer to several evidence-based publications, such as:

- *Best Practices for Comprehensive Tobacco Control Programs*[1]
- *Reducing Tobacco Use: A Report of the Surgeon General*[5]
- *The Guide to Community Preventive Services: Tobacco Use Prevention and Control*[6]
- *Treating Tobacco Use and Dependence: Clinical Practice Guideline*[7]

- *The Health Consequences of Smoking: A Report of the Surgeon General*[8]
- *Preventing Tobacco Use Among Young People: A Report of the Surgeon General*[9]
- *Women and Smoking: A Report of the Surgeon General*[10]
- *Tobacco Use Among U.S. Racial/Ethnic Minority Groups—African Americans, American Indians and Alaska Natives, Asian Americans and Pacific Islanders, and Hispanics: A Report of the Surgeon General*[12]

We also encourage managers and evaluators to contact their state's program consultant at CDC.

Step 6. Implement your selected intervention activities.

Program staff should implement intervention activities and monitor them to determine the degree to which activities have been implemented as intended.[11]

Step 7. Evaluate your progress toward achieving your selected outcomes.

Monitor indicators selected in step 4 to assess your program's progress over time and to compare your data with those of other states. Focus your evaluation design on answering your evaluation questions within your state context by creating program objectives. Good program objectives are SMART (i.e., they are specific, measurable, achievable, relevant, and time-bound). An example of a SMART objective is increasing the percentage of young people in a given state who have confirmed awareness of anti-tobacco messages on the dangers of secondhand smoke from 25% in January 2005 to 50% in January 2006. For more information on creating SMART objectives, see *Introduction to Program Evaluation for Comprehensive Tobacco Control Programs*.[2]

The Importance of Merging Program and Evaluation Planning Early in the Program Planning Process

When a program is organized and planned on the basis of the goal area's logic model, managers and evaluators essentially have an outline of their outcome evaluation plan early in the program planning process. As the program evolves, managers and staff can make adjustments to program activities and, at the same time, the evaluation plan. Evaluation data can be used to show the program's effect and to inform planning and implementation of program activities.

For information on program planning, see the publications listed in step 5 (page 10).

Steps for Planning and Evaluating a State Tobacco Control Program

1. Select the NTCP goal area that suits your program best.
2. Select long-term outcomes for your program.
3. Select short-term and intermediate outcomes for your program.
4. Select indicators of progress toward your selected short-term, intermediate, and long-term outcomes.
5. Select or design activities to achieve your selected outcomes.
6. Implement your selected intervention activities.
7. Evaluate your progress toward achieving your selected outcomes.

**Planning an Evaluation of a State Tobacco Control Program:
A Hypothetical Example**

In this example, assume that recent data from a state's adult tobacco survey show an increase in nonsmokers' exposure to secondhand smoke among adults, and state legislators are concerned about this increase. The legislators let it be known that new funds may become available if the state tobacco program can show that it is effective in reducing nonsmokers' exposure to secondhand smoke.

On the basis of these factors, the state tobacco control program follows the steps described above:

Step 1. Select the NTCP goal area that suits your program best.

The legislature is providing funds specifically to eliminate nonsmokers' exposure to secondhand smoke. Therefore, the state tobacco control program chooses NTCP goal area 2: Eliminating nonsmokers' exposure to secondhand smoke.

Step 2. Select long-term outcomes for your program.

Program staff and evaluators review the logic model for NTCP goal area 2 (page 123) and select two long-term outcomes that they aim to achieve:

    Outcome 7. Reduced exposure to secondhand smoke

    Outcome 8. Reduced tobacco consumption

To learn about these long-term outcomes, they study the relevant outcome component overviews (pages 174 and 184) and read several articles listed after the references for each overview in the section titled "For Further Reading."

Step 3. Select short-term and intermediate outcomes for your program.

Following our recommendations, the program planners and evaluators read the logic model for NTCP goal area 2 backward (starting at long-term outcomes) to select intermediate and short-term outcomes. They select one intermediate outcome:

    Outcome 6. Compliance with tobacco-free policies

This outcome serves as a funnel between the long-term outcomes (selected in step 2) and three short-term outcomes in the logic model of NTCP goal area 2:

    Outcome 3. Increased knowledge of, improved attitudes toward, and increased support for the creation and active enforcement of tobacco-free policies

    Outcome 4. Creation of tobacco-free policies

    Outcome 5. Enforcement of tobacco-free public policies

The program planners and evaluators understand that achieving one or more of these short-term and intermediate outcomes will lead to achieving the selected long-term outcomes and then to the distal outcomes of reducing tobacco-related morbidity and mortality and decreasing tobacco-related disparities. The planners and evaluators select the suggested short-term and intermediate outcomes with the intention of learning more about them before making a final decision about which outcomes are most relevant to their program.

The planners and evaluators read the outcome component overviews on the candidate short-term outcomes (pages 127, 147, 159) and intermediate outcome (page 165). They also read several of the articles listed after the references for each outcome component overview in the section titled "For Further Reading" to determine the degree to which selected outcomes are relevant to their program.

Step 4. Select indicators of progress toward your selected short-term, intermediate, and long-term outcomes.

Next, the planners and evaluators look at the list of indicators associated with each selected outcome component (3–8), and they begin with outcome 3.

First the planners and evaluators examine the indicator rating table for outcome 3 (page 131). By doing so, they can assess which indicators meet the criteria (e.g., overall quality, resources needed, strength of evaluation evidence, utility, face validity, and accepted practice) that are most important to the program. Because the available funds are not sufficient for an expensive evaluation, the planners pay special attention to the "resources needed" criterion in the indicator rating table to avoid selecting indicators that are too costly to measure. In addition, since the state legislature expressed an interest in this effort, program managers want to select indicators that have a high rating for face validity to policy makers.

Before making a decision about which indicators to select, however, the planners and evaluators read the information in the indicator profiles associated with outcome component 3 (pages 132–146).

The planners and evaluators realize that data collection for all the indicators would be equally expensive if they were to design and implement a new survey. But, because they have studied the indicator information carefully, they realize that three indicators associated with outcome component 3 can be measured using CDC Recommended Questions in the State's Adult Tobacco Survey:

2.3.5   Proportion of the population that thinks secondhand smoke is harmful

2.3.6   Proportion of the population that thinks secondhand smoke is harmful to children and pregnant women

2.3.7   Level of support for creating tobacco-free policies in public places and workplaces

Another indicator can be measured using CDC's Recommended Questions in Supplemental Section D: Environmental Tobacco Smoke in the State's Adult Tobacco Survey:

> 2.3.4 Proportion of the population willing to ask someone not to smoke in their presence

In addition, another indicator can be measured using the CDC's Recommended Questions in Supplemental Section F: Policy Issues in the State's Adult Tobacco Survey:

> 2.3.10[NR] Level of support for creating policies in schools

The planners and evaluators also understand that short-term changes in the knowledge and attitudes of young people are important contributors to successful enforcement of, and compliance with, tobacco-free policies. They therefore decide to monitor indicator 2.3.5, which can be measured using CDC's Recommended Core Questions in the State's Youth Tobacco Survey:

> 2.3.5. Proportion of the population that thinks secondhand smoke is harmful

The planners and evaluators use the same process to select indicators for each of the other selected outcome components (4, 5, 6, 7, and 8).

Step 5. Select or design activities to achieve your selected outcomes.

The program planners select and design evidence based interventions, such as countermarketing campaigns focused on the dangers of secondhand smoke; activities to create tobacco-free school, home, and workplace policies; and activities to mobilize decision makers to promote bans on secondhand smoke. See Appendix A for more information on program strategies.

Step 6. Implement your selected intervention activities.

The program staff implements the intervention activities and continuously monitors (1) whether the activities are being implemented as intended and (2) the extent to which the program is reaching its target audiences.

Step 7. Evaluate your progress toward achieving your selected outcomes.

The planners and evaluators translate indicators into SMART program objectives. For example, for indicator 2.3.7 (level of support for creating tobacco-free policies in public places and workplaces), they create the following objective: Increase the percentage of adults in the state who believe that smoking should not be allowed at all in indoor workplaces from 20% in January 2005 to at least 50% in June 2006. In addition, the planners and evaluators measure the selected indicators, track changes over time, and compare their data to data from similar states.

References

1. Centers for Disease Control and Prevention. *Best practices for comprehensive tobacco control programs.* Atlanta, GA: Centers for Disease Control and Prevention; 1999.

2. MacDonald G, Starr G, Schooley M, Yee SL, Klimowski K, Turner K. *Introduction to program evaluation for comprehensive tobacco control programs.* Atlanta, GA: Centers for Disease Control and Prevention; 2001.

3. Yee SL, Schooley M. *Surveillance and evaluation data resources for comprehensive tobacco control programs.* Atlanta, GA: Centers for Disease Control and Prevention; 2001.

4. United Way of America. *Measuring program outcomes: a practical approach.* Alexandria, VA: United Way of America; 1996.

5. U.S. Department of Health and Human Services. *Reducing tobacco use: a report of the Surgeon General.* Atlanta, GA: Centers for Disease Control and Prevention; 2000.

6. Task Force on Community Preventive Services. The guide to community preventive services: tobacco use prevention and control. *American Journal of Preventive Medicine.* 2001;20(Suppl 2):1–88.

7. Fiore M, Bailey W, Cohen S, Dorfman S, Goldstein M, Gritz E, Heyman RB, Jaén CR, Kottke TE, Lando HA, Micklenburg RE, Mullen PD, Nett LM, Robinson L, Stitzer ML, Tommasello AC, Villejo L, Wewers ME. *Treating tobacco use and dependence: clinical practice guideline.* Rockville, MD: U.S. Department of Health and Human Services; 2000.

8. U.S. Department of Health and Human Services. *The health consequences of smoking: a report of the Surgeon General.* Atlanta, GA: Centers for Disease Control and Prevention; 2004.

9. U.S. Department of Health and Human Services. *Preventing tobacco use among young people: a report of the Surgeon General.* Atlanta, GA: Centers for Disease Control and Prevention; 1994.

10. U.S. Department of Health and Human Services. *Women and smoking: a report of the Surgeon General.* Rockville, MD: U.S. Department of Health and Human Services, Public Health Service, Office of the Surgeon General; Washington, DC: Government Printing Office; 2001.

11. Patton M. *Utilization-focused evaluation.* 3rd edition. Thousand Oaks, CA: Sage; 1997.

12. U.S. Department of Health and Human Services. *Tobacco Use Among U.S. Racial/Ethnic Minority Groups—African Americans, American Indians and Alaska Natives, Asian Americans and Pacific Islanders, and Hispanics: A Report of the Surgeon General.* Atlanta, GA: Centers for Disease Control and Prevention; 1998.

CHAPTER 2

Goal Area 1: Preventing Initiation of Tobacco Use Among Young People

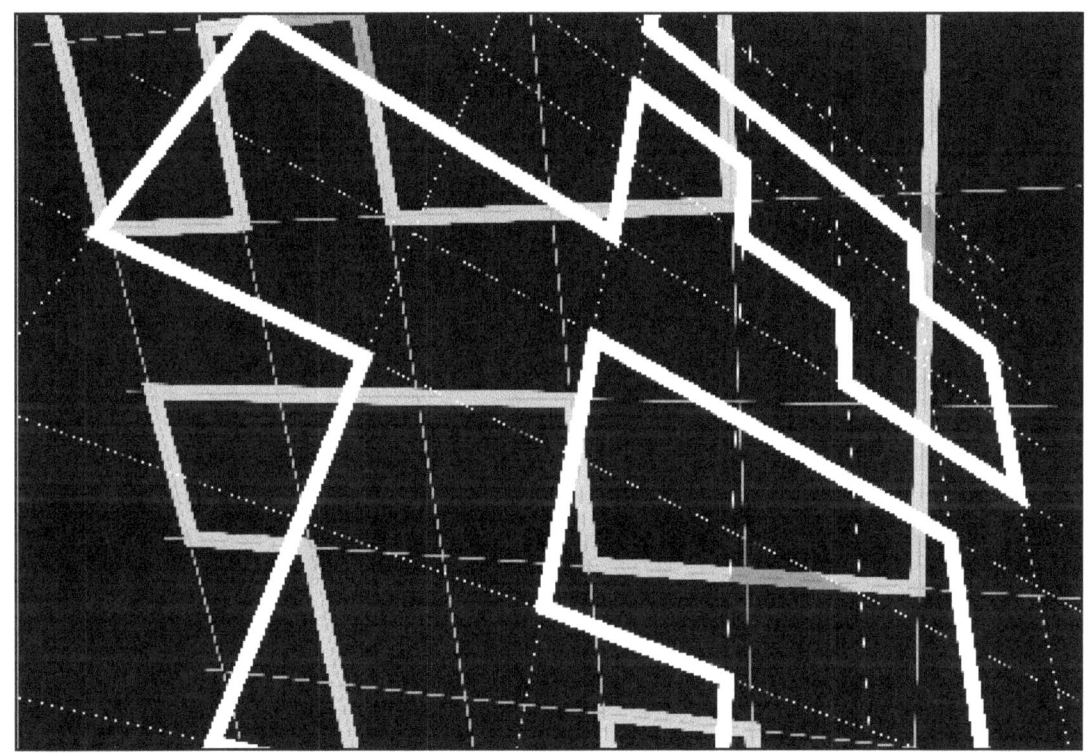

Goal Area 1

Preventing Initiation of Tobacco Use Among Young People

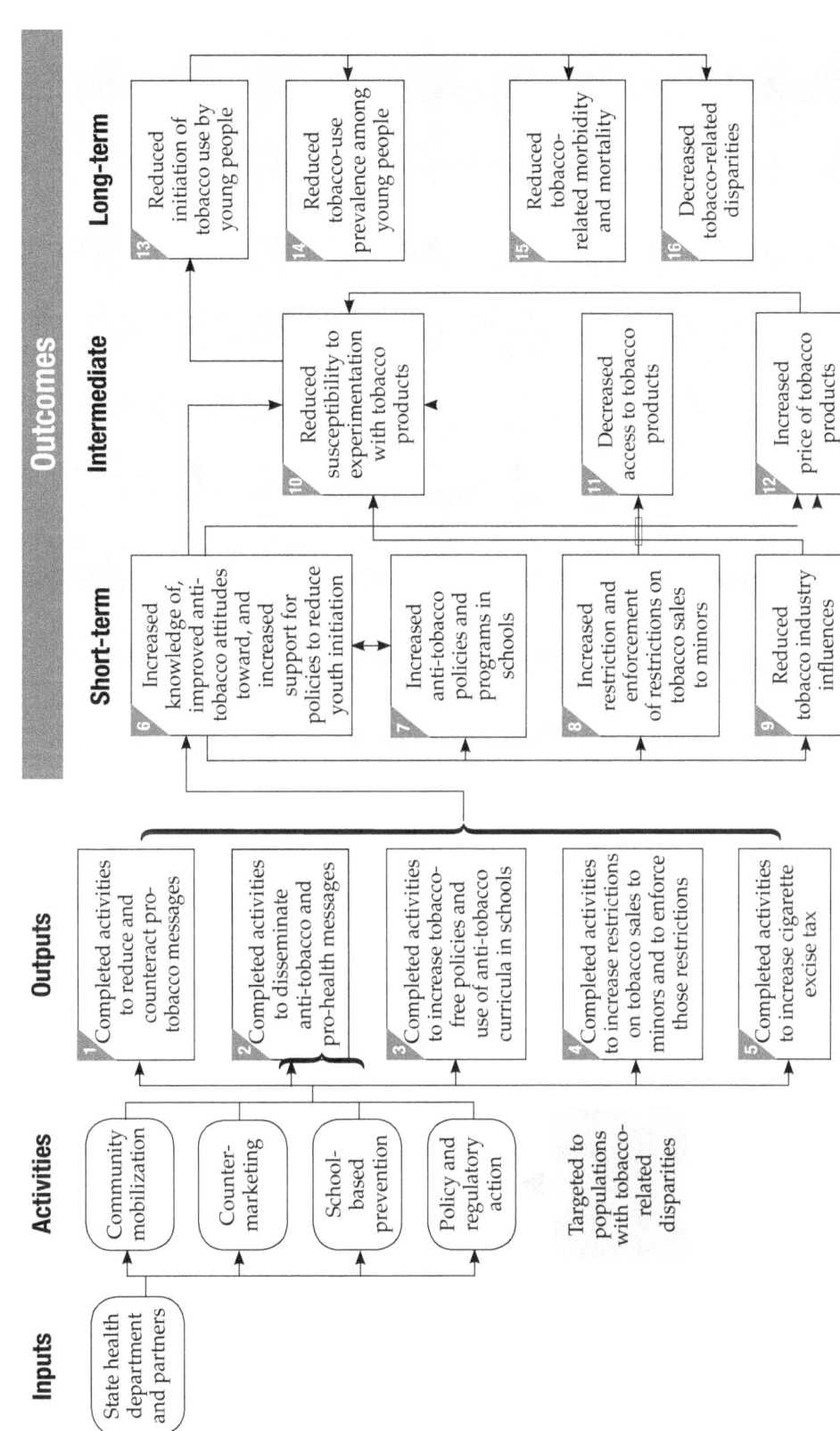

CHAPTER 2 · *Goal Area 1: Preventing Initiation of Tobacco Use Among Young People* | 19

Goal Area 1

Preventing Initiation of Tobacco Use Among Young People

Short-term Outcomes

- Outcome 6: Increased knowledge of, improved anti-tobacco attitudes toward, and increased support for policies to reduce youth initiation

    - 1.6.1   Level of confirmed awareness of anti-tobacco media messages
    - 1.6.2   Level of receptivity to anti-tobacco media messages
    - 1.6.3   Proportion of students who would ever wear or use something with a tobacco company name or picture
    - 1.6.4   Level of support for policies, and enforcement of policies, to decrease young people's access to tobacco
    - 1.6.5   Level of support for increasing excise tax on tobacco products
    - 1.6.6   Level of awareness among parents about the importance of discussing tobacco use with their children
    - 1.6.7[NR]   Level of support for creating policies in schools
    - 1.6.8[NR]   Proportion of young people who think that the cigarette companies try to get young people to smoke

- Outcome 7: Increased anti-tobacco policies and programs in schools

    - 1.7.1   Proportion of schools or school districts reporting the implementation of 100% tobacco-free policies
    - 1.7.2   Proportion of schools or school districts that provide instruction on tobacco-use prevention that meets CDC guidelines
    - 1.7.3   Proportion of schools or school districts that provide tobacco-use prevention education in grades K–12
    - 1.7.4   Proportion of schools or school districts that provide program-specific training for teachers
    - 1.7.5   Proportion of schools or school districts that involve families in support of school-based programs
    - 1.7.6   Proportion of schools or school districts that support cessation interventions for students and staff who use tobacco
    - 1.7.7   Proportion of schools or school districts that assess their tobacco-use prevention program at regular intervals
    - 1.7.8   Proportion of students who participate in tobacco-use prevention activities

1.7.9 Level of reported exposure to school-based tobacco-use prevention curricula that meet CDC guidelines

1.7.10 Perceived compliance with tobacco-free policies in schools

1.7.11 Proportion of schools or school districts with policies that regulate display of tobacco industry promotional items

- **Outcome 8: Increased restriction and enforcement of restrictions on tobacco sales to minors**

    1.8.1 Proportion of jurisdictions with policies that ban tobacco vending machine sales in places accessible to young people

    1.8.2 Proportion of jurisdictions with policies that require retail licenses to sell tobacco products

    1.8.3 Proportion of jurisdictions with policies that control the location, number, and density of retail outlets

    1.8.4 Proportion of jurisdictions with policies that control self-service tobacco sales

    1.8.5 Number of compliance checks conducted by enforcement agencies

    1.8.6 Number of warnings, citations, and fines issued for infractions of public policies against young people's access to tobacco products

    1.8.7 Changes in state tobacco control laws that preempt stronger local tobacco control laws

- **Outcome 9: Reduced tobacco industry influences**

    1.9.1 Extent and type of retail tobacco advertising and promotions

    1.9.2 Proportion of jurisdictions with policies that regulate the extent and type of retail tobacco advertising and promotions

    1.9.3 Extent of tobacco advertising outside of stores

    1.9.4 Proportion of jurisdictions with policies that regulate the extent of tobacco advertising outside of stores

    1.9.5 Extent of tobacco industry sponsorship of public and private events

    1.9.6 Proportion of jurisdictions with policies that regulate tobacco industry sponsorship of public events

    1.9.7 Extent of tobacco advertising on school property, at school events, and near schools

    1.9.8 Extent of tobacco advertising in print media

- 1.9.9 Amount and quality of news media stories about tobacco industry practices and political lobbying
- 1.9.10 Number and type of Master Settlement Agreement violations by tobacco companies
- 1.9.11 Extent of tobacco industry contributions to institutions and groups
- 1.9.12 Amount of tobacco industry campaign contributions to local and state politicians

Intermediate Outcomes

Outcome 10: Reduced susceptibility to experimentation with tobacco products

- 1.10.1 Proportion of young people who think that smoking is cool and helps them fit in
- 1.10.2 Proportion of young people who think that young people who smoke have more friends
- 1.10.3 Proportion of young people who report that their parents have discussed not smoking with them
- 1.10.4 Proportion of parents who report that they have discussed not smoking with their children
- 1.10.5 Proportion of young people who are susceptible never-smokers

Outcome 11: Decreased access to tobacco products

- 1.11.1 Proportion of successful attempts to purchase tobacco products by young people
- 1.11.2 Proportion of young people reporting that they have been sold tobacco products by a retailer
- 1.11.3 Proportion of young people reporting that they have been unsuccessful in purchasing tobacco products from a retailer
- 1.11.4 Proportion of young people reporting that they have received tobacco products from a social source
- 1.11.5 Proportion of young people reporting that they purchased cigarettes from a vending machine
- 1.11.6[NR] Proportion of young people who believe that it is easy to obtain tobacco products

Outcome 12: Increased price of tobacco products

- 1.12.1 Amount of tobacco product excise tax

Long-term Outcomes

■ **Outcome 13: Reduced initiation of tobacco use by young people**

　1.13.1　Average age at which young people first smoked a whole cigarette

　1.13.2　Proportion of young people who report never having tried a cigarette

■ **Outcome 14: Reduced tobacco-use prevalence among young people**

　1.14.1　Prevalence of tobacco use among young people

　1.14.2　Proportion of established young smokers

Outcome 6

Increased Knowledge of, Improved Anti-tobacco Attitudes Toward, and Increased Support for Policies to Reduce Youth Initiation

The theory of change associated with preventing young people from starting to use tobacco begins with increasing their knowledge of the dangers of tobacco use, changing their attitudes toward tobacco use, and increasing public support for policies that reduce the likelihood that young people will use tobacco. The tobacco industry spends more than $12.5 billion per year on marketing.[1] Adolescents are bombarded with pro-tobacco messages in and around retail stores, in magazines, in movies, and by smokers around them. Evidence shows that anti-tobacco media campaigns, when combined with other interventions, are effective in reducing tobacco use by adolescents.[2] For example, the "truth" anti-tobacco media campaign in Florida achieved nearly 93% confirmed awareness of the message among young people and was associated with improved anti-tobacco attitudes.[3] After one year, both susceptibility to smoking and cigarette use declined more among Florida's young people than among young people in the rest of the nation.[3]

In addition to changing young people's attitudes toward tobacco use, it is necessary to increase adult support for implementing and enforcing policies that reduce the likelihood that young people will begin smoking. Such policies include increasing tobacco excise taxes, passing and enforcing strong laws that decrease young people's access to tobacco, and implementing tobacco-free school policies. Policies such as these eventually create an environment that supports a smoke-free lifestyle among young people.

Listed below are the indicators associated with this outcome:

- **1.6.1** Level of confirmed awareness of anti-tobacco media messages
- **1.6.2** Level of receptivity to anti-tobacco media messages
- **1.6.3** Proportion of students who would ever wear or use something with a tobacco company name or picture
- **1.6.4** Level of support for policies, and enforcement of policies, to decrease young people's access to tobacco
- **1.6.5** Level of support for increasing excise tax on tobacco products
- **1.6.6** Level of awareness among parents about the importance of discussing tobacco use with their children
- **1.6.7**[NR] Level of support for creating policies in schools
- **1.6.8**[NR] Proportion of young people who think that the cigarette companies try to get young people to smoke

References

1. Federal Trade Commission. *Cigarette report for 2002.* Washington, DC: Federal Trade Commission; 2004.

2. Task Force on Community Preventive Services. The guide to community preventive services: tobacco use prevention and control. *American Journal of Preventive Medicine.* 2001;20(Suppl 2):1–88.

3. Sly DF, Heald GR, Ray S. The Florida "truth" anti-tobacco media evaluation: design, first year results, and implications for planning future state media evaluations. *Tobacco Control.* 2001;10(1):9–15.

For Further Reading

Alcaraz R, Klonoff EA, Landrine H. The effects on children of participating in studies of minors' access to tobacco. *Preventive Medicine.* 1997;26(2):236–40.

Brown J, Caston M, Pollard J. Students and substances: social power in drug education. *Educational Evaluation and Policy Analysis.* 1997;19(1):65–82.

Centers for Disease Control and Prevention. Effectiveness of school-based programs as a component of a statewide tobacco control initiative. *Morbidity and Mortality Weekly Report.* 2001;50(31):663–6.

Centers for Disease Control and Prevention. Guidelines for school health programs to prevent tobacco use and addiction. *Morbidity and Mortality Weekly Report Recommendations and Reports.* 1994;43(RR-2):1–18.

Eischen MH, Brownson RC, Davis JR, Cooperstock LR, Crawford R, Freeman D, Howard G, Michael MJ. Grassroots efforts to promote tobacco-free schools in rural Missouri. *American Journal of Public Health.* 1994;84(8):1336–7.

Elder JP, Perry CL, Stone EJ, Johnson CC, Yang M, Edmundson EW, Smyth MH, Galati T, Feldman H, Cribb P, Parcel GS. Tobacco-use measurement, prediction, and intervention in elementary schools in four states: the CATCH Study. *Preventive Medicine.* 1996;25(4):486–94.

Flay BR, Brannon BR, Johnson CA, Hansen WB, Ulene AL, Whitney-Saltiel DA, et al. The television school and family smoking prevention and cessation project. 1. Theoretical basis and program development. *Preventive Medicine.* 1988;17(5): 585–607.

Lantz PM, Jacobson PD, Warner KE, Wasserman J, Pollack HA, Berson J, Ahlstrom A. Investing in youth tobacco control: a review of smoking prevention and control strategies. *Tobacco Control.* 2000;9(1):47–63.

Lee DJ, Trapido E, Weatherby N, Rodriguez R. Correlates of participation and willingness to participate in anti-tobacco activities among 4th–7th graders. *Journal of Community Health.* 2001;26(6):447–57.

Lynch BS, Bonnie RJ. *Growing up tobacco free: preventing nicotine addiction in children and youths.* Washington, DC: National Academy Press; 1994.

National Cancer Institute. Smoking and Tobacco Control Monograph, No. 14. *Changing adolescent smoking prevalence: where it is and why.* Bethesda, MD: National Cancer Institute; 2001. NIH Publication No. 02-5086.

Pentz M. *Primary prevention of adolescent drug abuse: applied developmental psychology.* Columbus, OH: McGraw-Hill; 1994. pp. 435–74.

Pentz MA, Brannon BR, Charlin VL, Barrett EJ, MacKinnon DP, Flay BR. The power of policy: the relationship of smoking policy to adolescent smoking. *American Journal of Public Health.* 1989;79(7):857–62.

Peterson AV Jr, Kealey KA, Mann SL, Marek PM, Sarason IG. Hutchinson Smoking Prevention Project: long-term randomized trial in school-based tobacco use prevention—results on smoking. *Journal of the National Cancer Institute.* 2000;92(24):1979–91.

Thomas R. School-based programmes for preventing smoking. *The Cochrane Database of Systematic Reviews*, 2002;(4):CD001293. DOI: 10.1002/14651858.CD001293.

U.S. Department of Health and Human Services. *Preventing tobacco use among young people: a report of the Surgeon General.* Atlanta, GA: Centers for Disease Control and Prevention; 1994.

Unger JB, Rohrbach LA, Howard KA, Boley Cruz T, Johnson CA, Chen X. Attitudes toward anti-tobacco policy among California youth: associations with smoking status, psychosocial variables and advocacy actions. *Health Education Research.* 1999;14(6):751–63.

Winkleby MA, Feighery EC, Altman DA, Kole S, Tencati E. Engaging ethnically diverse teens in a substance use prevention advocacy program. *American Journal of Health Promotion.* 2001;15(6):433–6.

Outcome 6

Increased Knowledge of, Improved Anti-tobacco Attitudes Toward, and Increased Support for Policies to Reduce Youth Initiation

Indicator Rating
← ○ ◔ ◐ ● → better

Number	Indicator	Overall quality (low → high)	Resources needed	Strength of evaluation evidence	Utility	Face validity	Accepted practice
1.6.1	Level of confirmed awareness of anti-tobacco media messages	▬▬▬▬	$$	●	●	●	●
1.6.2	Level of receptivity to anti-tobacco media messages	▬▬▬▬	$$	●	●	●	●
1.6.3	Proportion of students who would ever wear or use something with a tobacco company name or picture	▬▬▬▬ †	$$	●	●	●	●
1.6.4	Level of support for policies, and enforcement of policies, to decrease young people's access to tobacco	▬▬▬▬	$$	⊘	●	●	●
1.6.5	Level of support for increasing excise tax on tobacco products	▬▬▬▬	$$†	⊘	●	●	●
1.6.6	Level of awareness among parents about the importance of discussing tobacco use with their children	▬▬▬▬ †	$$	●	◐	◐†	◔
1.6.7[NR]	Level of support for creating policies in schools	▬▬▬▬	⊘	⊘	⊘	⊘	⊘
1.6.8[NR]	Proportion of young people who think that the cigarette companies try to get young people to smoke	▬▬▬▬	⊘	⊘	⊘	⊘	⊘

† Denotes low agreement among reviewers: that is, fewer than 75% of the valid ratings for this indicator were within one point of each other (see Appendix B for an explanation).
⊘ Denotes no data.
[NR] Denotes an indicator that is not rated (see Appendix B for an explanation).

Indicator 1.6.1

Level of Confirmed Awareness of Anti-tobacco Media Messages

Goal area 1	Preventing initiation of tobacco use among young people
Outcome 6	Increased knowledge of, improved anti-tobacco attitudes toward, and increased support for policies to reduce youth initiation
What to measure	Proportion of the target population that can accurately recall a media message
Why this indicator is useful	Evaluators should measure exposure to anti-tobacco media messages to confirm awareness of these messages by asking respondents to provide specific information about the message.[1]
Example data source(s)	Legacy Media Tracking Survey (LMTS), 2003 Information on LMTS available at: http://tobacco.rti.org/data/lmts.cfm
Population group(s)	Young people aged less than 18 years
Example survey question(s)	**From LMTS** Have you recently seen an anti-smoking or anti-tobacco ad on TV that shows _____? ☐ Yes ☐ Maybe, not sure ☐ No ☐ Refused to answer What happens in this advertisement? (DO NOT READ RESPONSE CATEGORIES) What do you think the main message of this ad was? (DO NOT READ RESPONSE CATEGORIES)
Comments	The example questions could be asked of adults. Evaluators may want to categorize awareness of the medium (e.g., billboard, television, print) through which respondents learned of the anti-tobacco message. Programs may want to evaluate confirmed awareness of an advertisement by respondents' smoking status (current, former, or never) and addiction level (e.g., light, moderate, or heavy), because awareness levels may differ significantly among groups with different levels of addiction. Evaluators should work closely with countermarketing campaign managers to (1) develop a separate series of questions for each main media message and (2) coordinate data collection with the timing of the media campaign.

Rating	Overall quality low ←———→ high	Resources needed	Strength of evaluation evidence	Utility	Face validity	Accepted practice
	███████████	$$	●	●	●	●

← ○ ◐ ● ● → better

Reference
1. Sly DF, Heald GR, Ray S. The Florida "truth" anti-tobacco media evaluation: design, first year results, and implications for planning future state media evaluations. *Tobacco Control.* 2001;10(1):9–15.

Indicator 1.6.2

Level of Receptivity to Anti-tobacco Media Messages

Goal area 1	Preventing initiation of tobacco use among young people
Outcome 6	Increased knowledge of, improved anti-tobacco attitudes toward, and increased support for policies to reduce youth initiation
What to measure	The level of receptivity to media messages by the intended audience. Receptivity is generally defined as the extent to which people are willing to listen to a persuasive message. In tobacco control evaluation, however, the definition is narrower; receptivity is the extent to which people believe that the message was convincing, made them think about their behavior, and stimulated discussion with others.[1]
Why this indicator is useful	Message awareness is necessary but not sufficient to change the knowledge, attitudes, and intentions of young people. Media campaigns are effective only if their messages reach and resonate with the intended audience. A well-received message helps ensure campaign effectiveness.[2-5] One study found that receptivity to anti-tobacco messages was a significant predictor of lower rates of intention to smoke.[6]
Example data source(s)	Legacy Media Tracking Survey (LMTS), 2003 Information on LMTS available at: http://tobacco.rti.org/data/lmts.cfm
Population group(s)	Young people aged less than 18 years
Example survey question(s)	**From LMTS** Tell me how much you agree or disagree with the following statement: This ad is convincing. Would you say you: ☐ Strongly agree ☐ Agree ☐ Disagree ☐ Strongly disagree ☐ Have no opinion ☐ Don't know Would you say the ad gave you good reasons not to smoke? ☐ Yes ☐ No ☐ Don't know Did you talk to your friends about this ad? ☐ Yes ☐ No ☐ Don't know
Comments	The example questions could be asked of adults. Evaluators may want to assess receptivity by the medium through which respondents learned of the media message (e.g., television, print, or radio). Evaluators should work closely with countermarketing campaign managers to (1) develop a separate series of questions for each main media message and (2) coordinate data collection with the timing of the media campaign.

Rating

Overall quality low ◄──► high	Resources needed	Strength of evaluation evidence	Utility	Face validity	Accepted practice
▬▬▬▬▬	$$	◐	◐	◐	●

◄ ○ ◔ ◐ ● ► better

References
1. Sly DF, Heald GR, Ray S. The Florida "truth" anti-tobacco media evaluation: design, first-year results, and implications for planning future state media evaluations. *Tobacco Control.* 2001;10:9–15.
2. McGuire WJ. Public communication as a strategy for inducing health-promoting behavioral change. *Preventive Medicine.* 1984;13(3):299–319.
3. Kotler P, Armstrong G. *Principles of marketing,* 9th ed. Upper Saddle River, NJ: Prentice-Hall; 2001.
4. Carter WB. Health behavior as a rational process: theory of reasoned action and multiattribute utility theory. In: Glanz K, Lewis F, Rimer B, editors. *Health behavior and health education: theory, research, and practice.* San Francisco, CA: Jossey-Bass; 1990. p. 63–91.
5. Maibach E, Parrott RL, editors. *Designing health messages: approaches from communication theory and public health practice.* Thousand Oaks, CA: Sage; 1995.
6. Straub DM, Hills NK, Thompson PJ, Moscicki AB. Effects of pro- and anti-tobacco advertising on nonsmoking adolescents' intentions to smoke. *Journal of Adolescent Health.* 2003;32(1):36–43.

Indicator 1.6.3

Proportion of Students Who Would Ever Wear or Use Something with a Tobacco Company Name or Picture

Goal area 1	Preventing initiation of tobacco use among young people
Outcome 6	Increased knowledge of, improved anti-tobacco attitudes toward, and increased support for policies to reduce youth initiation
What to measure	Proportion of students who are willing to buy or receive a cigarette promotional item (e.g., sports gear, clothing, lighters, or sunglasses)
Why this indicator is useful	Evidence suggests a causal relationship between adolescents' willingness to wear or use tobacco promotional items and the likelihood that they will experiment with cigarettes.[1-5] Young people who are highly receptive to tobacco marketing are more than twice as likely to become established smokers as those with a low level of receptivity to tobacco marketing.[3]
Example data source(s)	Youth Tobacco Survey (YTS): CDC Recommended Questions: Core, 2004
Population group(s)	Young people aged less than 18 years
Example survey question(s)	**From YTS** Would you ever use or wear something that has a tobacco company name or picture on it, such as a lighter, t-shirt, hat, or sunglasses? ☐ Definitely yes ☐ Probably yes ☐ Probably not ☐ Definitely not
Comments	None

Rating

Overall quality low ⟵⟶ high	Resources needed	Strength of evaluation evidence	Utility	Face validity	Accepted practice
▬▬▬▬▬†	$$	●	◐	●	●

⟵ ○ ◔ ◐ ● ⟶ better

† Denotes low agreement among reviewers: that is, fewer than 75% of the valid ratings for this indicator were within one point of each other (see Appendix B for an explanation).

References
1. U.S. Department of Health and Human Services. *Preventing tobacco use among young people: a report of the Surgeon General.* Atlanta, GA: Centers for Disease Control and Prevention; 1994.
2. Gilpin EA, Pierce JP, Rosbrook B. Are adolescents receptive to current sales promotion practices of the tobacco industry? *Preventive Medicine.* 1997;26(1):14–21.
3. Biener L, Siegel M. Tobacco marketing and adolescent smoking: more support for a causal inference. *American Journal of Public Health.* 2000;90(3):407–11.
4. Sargent JD, Dalton M, Beach M, Bernhardt A, Heatherton T, Stevens M. Effect of cigarette promotions on smoking uptake among adolescents. *Preventive Medicine.* 2000;30(4):320–7.
5. Feighery EC, Borzekowski DL, Schooler C, Flora J. Seeing, wanting, owning: the relationship between receptivity to tobacco marketing and smoking susceptibility in young people. *Tobacco Control.* 1998;7:123–8.

Indicator 1.6.4

Level of Support for Policies, and Enforcement of Policies, to Decrease Young People's Access to Tobacco

Goal area 1	Preventing initiation of tobacco use among young people
Outcome 6	Increased knowledge of, improved anti-tobacco attitudes toward, and increased support for policies to reduce youth initiation
What to measure	Proportion of adults who support policies and enforcement of policies restricting young people's access to tobacco products
Why this indicator is useful	Tobacco-free policies are unlikely to be adopted without support from business owners, policy makers, and the general public.[1-4] In California, for example, public support for retail tobacco sales licensing policies has grown since 1990, and this has contributed to the passage of local tobacco licensing ordinances in several jurisdictions.[5]
Example data source(s)	Adult Tobacco Survey (ATS): CDC Recommended Questions: Supplemental Section F: Policy Issues, 2003
Population group(s)	Adults aged 18 years or older
Example survey question(s)	**From ATS** How important is it that communities keep stores from selling tobacco products to teenagers? Would you say it is ☐ Very important ☐ Somewhat important ☐ Not very important ☐ Not important at all ☐ No opinion/Don't know ☐ Refused How strongly do you agree or disagree with the following statement: Store owners should be required to have a license to sell tobacco products, similar to alcohol, so that teens can't buy tobacco products. Would you say it is ☐ Very important ☐ Somewhat important ☐ Not very important ☐ Not important at all ☐ No opinion/Don't know ☐ Refused
Comments	The example questions could be asked of decision makers or retailers. Evaluators may want to analyze the level of support for creating policies to decrease access to tobacco by respondent's tobacco use.

Rating

Overall quality low ←→ high	Resources needed	Strength of evaluation evidence	Utility	Face validity	Accepted practice
▬▬▬▬	$$	⊘	●	●	●

←○ ◐ ● ●→ better

⊘ Denotes no data.

References
1. U.S. Department of Health and Human Services. *Reducing tobacco use: a report of the Surgeon General.* Atlanta. GA: Centers for Disease Control and Prevention; 2000.
2. U.S. Department of Health and Human Services. *Women and smoking: a report of the Surgeon General.* Rockville, MD: U.S. Department of Health and Human Services, Public Health Service, Office of the Surgeon General; 2001.
3. Thompson GW, Wilson N. Public attitudes about tobacco smoke in workplaces: the importance of workers' rights in survey questions. *Tobacco Control.* 2003;13:206–8.
4. Howard KA, Rogers T, Howard-Pitney B, Flora JA, Norman GJ, Ribisl KM. Opinion leaders' support for tobacco control policies and participation in tobacco control activities. *American Journal of Public Health.* 2000;90(8):1283–7.
5. Gilpin EA, Emery SL, Farkas AJ, Distefan JM, White MM, Pierce JP. *The California Tobacco Control Program: a decade of progress, results from the California tobacco surveys, 1990–1998.* La Jolla, CA: University of California, San Diego; 2001. Available from: http://repositories.cdlib.org/tc/surveys/CTS1999/. Accessed December 2004.

Indicator 1.6.5

Level of Support for Increasing Excise Tax on Tobacco Products

Goal area 1	Preventing initiation of tobacco use among young people
Outcome 6	Increased knowledge of, improved anti-tobacco attitudes toward, and increased support for policies to reduce youth initiation
What to measure	Proportion of adults who support an increase in excise tax on cigarettes and the amount of tax increase they support
Why this indicator is useful	Public opinion is a major determinant of the feasibility of enacting an excise tax increase on tobacco products. Tobacco policies are unlikely to be adopted without support from business owners, policy makers, and the general public.[1-4] Measuring policy makers' support for a tax increase will assess their willingness to support legislation for a tax increase.[5]
Example data source(s)	Adult Tobacco Survey (ATS): CDC Recommended Questions: Supplemental Section F: Policy Issues, 2003
Population group(s)	Adults aged 18 years or older
Example survey question(s)	**From ATS** How much additional tax on a pack of cigarettes would you be willing to support if some or all the money raised was used to support tobacco control programs? ☐ More than two dollars a pack ☐ Less than fifty cents a pack ☐ Two dollars a pack ☐ No tax increase ☐ One dollar a pack ☐ Don't know/Not sure ☐ Fifty to ninety-nine cents a pack ☐ Refused
Comments	The example questions could be asked of decision makers or opinion leaders. Evaluators may want to analyze the level of support for increasing an excise tax on tobacco products according to the smoking status of the respondent. To gather more complete data on tobacco use, evaluators can also ask questions about the use of other tobacco products such as spit tobacco (smokeless), bidis, small cigars, and loose tobacco (roll-your-own).

Rating

Overall quality low ←——→ high	Resources needed	Strength of evaluation evidence	Utility	Face validity	Accepted practice
■■■■■	$$†	⊘	◕	●	●

← ○ ◔ ◕ ● → better

† Denotes low agreement among reviewers: that is, fewer than 75% of the valid ratings for this indicator were within one point of each other (see Appendix B for an explanation).
⊘ Denotes no data.

References
1. U.S. Department of Health and Human Services. *Reducing tobacco use: a report of the Surgeon General.* Atlanta, GA: Centers for Disease Control and Prevention; 2000.
2. U.S. Department of Health and Human Services. *Women and smoking: a report of the Surgeon General.* Rockville, MD: U.S. Department of Health and Human Services, Public Health Service, Office of the Surgeon General; 2001.
3. Thompson GW, Wilson N. Public attitudes about tobacco smoke in workplaces: the importance of workers' rights in survey questions. *Tobacco Control.* 2003;13:206–8.
4. Howard KA, Rogers T, Howard-Pitney B, Flora JA, Norman GJ, Ribisl KM. Opinion leaders' support for tobacco control policies and participation in tobacco control activities. *American Journal of Public Health.* 2000;90(8):1283–7.
5. O'Connell P. Tobacco control in the land of the golden leaf. Has political perception kept pace with reality? *North Carolina Medical Journal.* 2002;63(3):175–6.

GOAL AREA 1
Outcome 6

Indicator 1.6.6

Level of Awareness Among Parents About the Importance of Discussing Tobacco Use with Their Children

Goal area 1	Preventing initiation of tobacco use among young people
Outcome 6	Increased knowledge of, improved anti-tobacco attitudes toward, and increased support for policies to reduce youth initiation
What to measure	Proportion of parents who believe that discussing tobacco use with their children is important
Why this indicator is useful	Although studies show that parental discussion about tobacco can reduce young people's tobacco use, many parents do not discuss tobacco use with their children.[1-3] Increasing awareness among parents of the importance of discussing tobacco use with their children is an important step in reducing tobacco initiation and use.
Example data source(s)	No commonly used data sources were found
Population group(s)	Parents of young people aged less than 18 years
Example survey question(s)	How important is it that you discuss tobacco use with your child(ren)? Would you say it is ☐ Very important ☐ Somewhat important ☐ Not very important ☐ Not important at all ☐ No opinion/Don't know ☐ Refused to answer
Comments	The authors created this example question. It does not come from any commonly used data source.
Rating	Overall quality: low→high (marked low)[†]; Resources needed: $$; Strength of evaluation evidence: ●; Utility: ○; Face validity: ○[†]; Accepted practice: ◐ ←○ ◐ ● ●→ better

† Denotes low agreement among reviewers: that is, fewer than 75% of the valid ratings for this indicator were within one point of each other (see Appendix B for an explanation).

References
1. Clark PI, Scarisbrick-Hauser A, Gautam SP, Wirk SJ. Anti-tobacco socialization in homes of African-American and white parents, and smoking and nonsmoking parents. *Journal of Adolescent Health*. 1999;24:329–39.
2. Jackson C, Henriksen L. Do as I say: parent smoking, antismoking socialization, and smoking onset among children. *Addictive Behaviors*. 1997;22(1):107–14.
3. U.S. Department of Health and Human Services. *Preventing tobacco use among young people: a report of the Surgeon General*. Atlanta, GA: Centers for Disease Control and Prevention; 1994.

Indicator 1.6.7[NR]

Level of Support for Creating Policies in Schools

Goal area 1	Preventing initiation of tobacco use among young people
Outcome 6	Increased knowledge of, improved anti-tobacco attitudes toward, and increased support for policies to reduce youth initiation
What to measure	Proportion of adults who support creating and actively enforcing tobacco-free policies in schools
Why this indicator is useful	Young people's attitudes about the acceptability of smoking are influenced by what they see their peers and educators doing at school. Strong school anti-tobacco policies require the support of parents, teachers, principals, policy makers, and the general public.[1]
Example data source(s)	▸ Adult Tobacco Survey (ATS): CDC Recommended Questions: Supplemental Section F: Policy Issues, 2003 ▸ University of California at San Diego, California Tobacco Survey (CTS): Adult Attitudes and Practices, 1996 Information on CTS available at: • http://ssdc.ucsd.edu/tobacco • http://www.dhs.ca.gov/ps/cdic/ccb/TCS/html/Evaluation_Resources.htm ▸ Behavioral Risk Factor Surveillance System (BRFSS), Tobacco Use Prevention Module, 2000
Population group(s)	Adults aged 18 years or older
Example survey question(s)	**From ATS** How strongly do you agree or disagree with the following statement: Tobacco use by adults should not be allowed on school grounds or at any school events. ☐ Strongly agree ☐ Agree ☐ Disagree ☐ Strongly disagree ☐ No opinion/Don't know ☐ Refused **From CTS** Do you think schools should prohibit students from wearing clothing or bringing gear with tobacco brand logos to school? ☐ Yes ☐ No **From BRFSS** Do you think that smoking should be allowed in all areas of schools, restaurants, day care, and indoor work areas, some areas, or not allowed at all? ☐ All areas ☐ Some areas ☐ Not allowed ☐ Refused to answer
Comments	The example questions could also be asked of decision makers. Evaluators may want to analyze the level of support for creating tobacco-free policies in schools based on the respondent's tobacco use. This indicator was not rated by the panel of experts and, therefore, no rating information is provided. See Appendix B for an explanation.

Rating	Overall quality low ⟷ high	Resources needed	Strength of evaluation evidence	Utility	Face validity	Accepted practice
	▬▬▬▬▬	⊘	⊘	⊘	⊘	⊘

←○◐●●→ better

⊘ Denotes no data.

NR Denotes an indicator that is not rated (see Appendix B for an explanation).

Reference
1. Task Force on Community Preventive Services Meeting. February 25, 2004. Meeting minutes available at www.thecommunityguide.org.

Indicator 1.6.8[NR]

Proportion of Young People Who Think That the Cigarette Companies Try to Get Young People to Smoke

Goal area 1	Preventing initiation of tobacco use among young people
Outcome 6	Increased knowledge of, improved anti-tobacco attitudes toward, and increased support for policies to reduce youth initiation
What to measure	Proportion of young people who believe that cigarette companies try to get young people to start smoking
Why this indicator is useful	If young people are aware of the tobacco industry's attempts to persuade them to start smoking, they may become less susceptible to the tobacco industry's marketing tactics.[1]
Example data source(s)	California Independent Evaluation: Youth Survey, 2000 Information available at: http://www.dhs.ca.gov/ps/cdic/ccb/TCS/html/Evaluation_Resources.htm
Population group(s)	Young people aged less than 18 years
Example survey question(s)	**From California Independent Evaluation: Youth Survey** Do tobacco companies try to get young people to start smoking by using advertisements that are attractive to young people? ☐ Yes, definitely ☐ Yes, maybe ☐ Probably not ☐ Not sure
Comments	This indicator was not rated by the panel of experts and, therefore, no rating information is provided. See Appendix B for an explanation.

Rating

Overall quality low ⟷ high	Resources needed	Strength of evaluation evidence	Utility	Face validity	Accepted practice
▬▬▬▬▬	⊘	⊘	⊘	⊘	⊘

← ○ ◔ ◉ ● → better

⊘ Denotes no data.

[NR] Denotes an indicator that is not rated (see Appendix B for an explanation).

Reference
1. Evans N, Farkas A, Gilpin E, Berry C, Pierce JP. Influence of tobacco marketing and exposure to smokers on adolescent susceptibility to smoking. *Journal of the National Cancer Institute.* 1995;87(20):1538–45.

Outcome 7

Increased Anti-tobacco Policies and Programs in Schools

To prevent and reduce tobacco use by young people, schools should implement comprehensive anti-tobacco policies and programs that reinforce tobacco-free norms. Young people spend much of their time in school and are influenced by school policies and programs and by the actions of their peers and of adults.[1] Evidence shows that education programs that include instruction on the short- and long-term physiologic and social consequences of tobacco use, social influences on tobacco use, peer norms, and life skills can prevent or reduce tobacco use among students.[2,3] School-based interventions that are combined with mass media campaigns and additional community-wide educational anti-tobacco activities show evidence of effectiveness in reducing tobacco use among young people.[3] The Community Guide to Preventive Services Task Force, however, states that insufficient evidence is available to indicate that either school-based education programs (e.g., classroom programs) or student-delivered community education (e.g., Students Working Against Tobacco [SWAT]) are effective when implemented alone, without other community activities to supplement or reinforce them.[3]

The demand for effective tobacco-use cessation interventions for young people has been growing.[4] As with all public health programs, such interventions must be based on evidence that proves that they work. Unfortunately, few rigorous scientific studies exist on which to base recommendations that would help young smokers quit.[4]

CDC provides guidelines for school health programs to prevent tobacco use and addiction.[2] The guidelines include recommendations on policies, curricula and instruction, teacher training, parental involvement, tobacco-use cessation, and evaluation. The guidelines are based on research, scientific theory, and practice.

Listed below are the indicators associated with this outcome:

1.7.1 Proportion of schools or school districts reporting the implementation of 100% tobacco-free policies

1.7.2 Proportion of schools or school districts that provide instruction on tobacco-use prevention that meets CDC guidelines

1.7.3 Proportion of schools or school districts that provide tobacco-use prevention education in grades K–12

1.7.4 Proportion of schools or school districts that provide program-specific training for teachers

1.7.5 Proportion of schools or school districts that involve families in support of school-based programs

1.7.6 Proportion of schools or school districts that support cessation interventions for students and staff who use tobacco

1.7.7 Proportion of schools or school districts that assess their tobacco-use prevention program at regular intervals

- **1.7.8** Proportion of students who participate in tobacco-use prevention activities
- **1.7.9** Level of reported exposure to school-based tobacco-use prevention curricula that meet CDC guidelines
- **1.7.10** Perceived compliance with tobacco-free policies in schools
- **1.7.11** Proportion of schools or school districts with policies that regulate display of tobacco industry promotional items

References

1. U.S. Department of Health and Human Services. *Preventing tobacco use among young people: a report of the Surgeon General.* Atlanta, GA: Centers for Disease Control and Prevention; 1994.
2. Centers for Disease Control and Prevention. Guidelines for school health programs to prevent tobacco use and addiction. *Morbidity and Mortality Weekly Report Recommendations and Reports.* 1994;43(RR-2):1–18. Available from: http://www.cdc.gov/mmwr/PDF/RR/RR4302.pdf. Accessed March 2005.
3. Task Force on Community Preventive Services Meeting. February 25, 2004. Meeting minutes available at www.thecommunityguide.org.
4. Milton MH, Maule CO, Yee SL, Backinger C, Malarcher AM, Husten CG. *Youth tobacco cessation: a guide for making informed decisions.* Atlanta, GA: Centers for Disease Control and Prevention; 2004.

For Further Reading

Alcaraz R, Klonoff EA, Landrine H. The effects on children of participating in studies of minors' access to tobacco. *Preventive Medicine.* 1997;26(2):236–40.

Epstein JA, Griffin KW, Botvin GJ. Competence skills help deter smoking among inner city adolescents. *Tobacco Control.* 2000;9(1):33–9.

Farrelly MC, Healton CG, Davis KC, Messeri P, Hersey JC, Haviland ML. Getting to the truth: evaluating national tobacco countermarketing campaigns. *American Journal of Public Health.* 2002;92(6):901–7. Erratum in: *American Journal of Public Health.* 2003;93(5):703.

Glantz SA, Begay ME. Tobacco industry campaign contributions are affecting tobacco control policymaking in California. *Journal of the American Medical Association.* 1994; 272(15):1176–82.

Huang TT, Unger JB, Rohrbach LA. Exposure to, and perceived usefulness of, school-based tobacco-prevention programs: associations with susceptibility to smoking among adolescents. *Journal of Adolescent Health.* 2000;27(4):248–54.

Lee DJ, Trapido E, Weatherby N, Rodriguez R. Correlates of participation and willingness to participate in anti-tobacco activities among 4th–7th graders. *Journal of Community Health*. 2001;26(6):447–57.

Lewit EM, Hyland A, Kerrebrock N, Cummings KM. Price, public policy, and smoking in young people. *Tobacco Control*. 1997;6(Suppl 2):S17–24.

National Cancer Institute. Smoking and Tobacco Control Monograph, No. 14. *Changing adolescent smoking prevalence: where it is and why.* Bethesda, MD: National Cancer Institute; 2001. NIH Publication No. 02-5086.

Pierce JP, Gilpin EA, Emery SL, White MM, Rosbrook B, Berry CC, Farkas AJ. Has the California tobacco control program reduced smoking? *Journal of the American Medical Association*. 1998;280(10):893–9.

Rohrbach LA, Howard-Pitney B, Unger JB, Dent CW, Howard KA, Cruz TB, Ribisl KM, Norman GJ, Fishbein H, Johnson CA. Independent evaluation of the California Tobacco Control Program: relationships between program exposure and outcomes, 1996–1998. *American Journal of Public Health*. 2002;92(6):975–83.

Sargent JD, Dalton MA, Beach M, Bernhardt A, Pullin D, Stevens M. Cigarette promotional items in public schools. *Archives of Pediatrics & Adolescent Medicine*. 1997;151(12):1189–96.

Siegel M, Biener L. The impact of an antismoking media campaign on progression to established smoking: results of a longitudinal youth study. *American Journal of Public Health*. 2000;90(3):380–6.

Sly DF, Heald GR, Ray S. The Florida "truth" anti-tobacco media evaluation: design, first year results, and implications for planning future state media evaluations. *Tobacco Control*. 2001;10(1):9–15.

Sly DF, Trapido E, Ray S. Evidence of the dose effects of an antitobacco counter-advertising campaign. *Preventive Medicine*. 2002;35(5):511–8.

Straub DM, Hills NK, Thompson PJ, Moscicki AB. Effects of pro- and anti-tobacco advertising on nonsmoking adolescents' intentions to smoke. *Journal of Adolescent Health*. 2003;32(1):36–43.

Task Force on Community Preventive Services. The guide to community preventive services: tobacco use prevention and control. *American Journal of Preventive Medicine*. 2001;20(Suppl 2):1–88.

U.S. Department of Health and Human Services. *Preventing tobacco use among young people: a report of the Surgeon General.* Atlanta, GA: Centers for Disease Control and Prevention; 1994.

Unger JB, Rohrbach LA, Howard KA, Boley Cruz T, Johnson CA, Chen X. Attitudes toward anti-tobacco policy among California youth: associations with smoking status, psychosocial variables and advocacy actions. *Health Education Resources.* 1999;14(6):751–63.

Winkleby MA, Feighery EC, Altman DA, Kole S, Tencati E. Engaging ethnically diverse teens in a substance-use prevention advocacy program. *American Journal of Health Promotion.* 2001;15(6):433–6.

Zucker D, Hopkins R, Sly D, Urich J, Mendoza Kershaw J, Solari S. Florida's "truth" campaign: a counter-marketing, anti-tobacco media campaign. *Journal of Public Health Management and Practice.* 2000;6(3):1–6.

Outcome 7

Increased Anti-tobacco Policies and Programs in Schools

Indicator Rating
← ○ ◐ ● ● → better

Number	Indicator	Overall quality (low → high)	Resources needed	Strength of evaluation evidence	Utility	Face validity	Accepted practice
1.7.1	Proportion of schools or school districts reporting the implementation of 100% tobacco-free policies	▬▬▬▬†	$$	●	◐	●	●
1.7.2	Proportion of schools or school districts that provide instruction on tobacco-use prevention that meets CDC guidelines	▬▬▬	$$	●	○	◐†	◐
1.7.3	Proportion of schools or school districts that provide tobacco-use prevention education in grades K–12	▬▬▬▬†	$$	◐	◐	◐	◐†
1.7.4	Proportion of schools or school districts that provide program-specific training for teachers	▬▬▬	$$	○	○	◐	◐
1.7.5	Proportion of schools or school districts that involve families in support of school-based programs	▬▬▬▬†	$$	○	○	◐	◐
1.7.6	Proportion of schools or school districts that support cessation interventions for students and staff who use tobacco	▬▬▬	$$	○	○	◐	◐
1.7.7	Proportion of schools or school districts that assess their tobacco-use prevention program at regular intervals	▬▬▬▬†	$$$	○	◐	◐†	○
1.7.8	Proportion of students who participate in tobacco-use prevention activities	▬▬▬▬†	$$	◐	◐	◐	◐
1.7.9	Level of reported exposure to school-based tobacco-use prevention curricula that meet CDC guidelines	▬▬▬	$$	◐	◐	◐	◐
1.7.10	Perceived compliance with tobacco-free policies in schools	▬▬▬	$$	⊘	◐	◐	●
1.7.11	Proportion of schools or school districts with policies that regulate display of tobacco industry promotional items	▬▬▬	$$	◐	◐	◐	◐

† Denotes low agreement among reviewers: that is, fewer than 75% of the valid ratings for this indicator were within one point of each other (see Appendix B for an explanation).
⊘ Denotes no data.

Indicator 1.7.1

Proportion of Schools or School Districts Reporting the Implementation of 100% Tobacco-free Policies

Goal area 1	Preventing initiation of tobacco use among young people
Outcome 7	Increased anti-tobacco policies and programs in schools
What to measure	Proportion of schools or school districts that report having a policy that prohibits anyone from using tobacco at all times on school grounds, at all school-sponsored functions, and in school vehicles
Why this indicator is useful	Young people spend much of their formative years in school. Their attitudes toward the acceptability of smoking in general are influenced by the actions of their peers and educators at school.[1,2]
Example data source(s)	CDC School Health Profiles: School Principal Questionnaire (Profiles), 2002
Population group(s)	School principals
Example survey question(s)	**From Profiles** Has this school adopted a policy prohibiting tobacco use? ☐ Yes ☐ No Does the tobacco prevention policy specifically prohibit use of each type of tobacco product for each for the following groups? Type of tobacco product — Students (Yes/No) — Faculty/Staff (Yes/No) — Visitors (Yes/No) • Cigarettes • Smokeless tobacco • Cigars • Pipes Does the tobacco prevention policy specifically prohibit use during each of the following times for each for the following groups? Time — Students (Yes/No) — Faculty/Staff (Yes/No) — Visitors (Yes/No) • During school hours • During non-school hours Does the tobacco prevention policy specifically prohibit tobacco use in each of the following locations for each of the following groups? Location — Students (Yes/No) — Faculty/Staff (Yes/No) — Visitors (Yes/No) • In school buildings • On school grounds • In school buses or other vehicles used to transport students • At off-campus, school-sponsored events

Comments	To measure this indicator fully, evaluators should use all four example questions, not just one or two.
	Evaluators could also collect information on school districts in order to measure the proportion of students in the district who attend schools with anti-tobacco policies.
	This indicator can be used to measure progress toward achieving Recommendation 1 of CDC's "Guidelines for School Health Programs to Prevent Tobacco Use and Addiction."[1]

Rating

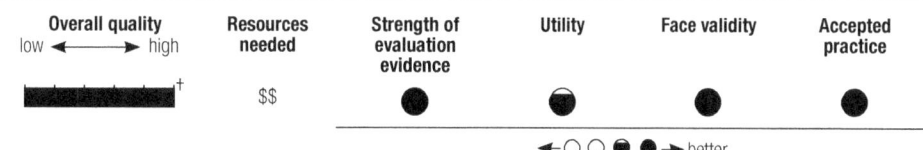

† Denotes low agreement among reviewers: that is, fewer than 75% of the valid ratings for this indicator were within one point of each other (see Appendix B for an explanation).

References
1. Centers for Disease Control and Prevention. Guidelines for school health programs to prevent tobacco use and addiction. *Morbidity and Mortality Weekly Report Recommendations and Reports.* 1994;43(RR-2):1–18.
2. U.S. Department of Health and Human Services. *Preventing tobacco use among young people: a report of the Surgeon General.* Atlanta, GA: Centers for Disease Control and Prevention; 1994.

Indicator 1.7.2

Proportion of Schools or School Districts That Provide Instruction on Tobacco-use Prevention That Meets CDC Guidelines

Goal area 1	Preventing initiation of tobacco use among young people
Outcome 7	Increased anti-tobacco policies and programs in schools
What to measure	Proportion of schools or school districts that report providing instruction on (1) the physiologic and social consequences of tobacco use and (2) the social influences on tobacco use, peer norms, and life skills
Why this indicator is useful	Evidence suggests that programs that include instruction on the short- and long-term physiologic and social consequences of tobacco use, social influences on tobacco use, peer norms, and life skills can prevent or reduce tobacco use among students.[1,2]
Example data source(s)	▹ CDC School Health Profiles: Lead Health Education Teacher Questionnaire (Profiles), 2002 ▹ California Tobacco Use Prevention Education Evaluation: Teacher Survey, 2003 Information available at: http://www.dhs.ca.gov/ps/cdic/ccb/TCS/html/Evaluation_Resources.htm
Population group(s)	▹ Health education teachers ▹ Teachers and school administrators

Example survey question(s)

From Profiles

During this school year, did teachers in this school teach each of the following tobacco use prevention topics in a required health education course for students in any of grades 6 through 12? Mark yes or no for each topic.

	Yes	No
a. Short- and long-term health consequences of cigarette smoking (such as stained teeth, bad breath, heart disease, and cancer)	☐	☐
b. Benefits of not smoking cigarettes (including long- and short-term health benefits, social benefits, environmental benefits, and financial benefits)	☐	☐
c. Risks of cigar or pipe smoking	☐	☐
d. Short- and long-term health consequences of using smokeless tobacco	☐	☐
e. Benefits of not using smokeless tobacco	☐	☐
f. Addictive effects of nicotine in tobacco products	☐	☐
g. How many young people use tobacco	☐	☐
h. The number of illnesses and deaths related to tobacco use	☐	☐
i. Influence of families on tobacco use	☐	☐
j. Influence of the media on tobacco use	☐	☐
k. Social or cultural influences on tobacco use	☐	☐
l. How to find valid information or services related to tobacco-use cessation	☐	☐
m. Making a personal commitment not to use tobacco	☐	☐
n. How students can influence or support others in efforts to prevent tobacco use	☐	☐
o. How students can influence or support others in efforts to quit using tobacco	☐	☐
p. How to say no to tobacco use	☐	☐
q. The health effects of environmental tobacco smoke (ETS) or second-hand smoke	☐	☐

Example survey question(s) (cont.)

From California Tobacco Use Prevention Education Evaluation: Teacher Survey

During the last school year (2002–2003), which of the following topics did you cover in your tobacco use prevention lessons? (Mark all that apply).

☐ I did not teach tobacco prevention lessons
☐ Effects of tobacco on health
☐ How many young people smoke
☐ Reasons why young people smoke
☐ Social consequences of using tobacco
☐ Secondhand smoke
☐ Social influences that promote tobacco use
☐ Behavioral skills for resisting tobacco offers
☐ General personal and social skills (e.g., problem solving, assertiveness, communication, and goal setting)
☐ Tobacco cessation
☐ Tobacco advertising and marketing
☐ Cigar use
☐ Other (specify):_____

Comments

It would be useful for evaluators to obtain information on the specific curriculum taught. Further information on the anti-tobacco curriculum being taught could be collected using a student survey.

This indicator can be used to measure progress toward achieving Recommendation 2 of CDC's "Guidelines for School Health Programs to Prevent Tobacco Use and Addiction."[2]

Rating

Overall quality low ◄——► high	Resources needed	Strength of evaluation evidence	Utility	Face validity	Accepted practice
▮▮▮▮	$$	●	○	●[†]	◐

◄ ○ ◔ ◑ ● ► better

† Denotes low agreement among reviewers: that is, fewer than 75% of the valid ratings for this indicator were within one point of each other (see Appendix B for an explanation).

References

1. U.S. Department of Health and Human Services. *Preventing tobacco use among young people: a report of the Surgeon General.* Atlanta, GA: Centers for Disease Control and Prevention; 1994.
2. Centers for Disease Control and Prevention. Guidelines for school health programs to prevent tobacco use and addiction. *Morbidity and Mortality Weekly Report Recommendations and Reports.* 1994;43(RR-2):1–18.

Indicator 1.7.3

Proportion of Schools or School Districts That Provide Tobacco-use Prevention Education in Grades K–12

Goal area 1	Preventing initiation of tobacco use among young people
Outcome 7	Increased anti-tobacco policies and programs in schools
What to measure	Proportion of schools or school districts that report providing tobacco-use prevention education in grades K–12
Why this indicator is useful	Research, theory, and current practice demonstrate that the success of school-based prevention programs dissipates over time. CDC's "Guidelines for School Health Programs to Prevent Tobacco Use and Addiction," therefore, calls for tobacco use prevention to be taught in each grade, with increasing intensity in middle school and reinforcement in high school grades.[1]
Example data source(s)	CDC School Health Profiles: Lead Health Education Teacher Questionnaire (Profiles), 2002
Population group(s)	Health education teachers

Example survey question(s)	**From Profiles**
	
	During the school year, in which of the following grades was information on tobacco-use prevention provided?
	
	                                                  Yes No
	    Grade 6 ☐ ☐
	    Grade 7 ☐ ☐
	    Grade 8 ☐ ☐
	    Grade 9 ☐ ☐
	    Grade 10 ☐ ☐
	    Grade 11 ☐ ☐
	    Grade 12 ☐ ☐
	
	Are required tobacco-use prevention units or lessons taught in each of the following courses in the school?
	
	    Course Yes No
	    a. Science ☐ ☐
	    b. Home economics or family
	        and consumer education ☐ ☐
	    c. Physical education ☐ ☐
	    d. Family life education
	        or life skills ☐ ☐
	    e. Special education ☐ ☐

Comments	This indicator can be used to measure progress toward achieving Recommendation 3 of CDC's "Guidelines for School Health Programs to Prevent Tobacco Use and Addiction."[1]

Rating	Overall quality low ←——→ high	Resources needed	Strength of evaluation evidence	Utility	Face validity	Accepted practice
	▬▬▬▬▬†	$$	●	●	●	●†

←○◐●●→ better

† Denotes low agreement among reviewers: that is, fewer than 75% of the valid ratings for this indicator were within one point of each other (see Appendix B for an explanation).

Reference
1. Centers for Disease Control and Prevention. Guidelines for school health programs to prevent tobacco use and addiction. *Morbidity and Mortality Weekly Report Recommendations and Reports.* 1994;43(RR-2):1–18.

Indicator 1.7.4

Proportion of Schools or School Districts That Provide Program-specific Training for Teachers

Goal area 1	Preventing initiation of tobacco use among young people
Outcome 7	Increased anti-tobacco policies and programs in schools
What to measure	Proportion of schools or school districts that report providing tobacco-use prevention education training for school educators
Why this indicator is useful	CDC's "Guidelines for School Health Programs to Prevent Tobacco Use and Addiction" state that curriculum implementation and overall program effectiveness are improved when teachers are trained to deliver the program as designed.[1]
Example data source(s)	▹ CDC School Health Profiles: Lead Health Education Teacher Questionnaire, (Profiles), 2002 ▹ California Tobacco Use Prevention Education Evaluation: Teacher Survey, 2003 Information available at: http://www.dhs.ca.gov/ps/cdic/ccb/TCS/html/Evaluation_Resources.htm ▹ California Tobacco Use Prevention Education Evaluation: District Coordinator Survey, 2003 Information available at: http://www.dhs.ca.gov/ps/cdic/ccb/TCS/html/Evaluation_Resources.htm
Population group(s)	▹ Health education teachers ▹ Teachers ▹ District coordinators
Example survey question(s)	**From Profiles** During the past two years, did you receive staff development (such as workshops, conferences, continuing education, or any other kind of in-service training) on each of the following topics? [22 health topics (letters a–v) are listed; tobacco-use prevention is one topic] Mark yes or no for each topic. Would you like to receive staff development on each of these [22] health education topics? Mark yes or no for each topic. **From California Tobacco Use Prevention Education Evaluation: Teacher Survey** During the past five years, how much tobacco use prevention training have you received? ☐ None ☐ More than one full day of in-service training ☐ One full-day of in-service training ☐ Less than a full-day of in-service training ☐ I don't remember During the past five years, were you trained to deliver a specific published tobacco-use prevention curriculum? ☐ Yes ☐ No ☐ I don't remember

GOAL AREA 1
Outcome 7

Example survey question(s) (cont.)	Overall, to what extent do you feel you are prepared to teach tobacco use prevention lessons? ☐ A great deal ☐ Somewhat ☐ Not too much ☐ Not at all ☐ Does not apply **From California Tobacco Use Prevention Education Evaluation: District Coordinator Survey** During the 2002–2003 school year, how many tobacco-specific in-service trainings, workshops, or staff development sessions has your school district sponsored or attended? _____ Number of trainings, workshops, or staff development sessions. ☐ I do not know/I'm not sure If your district did sponsor or attend tobacco-specific in-service trainings, workshops, or staff development sessions during the last school year (2002–2003), how many schools were represented? Number of schools represented: _____
Comments	This indicator can be used to measure progress toward achieving Recommendation 4 of CDC's "Guidelines for School Health Programs to Prevent Tobacco Use and Addiction."[1]
Rating	Overall quality: low ◄────► high (high) Resources needed: $$ Strength of evaluation evidence: ◐ Utility: ◐ Face validity: ● Accepted practice: ● ←○ ◐ ● ●→ better

Reference
1. Centers for Disease Control and Prevention. Guidelines for school health programs to prevent tobacco use and addiction. *Morbidity and Mortality Weekly Report Recommendations and Reports.* 1994;43(RR-2):1–18.

Indicator 1.7.5

Proportion of Schools or School Districts That Involve Families in Support of School-based Programs

Goal area 1	Preventing initiation of tobacco use among young people
Outcome 7	Increased anti-tobacco policies and programs in schools
What to measure	Proportion of schools or school districts that attempt to get students' parents or families involved in school-based tobacco-use prevention or cessation programs
Why this indicator is useful	CDC's "Guidelines for School Health Programs to Prevent Tobacco Use and Addiction" recognizes the important role that parents and families play in providing social and environmental support that will help young people remain tobacco-free. Families are part of the greater community to which schools should be connecting their programs.[1,2]
Example data source(s)	▹ CDC School Health Profiles: Lead Health Education Teacher Questionnaire (Profiles), 2002 ▹ California Tobacco Use Prevention Education Evaluation: Teacher Survey, 2003 Information available at: http://www.dhs.ca.gov/ps/cdic/ccb/TCS/html/Evaluation_Resources.htm
Population group(s)	▹ Health education teachers ▹ Teachers

Example survey question(s)

From Profiles

During this school year, has this school done each of the following activities? Mark yes or no for each activity.

	Yes	No
• Provided families with information on the health education program	☐	☐
• Met with a parents' organization such as the PTA or PTO to discuss the health education program	☐	☐
• Invited family members to attend a health education class	☐	☐

From California Tobacco Use Prevention Education Evaluation: Teacher Survey

To what extent have you tried to get students' parents involved in tobacco use prevention education?

Type of Involvement	Not at all	Very small extent	Small extent	Modest extent	Great extent	Very great extent
• Included parents in homework assignments	☐	☐	☐	☐	☐	☐
• Held meeting with parents of student smokers	☐	☐	☐	☐	☐	☐
• Distributed parent-student handbook that included description of tobacco-free school policy	☐	☐	☐	☐	☐	☐
• Distributed newsletters or educational materials to parents	☐	☐	☐	☐	☐	☐
• Provided information on smoking cessation to parents	☐	☐	☐	☐	☐	☐
• Had tobacco education displays or discussions at open houses, meetings, health fairs	☐	☐	☐	☐	☐	☐
• Invited parents to be guest speakers on tobacco issues	☐	☐	☐	☐	☐	☐
• Involved parents in school-related activities (e.g., as judges of poster essay contests)	☐	☐	☐	☐	☐	☐
• Other (describe)_____						

(Please mark a response for each)

Comments	The example survey questions are limited to the perspective of educators. They cannot be used to assess parents' actual involvement or desire to be involved in school-based tobacco control activities.
	This indicator can be used to measure progress toward achieving Recommendation 5 of CDC's "Guidelines for School Health Programs to Prevent Tobacco Use and Addiction."[1]

Rating	Overall quality low ←——→ high	Resources needed	Strength of evaluation evidence	Utility	Face validity	Accepted practice
	▬▬▬▬[†]	$$	◐	◐	◕	●

←○◔◑◕●→ better

† Denotes low agreement among reviewers: that is, fewer than 75% of the valid ratings for this indicator were within one point of each other (see Appendix B for an explanation).

References

1. Centers for Disease Control and Prevention. Guidelines for school health programs to prevent tobacco use and addiction. *Morbidity and Mortality Weekly Report Recommendations and Reports*. 1994;43(RR-2):1–18.
2. Task Force on Community Preventive Services Meeting. February 25, 2004. Meeting minutes available at www.thecommunityguide.org.

Indicator 1.7.6

Proportion of Schools or School Districts That Support Cessation Interventions for Students and Staff Who Use Tobacco

Goal area 1	Preventing initiation of tobacco use among young people
Outcome 7	Increased anti-tobacco policies and programs in schools
What to measure	Proportion of schools or school districts that report providing tobacco cessation support (e.g., counseling for students and staff who use tobacco or referrals to tobacco-cessation programs)
Why this indicator is useful	CDC's "Guidelines for School Health Programs to Prevent Tobacco Use and Addiction" recommends that schools support cessation for staff and students, either by providing referrals to cessation services or by sponsoring cessation programs.[1,2]
Example data source(s)	CDC School Health Profiles: School Principal Questionnaire (Profiles), 2002
Population group(s)	School principals
Example survey question(s)	**From Profiles** Does your school provide referrals to tobacco cessation programs for each of the following groups? Group Yes No • Faculty and staff ☐ ☐ • Students ☐ ☐
Comments	A survey question could be added regarding (1) the cessation services at the school or (2) the type of cessation programs to which students and faculty are referred. This indicator can be used to measure progress toward achieving Recommendation 6 of CDC's "Guidelines for School Health Programs to Prevent Tobacco Use and Addiction."[1]

Rating

Overall quality low ⟷ high	Resources needed	Strength of evaluation evidence	Utility	Face validity	Accepted practice
▬▬▬▬	$$	◐	◐	●	●

←○ ◐ ● ●→ better

References
1. Centers for Disease Control and Prevention. Guidelines for school health programs to prevent tobacco use and addiction. *Morbidity and Mortality Weekly Report Recommendations and Reports*. 1994;43(RR-2):1–18.
2. Milton MH, Maule CO, Yee SL, Backinger C, Malarcher AM, Husten CG. *Youth tobacco cessation: a guide for making informed decisions*. Atlanta, GA: Centers for Disease Control and Prevention; 2004.

GOAL AREA 1
Outcome 7

Indicator 1.7.7

Proportion of Schools or School Districts That Assess Their Tobacco-use Prevention Program at Regular Intervals

Goal area 1	Preventing initiation of tobacco use among young people
Outcome 7	Increased anti-tobacco policies and programs in schools
What to measure	Proportion of schools or school districts that report having an evaluation system in place and using it to assess their tobacco-use prevention program at regular intervals
Why this indicator is useful	CDC's "Guidelines for School Health Programs to Prevent Tobacco Use and Addiction" recommend that schools assess their tobacco-use prevention programs at regular intervals.[1]
Example data source(s)	No commonly used data sources were found
Population group(s)	School principals Health education teachers
Example survey question(s)	Does your school (or school district) assess your tobacco-use prevention program at regular intervals? ☐ Yes ☐ No ☐ Not sure
Comments	The authors created this example question. It does not come from any commonly used data source. This indicator can be used to measure progress toward achieving Recommendation 7 of CDC's "Guidelines for School Health Programs to Prevent Tobacco Use and Addiction."[1]

Rating

Overall quality low ← → high	Resources needed	Strength of evaluation evidence	Utility	Face validity	Accepted practice
[bar][†]	$$$	○	●	●[†]	◐

← ○ ◔ ◑ ● → better

† Denotes low agreement among reviewers: that is, fewer than 75% of the valid ratings for this indicator were within one point of each other (see Appendix B for an explanation).

Reference
1. Centers for Disease Control and Prevention. Guidelines for school health programs to prevent tobacco use and addiction. *Morbidity and Mortality Weekly Report Recommendations and Reports*. 1994;43(RR-2):1–18.

Indicator 1.7.8

Proportion of Students Who Participate in Tobacco-use Prevention Activities

Goal area 1	Preventing initiation of tobacco use among young people
Outcome 7	Increased anti-tobacco policies and programs in schools
What to measure	Proportion of students who report participating in at least one tobacco-use prevention activity in the past 12 months
Why this indicator is useful	An intervention with growing popularity is involving young people in anti-tobacco activities. These activities help reduce young people's susceptibility to experimenting with tobacco by changing the social norm regarding tobacco use.[1,2]
Example data source(s)	Youth Tobacco Survey (YTS): CDC Recommended Questions: Core, 2004
Population group(s)	Young people aged less than 18 years
Example survey question(s)	**From YTS** During the past 12 months, have you participated in any community activities to discourage people your age from using cigarettes, chewing tobacco, snuff, dip, or cigars? ☐ Yes ☐ No, I did not know about any activities
Comments	Evaluators may choose to categorize data by grade level and type of school (elementary, middle, high school, private, parochial, public). Evaluators may want to assess young people's awareness of anti-smoking activities at school and outside school.

Rating	Overall quality low ◄——► high	Resources needed	Strength of evaluation evidence	Utility	Face validity	Accepted practice
	▬▬▬▬▬[†]	$$	●	●	●	●

◄ ○ ◐ ● ● ► better

† Denotes low agreement among reviewers: that is, fewer than 75% of the valid ratings for this indicator were within one point of each other (see Appendix B for an explanation).

References
1. Unger JB, Rohrbach LA, Howard KA, Boley Cruz T, Johnson CA, Chen X. Attitudes toward anti-tobacco policy among California youth: associations with smoking status, psychosocial variables and advocacy actions. *Health Education Resources*. 1999;14(6):751–63.
2. Winkleby MA, Feighery E, Dunn M, Kole S, Ahn D, Killen JD. Effects of an advocacy intervention to reduce smoking among teenagers. *Archives of Pediatrics & Adolescent Medicine*. 2004;158(3):269–75.

Indicator 1.7.9

Level of Reported Exposure to School-based Tobacco-use Prevention Curricula That Meet CDC Guidelines

Goal area 1	Preventing initiation of tobacco use among young people
Outcome 7	Increased anti-tobacco policies and programs in schools
What to measure	Proportion of students who report receiving tobacco prevention education in class
Why this indicator is useful	Measuring students' recall of tobacco education helps verify curriculum delivery and saliency.[1]
Example data source(s)	Youth Tobacco Survey (YTS): CDC Recommended Questions: Core, 2004 California Independent Evaluation: Youth Survey, 2000 Information available at: http://www.dhs.ca.gov/ps/cdic/ccb/TCS/html/Evaluation_Resources.htm
Population group(s)	Young people aged less than 18 years
Example survey question(s)	**From YTS** During this school year, did you practice ways to say NO to tobacco in any of your classes (for example, by role-playing)? ☐ Yes ☐ No ☐ Not sure During this school year, were you taught in any of your classes about the dangers of tobacco use? ☐ Yes ☐ No ☐ Not sure **From California Independent Evaluation: Youth Survey** During the last year (12 months), did you discuss the reasons why people your age smoke during any of your classes? ☐ Yes ☐ No ☐ I don't know/I'm not sure During the last year (12 months), did you discuss how many people your age smoke during any of your classes? ☐ Yes ☐ No ☐ I don't know/I'm not sure
Comments	Evaluators may also choose to categorize data by grade level and type of school (elementary, middle, high school, private, parochial, public). Student perceptions of tobacco prevention education should also be evaluated; students who perceive the education as helpful are less susceptible to smoking than those who do not perceive it as useful.[2]

Rating

Overall quality low ⟵⟶ high	Resources needed	Strength of evaluation evidence	Utility	Face validity	Accepted practice
■■■■	$$	●	●	●	●

⟵ ○ ◐ ● ● ⟶ better

References
1. Centers for Disease Control and Prevention. Guidelines for school health programs to prevent tobacco use and addiction. *Morbidity and Mortality Weekly Report Recommendations and Reports.* 1994;43(RR-2):1–18.
2. Huang TTK, Unger JB, Rohrbach LA. Exposure to, and perceived usefulness of, school-based tobacco prevention programs: associations with susceptibility to smoking among adolescents. *Journal of Adolescent Health.* 2000;27(4):248–54.

Indicator 1.7.10

Perceived Compliance with Tobacco-free Policies in Schools

Goal area 1	Preventing initiation of tobacco use among young people
Outcome 7	Increased anti-tobacco policies and programs in schools
What to measure	Proportion of students who report that the school population is complying with the school's tobacco-free policy
Why this indicator is useful	Perceived compliance with tobacco-free policies is one measure of actual compliance with these policies.[1,2] If tobacco-free policies are not observed, they are not likely to be effective in changing social norms or inhibiting tobacco use among young people.
Example data source(s)	• Youth Tobacco Survey (YTS): CDC Recommended Questions: Core, 2004 • CDC Youth Risk Behavior Surveillance System (YRBSS), 2003 • California Independent Evaluation: Youth Survey, 2000 Information available at: http://www.dhs.ca.gov/ps/cdic/ccb/TCS/html/Evaluation_Resources.htm
Population group(s)	Young people aged less than 18 years
Example survey question(s)	**From YTS and YRBSS** During the past 30 days, on how many days did you smoke cigarettes on school property? ☐ 0 days ☐ 1 or 2 days ☐ 3 to 5 days ☐ 6 to 9 days ☐ 10 to 19 days ☐ 20 to 29 days ☐ All 30 days During the past 30 days, on how many days did you use chewing tobacco, snuff, or dip on school property? ☐ 0 days ☐ 1 or 2 days ☐ 3 to 5 days ☐ 6 to 9 days ☐ 10 to 19 days ☐ 20 to 29 days ☐ All 30 days **From California Independent Evaluation: Youth Survey** Is there a rule at your school that no one is allowed to smoke cigarettes in the school building or on the school yard? ☐ Yes ☐ No ☐ I don't know/I'm not sure Have you seen any students break that rule? ☐ Yes ☐ No ☐ My school does not have a no-smoking rule ☐ I don't know/I'm not sure How many students who are smokers break that rule? ☐ None ☐ A few ☐ Some ☐ Most ☐ All of them ☐ My school does not have a no-smoking rule ☐ I don't know/I'm not sure Have you seen adults break that rule? ☐ Yes ☐ No ☐ My school does not have a no-smoking rule ☐ I don't know/I'm not sure Is there a rule at your school that no one is allowed to use chewing tobacco or snuff in the school building or on the school yard? ☐ Yes ☐ No ☐ I don't know/I'm not sure

Comments	If students report on the YTS or YRBSS instruments (1) the existence of a tobacco-free school policy and (2) having personally used tobacco products more than 1 day on school property, they are considered noncompliant.
	Evaluators may categorize data by grade level and type of school (elementary, middle, high school, private, parochial, public).
	Evaluators should determine the scope of the tobacco-free policies before evaluating perceived compliance with them.
	The example survey questions could be asked of teachers and principals.

Rating	Overall quality (low ↔ high)	Resources needed	Strength of evaluation evidence	Utility	Face validity	Accepted practice
	high	$$	⊘	◑	◐	●

←○◔◑●→ better

⊘ Denotes no data.

References
1. Shopland DR, Anderson CM, Burns DM, Gerlach KK. Disparities in smoke-free workplace policies among food service workers. *Journal of Occupational and Environmental Medicine.* 2004;46(4):347–56.
2. Weber MD, Bagwell DA, Fielding JE, Glantz SA. Long-term compliance with California's smoke-free workplace law among bars and restaurants in Los Angeles County. *Tobacco Control.* 2003;12:269–73.

Indicator 1.7.11

Proportion of Schools or School Districts with Policies That Regulate Display of Tobacco Industry Promotional Items

Goal area 1	Preventing initiation of tobacco use among young people
Outcome 7	Increased anti-tobacco policies and programs in schools
What to measure	Proportion of schools and school districts that have policies that regulate the display of tobacco advertising in the school, on school grounds, on school vehicles, or in school publications. This policy should cover apparel and other merchandise showing tobacco logos.
Why this indicator is useful	Studies have consistently associated possession of or willingness to use tobacco industry promotional items with increased smoking among youth.[1,2] Restrictions on the display of these promotional items at school contribute to an anti-tobacco social norm.
Example data source(s)	CDC School Health Profiles: School Principal Questionnaire (Profiles), 2002
Population group(s)	School principals
Example survey question(s)	**From Profiles** Is tobacco advertising prohibited in each of the following locations? Location — Yes / No • In the school building • On the school grounds, including on the outside of the building, on playing fields, or other areas of the campus • On school buses or other vehicles used to transport students • In school publications Is tobacco advertising through sponsorship of school events prohibited? Are students at your school prohibited from wearing tobacco brand-name apparel or carrying merchandise with tobacco company names, logos, or cartoon characters on it? Does your school post signs marking a tobacco-free school zone (that is, a specified distance from school grounds where tobacco use by students, faculty and staff, and visitors is not allowed?)
Comments	Evaluators may also choose to categorize data by grade level and type of school (elementary, middle, high school, private, parochial, public).

Rating

Overall quality low ◄──► high	Resources needed	Strength of evaluation evidence	Utility	Face validity	Accepted practice
▮▮▮▮▮	$$	●	●	●	●

◄ ○ ◔ ● ● ► better

References
1. Sargent JD, Dalton MA, Beach M, Bernhardt A, Pullin D, Stevens M. Cigarette promotional items in public schools. *Archives of Pediatrics & Adolescent Medicine.* 1997;151(12):1189–96.
2. Centers for Disease Control and Prevention. Guidelines for school health programs to prevent tobacco use and addiction. *Morbidity and Mortality Weekly Report Recommendations and Reports.* 1994;43(RR-2):1–18.

Outcome 8

Increased Restriction and Enforcement of Restrictions on Tobacco Sales to Minors

Activities to decrease young people's access to tobacco products are recognized components of a comprehensive approach to reducing the number of young people who start smoking. Efforts to reduce young people's access to tobacco products are based on the rationale that making it more difficult for young people to obtain tobacco products will discourage them from beginning or continuing to use tobacco and thus reduce the prevalence of tobacco use. One strategy is to attempt to reduce retail tobacco sales to minors through activities such as (1) passing laws that restrict young people's access to tobacco (including laws barring the sale of tobacco products to minors, bans on self-service displays of tobacco products, and bans or restrictions on tobacco vending machines), (2) educating merchants about these laws, (3) enforcing compliance with these laws, (4) educating the community and the media about the value of these laws, and (5) mobilizing the community to support these laws.

Experience shows that adoption and sustained enforcement of strong laws are prerequisites for reducing young people's access to tobacco. Although this approach is necessary for success, it is not sufficient. Compliance checks show that laws against selling tobacco products to young people, when accompanied by retailer education and enforcement, can reduce the proportion of retailers who are willing to sell these products to minors. But, these reductions do not automatically translate into reductions in young people's self-reported or perceived access to tobacco products, or into reductions in their tobacco use—the ultimate goal of youth access interventions.[1] Some studies suggest that even if only a few retail outlets in a community sell tobacco to minors, young people who use tobacco are likely to know of these outlets and to frequent them.[2]

According to the *Guide to Community Preventive Services*, the most effective approach to preventing young people from gaining access to tobacco products (as measured by minors' self-reported tobacco purchase or use behaviors) consists of a combination of strong local and state laws, vigorous and sustained enforcement of these laws, retailer education, and—most importantly—community mobilization to generate community support for efforts to reduce youth access to tobacco products.[3] As with other aspects of tobacco control, community mobilization may play a particularly important role because of its ability to change social norms—in this case, norms regarding the social acceptability of selling or otherwise providing tobacco products to minors. The *Guide to Community Preventive Services* indicates that none of the interventions listed above have been shown to be effective when implemented in isolation, in particular when implemented without a strong link to community mobilization initiatives.[3]

Moreover, even if illegal sales to minors were eliminated completely, young people could still acquire tobacco products through other, noncommercial or social sources, including shoplifting, stealing from parents and other relatives, borrowing from friends and relatives, and asking older friends or strangers to buy tobacco products for them. In fact, younger children (who have less success than older children in purchasing tobacco products at retail outlets) often rely on these alternative sources to obtain tobacco products. Thus, even interventions that are successful in reducing young people's self-reported or perceived access to tobacco products through commercial sources will not necessarily reduce their overall access to or use of these products. Accordingly, as rates of retail sales to minors decline, interventions to address these other sources of access will become increasingly important.

Listed below are the indicators associated with this outcome:

- **1.8.1** Proportion of jurisdictions with policies that ban tobacco vending machine sales in places accessible to young people
- **1.8.2** Proportion of jurisdictions with policies that require retail licenses to sell tobacco products
- **1.8.3** Proportion of jurisdictions with policies that control the location, number, and density of retail outlets
- **1.8.4** Proportion of jurisdictions with policies that control self-service tobacco sales
- **1.8.5** Number of compliance checks conducted by enforcement agencies
- **1.8.6** Number of warnings, citations, and fines issued for infractions of public policies against young people's access to tobacco products
- **1.8.7** Changes in state tobacco control laws that preempt stronger local tobacco control laws

References

1. Rigotti NA, DiFranza JR, Chang Y, Tisdale T, Kemp B, Singer DE. The effect of enforcing tobacco-sales laws on adolescents' access to tobacco and smoking behavior. *New England Journal of Medicine.* 1997;337:1044–51.

2. DiFranza JR, Coleman M. Source of tobacco for youths in communities with strong enforcement of youth access laws. *Tobacco Control.* 2001;10(4):323–8.

3. Fielding JE, Briss PA, Carande-Kulis VG, Hopkins DP, Husten CG, Pechacek TF, et al. Tobacco. In: Briss PA, Zaza S, Harris KW, editors. *The guide to community preventive services.* New York: Oxford University Press; in press 2005.

For Further Reading

Castrucci BC, Gerlach KK, Kaufman NJ, Orleans CT. The association among adolescents' tobacco use, their beliefs and attitudes, and friends' and parents' opinions of smoking. *Maternal and Child Health Journal.* 2002;6(3):159–67.

Celebucki CC, Diskin K. A longitudinal study of externally visible cigarette advertising on retail storefronts in Massachusetts before and after the Master Settlement Agreement. *Tobacco Control.* 2002;11(Suppl 2):ii47–53.

Distefan JM, Gilpin EA, Choi WS, Pierce JP. Parental influences predict adolescent smoking in the United States, 1989–1993. *Journal of Adolescent Health*. 1998; 22(6):466–74.

Howard KA, Ribisl KM, Howard-Pitney B, Norman GJ, Rohrbach LA. What factors are associated with local enforcement of laws banning illegal tobacco sales to minors? A study of 182 law enforcement agencies in California. *Preventive Medicine*. 2001 Aug;33(2 Pt 1):63–70.

Jackson C, Dickinson D. Can parents who smoke socialise their children against smoking? Results from the Smoke-Free Kids intervention trial. *Tobacco Control*. 2003;12(1):52–9.

Jackson C, Henriksen L. Do as I say: parent smoking, antismoking socialization, and smoking onset among children. *Addictive Behaviors*. 1997;22(1):107–14.

Lantz PM, Jacobson PD, Warner KE, Wasserman J, Pollack HA, Berson J, Ahlstrom A. Investing in youth tobacco control: a review of smoking prevention and control strategies. *Tobacco Control*. 2000;9(1):47–63.

Pierce JP, Distefan JM, Jackson C, White MM, Gilpin EA. Does tobacco marketing undermine the influence of recommended parenting in discouraging adolescents from smoking? *American Journal of Preventive Medicine*. 2002;23(2):73–81.

Saffer H, Chaloupka F. The effect of tobacco advertising bans on tobacco consumption. *Journal of Health Economics*. 2000;19(6):1117–37.

Sargent JD, Dalton M. Does parental disapproval of smoking prevent adolescents from becoming established smokers? *Pediatrics*. 2001;108(6):1256–62.

Schooler C, Feighery E, Flora JA. Seventh graders' self-reported exposure to cigarette marketing and its relationship to their smoking behavior. *American Journal of Public Health*. 1996;86(9):1216–21.

Outcome 8

Increased Restriction and Enforcement of Restrictions on Tobacco Sales to Minors

Indicator Rating
← ○ ◐ ● ● → better

Number	Indicator	Overall quality (low → high)	Resources needed	Strength of evaluation evidence	Utility	Face validity	Accepted practice
1.8.1	Proportion of jurisdictions with policies that ban tobacco vending machine sales in places accessible to young people	▬▬▬▬	$$$	●	○	●	●†
1.8.2	Proportion of jurisdictions with policies that require retail licenses to sell tobacco products	▬▬▬▬	$$$	●	●	●	●
1.8.3	Proportion of jurisdictions with policies that control the location, number, and density of retail outlets	▬▬▬▬	$$$	◐	◐*	◐	◐*
1.8.4	Proportion of jurisdictions with policies that control self-service tobacco sales	▬▬▬▬	$$$	●	●	●	●
1.8.5	Number of compliance checks conducted by enforcement agencies	▬▬▬▬†	$$$	●	●	●	●
1.8.6	Number of warnings, citations, and fines issued for infractions of public policies against young people's access to tobacco products	▬▬▬▬†	$$$	●	●	●	●
1.8.7	Changes in state tobacco control laws that preempt stronger local tobacco control laws	▬▬▬▬†	$	⊘	●	●	●

* Denotes low reviewer response: that is, greater than 75% of the experts either did not rate the indicator, or gave the criterion an invalid rating (see Appendix B for an explanation).
† Denotes low agreement among reviewers: that is, fewer than 75% of the valid ratings for this indicator were within one point of each other (see Appendix B for an explanation).
⊘ Denotes no data.

GOAL AREA 1
Outcome 8

Indicator 1.8.1

Proportion of Jurisdictions with Policies That Ban Tobacco Vending Machine Sales in Places Accessible to Young People

Goal area 1	Preventing initiation of tobacco use among young people
Outcome 8	Increased restriction and enforcement of restrictions on tobacco sales to minors
What to measure	Proportion of local jurisdictions that have enforceable policies banning tobacco vending machine sales in locations accessible to minors
Why this indicator is useful	Accessible vending machines provide virtually unrestricted access to tobacco and can be used by even the youngest children. As of 2004, 46 states and the District of Columbia restricted minors' access to tobacco through vending machines, and 30 states and the District of Columbia banned vending machines in locations that are accessible to young people.[1]
Example data source(s)	Policy tracking system Americans for Nonsmokers' Rights (ANR) Information on ANR available at: http://www.no-smoke.org American Lung Association's State Legislated Actions on Tobacco Issues (SLATI) Information on SLATI available at: http://slati.lungusa.org
Population group(s)	Not applicable. This indicator is best measured by tracking and monitoring pertinent local tobacco laws, ordinances, or regulations.
Example survey question(s)	Not applicable
Comments	Evaluators may want to assess the levels of restrictions on tobacco vending machines (e.g., restrictions on placement of vending machines). Evaluators may also choose to gather data on the size and demographics of the population affected by the relevant laws or ordinances.

Rating

Overall quality low ◄──► high	Resources needed	Strength of evaluation evidence	Utility	Face validity	Accepted practice
	$$$	●	◐	●	●[†]

◄○◐●●► better

† Denotes low agreement among reviewers: that is, fewer than 75% of the valid ratings for this indicator were within one point of each other (see Appendix B for an explanation).

Reference
1. Centers for Disease Control and Prevention. *State Tobacco Activities Tracking and Evaluation (STATE) system.* Atlanta, GA: Centers for Disease Control and Prevention. Online database. Available from: http://www.cdc.gov/tobacco/statesystem. Accessed February 2005.

Indicator 1.8.2

Proportion of Jurisdictions with Policies That Require Retail Licenses to Sell Tobacco Products

Goal area 1	Preventing initiation of tobacco use among young people
Outcome 8	Increased restriction and enforcement of restrictions on tobacco sales to minors
What to measure	Proportion of local jurisdictions that have public policies requiring retailers to have a license in order to sell tobacco products
Why this indicator is useful	Licensing laws that include graduated penalties for illegal sales and provisions for suspension or revocation for repeated violations may be an incentive for merchants to obey the law.[1] Requiring licenses allows evaluators to develop a comprehensive list of tobacco merchants that can be used to conduct compliance checks. In addition, licensing fees can be used to support the cost of compliance checks. As of 2004, 39 states and the District of Columbia required tobacco retailers to obtain a license for over-the-counter tobacco sales and 27 states and the District of Columbia had laws in place identifying circumstances in which retail licenses can be suspended or revoked.[2]
Example data source(s)	▸ Policy tracking system ▸ Americans for Nonsmokers' Rights (ANR) Information on ANR available at: http://www.no-smoke.org
Population group(s)	Not applicable. This indicator is best measured by tracking and monitoring pertinent local tobacco laws, ordinances, or regulations.
Example survey question(s)	Not applicable
Comments	Evaluators may also choose to gather data on the size and demographics of the population affected by the relevant laws or ordinances.

Rating	Overall quality low ◄——► high	Resources needed	Strength of evaluation evidence	Utility	Face validity	Accepted practice
	███████████	$$$	●	●	●	●

◄ ○ ◐ ● ● ► better

References
1. Forster JL, Wolfson M. Youth access to tobacco: policies and politics. *Annual Review of Public Health.* 1998;19:203–35.
2. Centers for Disease Control and Prevention. *State Tobacco Activities Tracking and Evaluation (STATE) system.* Atlanta, GA: Centers for Disease Control and Prevention. Online database. Available from: http://www.cdc.gov/tobacco/statesystem. Accessed February 2005.

Indicator 1.8.3

Proportion of Jurisdictions with Policies That Control the Location, Number, and Density of Retail Outlets

Goal area 1	Preventing initiation of tobacco use among young people
Outcome 8	Increased restriction and enforcement of restrictions on tobacco sales to minors
What to measure	Proportion of local jurisdictions that have public policies controlling the location, number, and density of tobacco retail outlets
Why this indicator is useful	Limiting the number of retail tobacco outlets decreases the availability of tobacco products and the number of pro-tobacco messages in a community. It also means that fewer stores need to be monitored for compliance with laws that prohibit young people's access to tobacco.[1,2]
Example data source(s)	Policy tracking system Americans for Nonsmokers' Rights (ANR) Information on ANR available at: http://www.no-smoke.org
Population group(s)	Not applicable. This indicator is best measured by tracking and monitoring pertinent local tobacco laws, ordinances, or regulations.
Example survey question(s)	Not applicable
Comments	Evaluators may also choose to gather data on the size and demographics of the population affected by the relevant laws or ordinances.

Rating

Overall quality low ◄──► high	Resources needed	Strength of evaluation evidence	Utility	Face validity	Accepted practice
▬▬▬▬▬	$$$	◐	◐*	◐	◐*

◄─ ○ ◐ ● ● ─► better

* Denotes low reviewer response: that is, greater than 75% of the experts either did not rate the indicator, or gave the criterion an invalid rating (see Appendix B for an explanation).

References
1. Hyland A, Travers MJ, Cummings KM, Bauer J, Alford T, Wieczorek WF. Tobacco outlet density and demographics in Erie County, New York. *American Journal of Public Health*. 2003;93(7):1075–6.
2. Hyland A, Travers MJ, Cummings KM, Bauer J, Alford T, Wieczorek WF. Demographics and tobacco outlet density. [Letter]. *American Journal of Public Health*. 2003;93(11):1794.

Indicator 1.8.4

Proportion of Jurisdictions with Policies That Control Self-service Tobacco Sales

Goal area 1	Preventing initiation of tobacco use among young people
Outcome 8	Increased restriction and enforcement of restrictions on tobacco sales to minors
What to measure	Proportion of local jurisdictions that have public policies controlling self-service tobacco sales (i.e., sales that allow customers to handle tobacco products before purchasing them)
Why this indicator is useful	Self-service displays contribute to the visibility of tobacco and pro-tobacco messages in stores; they also make shoplifting tobacco products easier for minors. Illegal sales are more common when young people can access tobacco products directly through self-service displays rather than having to ask clerks for assistance.[1,2]
Example data source(s)	▹ Policy tracking system ▹ Americans for Nonsmokers' Rights (ANR) Information on ANR available at: http://www.no-smoke.org
Population group(s)	Not applicable. This indicator is best measured by tracking and monitoring pertinent local tobacco laws, ordinances, or regulations.
Example survey question(s)	Not applicable
Comments	Evaluators may also choose to gather data on the size and demographics of the population affected by the relevant laws or ordinances.

Rating

Overall quality low ◄────► high	Resources needed	Strength of evaluation evidence	Utility	Face validity	Accepted practice
▰▰▰▰▰▱▱	$$$	◕	●	◕	●

◄ ○ ◔ ◕ ● ► better

References
1. Lee RE, Feighery EC, Schleicher NC, Halvorson S. The relation between community bans of self-service tobacco displays and store environment and between tobacco accessibility and merchant incentives. *American Journal of Public Health.* 2001;91(12):2019–21.
2. Teall AM, Graham MC. Youth access to tobacco in two communities. *Journal of Nursing Scholarship.* 2001;33(2):175–8.

GOAL AREA 1
Outcome 8

Indicator 1.8.5

Number of Compliance Checks Conducted by Enforcement Agencies

Goal area 1	Preventing initiation of tobacco use among young people
Outcome 8	Increased restriction and enforcement of restrictions on tobacco sales to minors
What to measure	The number of checks conducted by enforcement agencies (e.g., police, health department inspectors, or building inspectors) to assess the level of retailer compliance with laws, regulations, or ordinances related to the sale of tobacco to minors
Why this indicator is useful	An effective means of enforcing tobacco-free public policies is to conduct regular compliance checks, which reduce illegal sales.[1] Compliance checks are also a method of assessing rates of compliance with laws regulating tobacco sales to minors. Such checks convey the message that policy makers and the public care about tobacco-free policies and are serious about enforcing them.[2,3]
Example data source(s)	Enforcement Agency Survey California Independent Evaluation: Policy Enforcement Survey: Youth Access to Tobacco, 2000 Information available at: http://www.dhs.ca.gov/ps/cdic/ccb/TCS/html/Evaluation_Resources.htm
Population group(s)	Agency representatives responsible for enforcement
Example survey question(s)	From California Independent Evaluation: Policy Enforcement Survey: Youth Access to Tobacco During the past 12 months, how many sting operations did your agency conduct to enforce PC §308(a) (illegal tobacco sales by merchants)?
Comments	Survey respondents may not have access to all requested information.

Rating

Overall quality low ←——→ high	Resources needed	Strength of evaluation evidence	Utility	Face validity	Accepted practice
▬▬▬▬▬ †	$$$	●	◐	◐	◐

←○◔●●→ better

† Denotes low agreement among reviewers: that is, fewer than 75% of the valid ratings for this indicator were within one point of each other (see Appendix B for an explanation).

References
1. Rigotti NA, DiFranza JR, Chang Y, Tisdale T, Kemp B, Singer DE. The effect of enforcing tobacco-sales laws on adolescents' access to tobacco and smoking behavior. *New England Journal of Medicine*. 1997;337(15):1044–51.
2. Kiser D, Boschert T. Eliminating smoking in bars, restaurants, and gaming clubs in California: BREATH, the California smoke-free bar program. *Journal of Public Health Policy*. 2001;22(i):81–7.
3. Weber MD, Bugwell DA, Fielding JE, Glantz SA. Long-term compliance with California's smoke-free workplace law among bars and restaurants in Los Angeles county. *Tobacco Control*. 2003;12:269–73.

Indicator 1.8.6

Number of Warnings, Citations, and Fines Issued for Infractions of Public Policies Against Young People's Access to Tobacco Products

Goal area 1	Preventing initiation of tobacco use among young people
Outcome 8	Increased restriction and enforcement of restrictions on tobacco sales to minors
What to measure	The number of warnings, citations, and fines issued to retailers for infractions of public policies against young people's access to tobacco
Why this indicator is useful	Studies show that aggressive enforcement of laws regulating tobacco sales to young people results in significantly reduced sales to minors and may also result in reduced smoking prevalence among teenagers.[1-3]
Example data source(s)	▷ Enforcement Agency Survey ▷ California Independent Evaluation: Policy Enforcement Survey: Youth Access to Tobacco, 2000 Information available at: http://www.dhs.ca.gov/ps/cdic/ccb/TCS/html/Evaluation_Resources.htm
Population group(s)	Agency representatives responsible for enforcement
Example survey question(s)	**From California Independent Evaluation: Policy Enforcement Survey: Youth Access to Tobacco** In the past year, how often has your agency conducted any of the following types of enforcement activities related to Penal Code §308? Never Rarely Very often Don't know • Responded to complaints about merchants selling tobacco products to minors ☐ ☐ ☐ ☐ • Issued warnings to merchants selling tobacco products to minors ☐ ☐ ☐ ☐ • Issued citations to merchants for illegal sales of tobacco products to minors ☐ ☐ ☐ ☐
Comments	Evaluators may want to assess the effects that different penalties (e.g., graduated fines, loss of license to sell tobacco) have on illegal tobacco sale to minors. Data must be interpreted in context. For example, a low number of citations may indicate either high levels of compliance or low levels of enforcement.
Rating	Overall quality: low ←——→ high † Resources needed: $$$ Strength of evaluation evidence: ● Utility: ● Face validity: ● Accepted practice: ● ← ○ ◐ ● ● → better † Denotes low agreement among reviewers: that is, fewer than 75% of the valid ratings for this indicator were within one point of each other (see Appendix B for an explanation).

References
1. Rigotti NA, DiFranza JR, Chang Y, Tisdale T, Kemp B, Singer DE. The effect of enforcing tobacco-sales laws on adolescents' access to tobacco and smoking behavior. *New England Journal of Medicine.* 1997;337(15):1044–51.
2. Jason LA, Berk M, Schnopp-Wyatt DL, Talbot B. Effects of enforcement of youth access laws on smoking prevalence. *American Journal of Community Psychology.* 1999;27(2):143–61.
3. Howard KA, Ribisl KM, Howard-Pitney B, Norman GJ, Rohrbach LA. What factors are associated with local enforcement of laws banning illegal tobacco sales to minors? A study of 182 law enforcement agencies in California. *Preventive Medicine.* 2001;33(2 Pt 1):63–70.

Indicator 1.8.7

Changes in State Tobacco Control Laws That Preempt Stronger Local Tobacco Control Laws

Goal area 1	Preventing initiation of tobacco use among young people
Outcome 8	Increased restriction and enforcement of restrictions on tobacco sales to minors
What to measure	Any change in legislation that prevents local jurisdictions from enacting restrictions that are more stringent than the state's restrictions on minors' access to tobacco or tobacco-related marketing
Why this indicator is useful	Preemptive legislation is the tobacco industry's chief strategy for eradicating local tobacco control ordinances.[1] Because of the striking increase in the number of local tobacco control ordinances from the mid-1980s to the mid-1990s, the tobacco industry aggressively pushed for states to pass legislation that preempted local regulation of tobacco in various areas, including minors' access, smoke-free indoor air, and marketing.[2] As of September 1998, 21 states preempted at least one provision of local minors' access restrictions.[3] As of December 31, 2004, only two states, Maine and Delaware, have successfully repealed preemption laws in their entirety in any area of tobacco control policy. Preemptive laws prevent communities from engaging in the process of public education, mobilization, and debate that occurs when a local ordinance is under consideration, a process that can increase awareness and change social norms. They also pose a barrier to local enforcement, because communities and local enforcement agencies may be less likely to enforce state laws that they were not directly involved in adopting than to enforce local ordinances.[2]
Example data source(s)	CDC State Tobacco Activities Tracking and Evaluation (STATE) system Data available at http://www.cdc.gov/tobacco/STATEsystem
Population group(s)	Not applicable. This indicator is best measured by tracking and monitoring state tobacco control laws.
Example survey question(s)	Not applicable
Comments	None

Rating

Overall quality low ◄──► high	Resources needed	Strength of evaluation evidence	Utility	Face validity	Accepted practice
▬▬▬▬▭ †	$	⊘	●	◐	●

◄─○◌●●─► better

† Denotes low agreement among reviewers: that is, fewer than 75% of the valid ratings for this indicator were within one point of each other (see Appendix B for an explanation).
⊘ Denotes no data.

References
1. National Cancer Institute. Smoking and Tobacco Control Monograph No. 11. *State and local legislative action to reduce tobacco use.* Bethesda, MD: National Cancer Institute; 2000. NIH Publication No. 00-4804.
2. Centers for Disease Control and Prevention. Preemptive state tobacco-control laws—United States, 1982–1998. *Morbidity and Mortality Weekly Report.* 1999;47(51 & 52):1112–4.
3. Centers for Disease Control and Prevention. State laws on tobacco control—United States, 1998. *Morbidity and Mortality Weekly Report CDC Surveillance Summaries.* 1999;48(SS-3):21–40.

Outcome 9

Reduced Tobacco Industry Influences

According to the most recent Federal Trade Commission tobacco report, the U.S. tobacco industry spent almost $12.5 billion in 2002 to advertise and promote its products.[1] It is not surprising, therefore, that studies show that a high percentage of young people are exposed to, aware of, and able to recall tobacco advertising.[2] Moreover, researchers have found that receptivity to tobacco industry marketing is associated with susceptibility towards tobacco use, that teenagers are three times more sensitive to cigarette advertising than adults, and that young people who approve of tobacco advertising and identify with the images portrayed in the advertisements are more likely than non-approving young people to start smoking.[2-8] In addition, tobacco advertising can distort young people's perceptions of tobacco use.[2,6-8] An indirect result of heavy tobacco industry advertising is the dampening effect it has on the number and quality of media stories about the health risks of smoking.[2] By promoting smoking, the tobacco industry undermines the ability of parents to prevent adolescents from starting to smoke.[9]

Many of the tobacco industry's advertising expenditures are in retail stores.[1] Retail stores are saturated with pro-tobacco signage, branded objects, and tobacco displays. Many of these objects are clustered around the cash registers, making it virtually impossible for anyone, including children, not to be exposed to pro-tobacco messages. Signage visible outside the stores exposes entire communities to tobacco marketing. The result is that many U.S. children grow up surrounded by pro-tobacco messages.[10]

The tobacco industry also spends considerable resources to sponsor or support public events, the arts, and other worthy causes.[1] It is clear that the tobacco industry influences policy makers through contributions and lobbying, which results in a more favorable, pro-tobacco policy environment.[11]

Listed below are the indicators associated with this outcome:

- **1.9.1** Extent and type of retail tobacco advertising and promotions
- **1.9.2** Proportion of jurisdictions with policies that regulate the extent and type of retail tobacco advertising and promotions
- **1.9.3** Extent of tobacco advertising outside of stores
- **1.9.4** Proportion of jurisdictions with policies that regulate the extent of tobacco advertising outside of stores
- **1.9.5** Extent of tobacco industry sponsorship of public and private events
- **1.9.6** Proportion of jurisdictions with policies that regulate tobacco industry sponsorship of public events
- **1.9.7** Extent of tobacco advertising on school property, at school events, and near schools

1.9.8   Extent of tobacco advertising in print media

1.9.9   Amount and quality of news media stories about tobacco industry practices and political lobbying

1.9.10 Number and type of Master Settlement Agreement violations by tobacco companies

1.9.11 Extent of tobacco industry contributions to institutions and groups

1.9.12 Amount of tobacco industry campaign contributions to local and state politicians

References

1. Federal Trade Commission. *Cigarette report for 2002.* Washington, DC: Federal Trade Commission; 2004.

2. U.S. Department of Health and Human Services. *Preventing tobacco use among young people: a report of the Surgeon General.* Atlanta, GA: Centers for Disease Control and Prevention; 1994.

3. Pollay RW, Siddarth S, Siegel M, Haddix A, Merritt RK, Giovino GA, et al. The last straw? Cigarette advertising and realized market shares among youths and adults. *Journal of Marketing.* 1996;60(2):1–16.

4. Schooler C, Feighery E, Flora JA. Seventh graders' self-reported exposure to cigarette marketing and its relationship to their smoking behavior. *American Journal of Public Health.* 1996;86(9):1216–21.

5. Feighery E, Borzekowski DL, Schooler C, Flora J. Seeing, wanting, owning: the relationship between receptivity to tobacco marketing and smoking susceptibility in young people. *Tobacco Control.* 1998;7(2):123–128.

6. Borzekowski DL, Flora JA, Feighery E, Schooler C. The perceived influence of cigarette advertisements and smoking susceptibility among seventh graders. *Journal of Health Communication.* 1999;4(2):105–118.

7. Evans N, Farkas A, Gilpin E, Berry C, Pierce JP. Influence of tobacco marketing and exposure to smokers on adolescent susceptibility to smoking. *Journal of the National Cancer Institute.* 1995;87(20):1538–45.

8. Henriksen L, Flora JA, Feighery E, Fortmann SP. Effects on youth of exposure to retail tobacco advertising. *Journal of Applied Social Psychology.* 2002;32(9):1771–89.

9. Pierce JP, Distefan JM, Jackson C, White MM, Gilpin EA. Does tobacco marketing undermine the influence of recommended parenting in discouraging adolescents from smoking? *American Journal of Preventive Medicine.* 2002;23(2):73–81.

10. Dewhirst T. POP goes the power wall? Taking aim at tobacco promotional strategies utilised at retail. *Tobacco Control.* 2004;13(2):209–10.

11. Monardi F, Glantz SA. Are tobacco industry campaign contributions influencing state legislative behavior? *American Journal of Public Health.* 1998;88(6):918–23.

For Further Reading

Biener L, Siegel M. Tobacco marketing and adolescent smoking: more support for a causal inference. *American Journal of Public Health.* 2000;90(3):407–11.

Celebucki CC, Diskin K. A longitudinal study of externally visible cigarette advertising on retail storefronts in Massachusetts before and after the Master Settlement Agreement. *Tobacco Control.* 2002;11(Suppl 2):ii47–53.

Forster JL, Murray DM, Wolfson M, Blaine TM, Wagenaar AC, Hennrikus DJ. The effects of community policies to reduce youth access to tobacco. *American Journal of Public Health.* 1998;88(8):1193–8.

Guthrie B. Tobacco advertising near schools. *British Medical Journal.* 1994 May 7;308(6929):658.

Lewit EM, Hyland A, Kerrebrock N, Cummings KM. Price, public policy, and smoking in young people. *Tobacco Control.* 1997;6(Suppl 2):S17–24.

Luke DA, Stamatakis KA, Brownson RC. State youth-access tobacco control policies and youth smoking behavior in the United States. *American Journal of Preventive Medicine.* 2000;19(3):180–7.

Morley CP, Cummings KM, Hyland A, Giovino GA, Horan JK. Tobacco Institute lobbying at the state and local levels of government in the 1990s. *Tobacco Control.* 2002;11(Suppl 1):i102–9.

Pucci L, Siegel M. Exposure to brand-specific cigarette advertising in magazines and its impact on youth smoking. *Preventive Medicine.* 1999;29(5):313–20.

Saffer H, Chaloupka F. The effect of tobacco advertising bans on tobacco consumption. *Journal of Health Economics.* 2000;19(6):1117–37.

Siegel M, Biener L, Rigotti NA. The effect of local tobacco sales laws on adolescent smoking initiation. *Preventive Medicine.* 1999;29(5):334–42.

Unger JB, Chen X. The role of social networks and media receptivity in predicting age of smoking initiation: a proportional hazards model of risk and protective factors. *Addictive Behaviors.* 1999;24(3):371–81.

Vaidya SG, Vaidya JS, Naik UD. Sports sponsorship by cigarette companies influences the adolescent children's mind and helps initiate smoking: results of a national study in India. *Journal of the Indian Medical Association.* 1999;97(9):354–6, 359.

Outcome 9

Reduced Tobacco Industry Influences

Indicator Rating

← ○ ◐ ● ●→ better

Number	Indicator	Overall quality (low ←→ high)	Resources needed	Strength of evaluation evidence	Utility	Face validity	Accepted practice
1.9.1	Extent and type of retail tobacco advertising and promotions		$$$$◊	◐	●	●	●
1.9.2	Proportion of jurisdictions with policies that regulate the extent and type of retail tobacco advertising and promotions		$$$	●	●	●	●
1.9.3	Extent of tobacco advertising outside of stores		$$$$◊	●	●	●	●
1.9.4	Proportion of jurisdictions with policies that regulate the extent of tobacco advertising outside of stores		$$$†	●	●	●	●
1.9.5	Extent of tobacco industry sponsorship of public and private events		$$$$◊	●	●	●	●
1.9.6	Proportion of jurisdictions with policies that regulate tobacco industry sponsorship of public events		$$$†	●	●	●	●
1.9.7	Extent of tobacco advertising on school property, at school events, and near schools		$$$	⊘	●	●	●
1.9.8	Extent of tobacco advertising in print media		$$$	●	●	●	●
1.9.9	Amount and quality of news media stories about tobacco industry practices and political lobbying		$$$	⊘	●	●	●
1.9.10	Number and type of Master Settlement Agreement violations by tobacco companies	†	$$$$◊	◐	●	●	●
1.9.11	Extent of tobacco industry contributions to institutions and groups		$◊	⊘	◐	●†	●
1.9.12	Amount of tobacco industry campaign contributions to local and state politicians	†	$◊	⊘	●	●	●

† Denotes low agreement among reviewers: that is, fewer than 75% of the valid ratings for this indicator were within one point of each other (see Appendix B for an explanation).
◊ Denotes that the experts' rating was modified (see Appendix B for an explanation).
⊘ Denotes no data.

Indicator 1.9.1

Extent and Type of Retail Tobacco Advertising and Promotions

Goal area 1	Preventing initiation of tobacco use among young people
Outcome 9	Reduced tobacco industry influences
What to measure	The level and type of tobacco advertising and promotion in and around retail stores and the extent of indoor and outdoor advertisements including promotions, price reductions, and strategic product placement
Why this indicator is useful	Retail stores have become the industry's primary communication channel to smokers and potential smokers. As a result, all shoppers, regardless of age or smoking status, are exposed to pro-tobacco messages.[1,2] Some studies show that young people who approve of tobacco advertising and identify with the image portrayed in the advertisements are more likely to start smoking.[3,4] Moreover, frequent (at least weekly) exposure to retail tobacco marketing among middle-school students is associated with a 50% increase in the odds of their ever smoking a cigarette, even after controlling for other known risk factors (e.g., parent smokes or friend smokes).[5]
Example data source(s)	▹ Environmental scan of tobacco advertising and promotional practices in retail outlets ▹ Operation Storefront: Youth Against Tobacco Advertising and Promotion Initiative Information available at: http://www.dhs.ca.gov/tobacco/html/Evaluation_Resources.htm
Population group(s)	Not applicable. This indicator is best measured by observation.
Example survey question(s)	Not applicable
Comments	Note that in *Lorillard v. Reilly* (533 U.S. 525 [2001]), the U.S. Supreme Court held that most regulations regarding cigarette advertising are preempted by the Federal Cigarette Labeling and Advertising Act, which makes it difficult for states and localities to regulate the extent and amount of retail tobacco advertising and promotion. Evaluators may choose to gather and report their findings by type of retailer (e.g., grocery store, convenience store, or gas station). States can track the price of tobacco products independently by collecting scanner data (obtained from scanning product bar codes), which provide information on brand and promotions. However, the cost of this type of data collection can be prohibitive.

Rating	Overall quality low ◄────► high	Resources needed	Strength of evaluation evidence	Utility	Face validity	Accepted practice
	███████	$$$$◊	◐	●	●	●

◄─○ ◔ ● ● ─► better

◊ Denotes that the experts' rating was modified (see Appendix B for an explanation).

References
1. Feighery EC, Ribisl KM, Clark PI, Haladjian HH. How tobacco companies ensure prime placement of their advertising and products in stores: interviews with retailers about tobacco company incentive programmes. *Tobacco Control.* 2003;12(2):184–8.
2. Centers for Disease Control and Prevention. Point-of-purchase tobacco environments and variation by store type—United States, 1999. *Morbidity and Mortality Weekly Report.* 2002; 51(9):184–7.
3. U.S. Department of Health and Human Services. *Preventing tobacco use among young people: a report of the Surgeon General.* Atlanta, GA: Centers for Disease Control and Prevention; 1994.
4. Schooler C, Feighery E, Flora JA. Seventh graders' self-reported exposure to cigarette marketing and its relationship to their smoking behavior. *American Journal of Public Health.* 1996;86(9):1216–21.
5. Henriksen L, Feighery EC, Wang Y, Fortmann SP. Association of retail tobacco marketing with adolescent smoking. *American Journal of Public Health.* 2004;94(12):2081–3.

Indicator 1.9.2

Proportion of Jurisdictions with Policies That Regulate the Extent and Type of Retail Tobacco Advertising and Promotions

Goal area 1	Preventing initiation of tobacco use among young people
Outcome 9	Reduced tobacco industry influences
What to measure	The proportion of local jurisdictions that have public policies that in some way regulate retail advertising and promotion of tobacco
Why this indicator is useful	The tobacco industry is increasingly shifting its advertising focus to retailer incentives including offering financial and trade benefits to retailers that sell and display tobacco products. Regulating retail advertising and promotions may significantly reduce young people's exposure to tobacco advertising.[1]
Example data source(s)	Policy tracking system
Population group(s)	Not applicable. This indicator is best measured by tracking and monitoring pertinent local tobacco laws, ordinances, or regulations.
Example survey question(s)	Not applicable
Comments	Note that in *Lorillard v. Reilly* (533 U.S. 525 [2001]), the U.S. Supreme Court held that most regulations regarding cigarette advertising are preempted by the Federal Cigarette Labeling and Advertising Act, which makes it difficult for states and localities to regulate the extent and amount of retail tobacco advertising and promotion. Evaluators may also choose to gather data on the size and demographics of the population affected by the relevant laws or ordinances.

Rating	Overall quality low ←→ high	Resources needed	Strength of evaluation evidence	Utility	Face validity	Accepted practice
	▬▬▬▬▬	$$$	◐	◐	◐	●

←○ ◐ ● ●→ better

Reference
1. Feighery EC, Ribisl KM, Clark PI, Haladjian HH. How tobacco companies ensure prime placement of their advertising and products in stores: interviews with retailers about tobacco company incentive programmes. *Tobacco Control.* 2003;12(2):184–8.

Indicator 1.9.3

Extent of Tobacco Advertising Outside of Stores

Goal area 1	Preventing initiation of tobacco use among young people
Outcome 9	Reduced tobacco industry influences
What to measure	The level and type of tobacco advertising on the exteriors of retail stores
Why this indicator is useful	Tobacco advertisements appear frequently outside U.S. stores. They can be on stores' outside walls and windows, in parking lots, or on the street.[1] The strategies for reducing tobacco advertising on the exteriors of retail establishments are often different from the strategies for reducing advertising and promotions inside stores.[2]
Example data source(s)	Environmental scan of tobacco advertising and promotional practices in retail outlets Operation Storefront: Youth Against Tobacco Advertising and Promotion Initiative Information available at: http://www.dhs.ca.gov/tobacco/html/Evaluation_Resources.htm
Population group(s)	Not applicable. This indicator is best measured by observation.
Example survey question(s)	Not applicable
Comments	None

Rating

Overall quality low ⟷ high	Resources needed	Strength of evaluation evidence	Utility	Face validity	Accepted practice
▬▬▬	$$$$◊	●	●	●	●

←○◐●●→ better

◊ Denotes that the experts' rating was modified (see Appendix B for an explanation).

References
1. Centers for Disease Control and Prevention. Point-of-purchase tobacco environments and variation by store type—United States, 1999. *Morbidity and Mortality Weekly Report.* 2002;51(9):184–7.
2. Rogers T, Feighery EC, Tencati EM, Butler JL, Weiner L. Community mobilization to reduce point-of-purchase advertising of tobacco products. *Health Education Quarterly.* 1995;22(4);427–42.

Indicator 1.9.4

Proportion of Jurisdictions with Policies That Regulate the Extent of Tobacco Advertising Outside of Stores

Goal area 1	Preventing initiation of tobacco use among young people
Outcome 9	Reduced tobacco industry influences
What to measure	The proportion of local jurisdictions that have public policies that in some way regulate tobacco advertising on the exteriors of retail outlets (for example, some jurisdictions limit the percentage of store windows that may be covered with advertisements)[1]
Why this indicator is useful	Reducing exterior tobacco-related retail signs and displays will reduce young people's exposure to tobacco advertising.[2]
Example data source(s)	Policy tracking system
Population group(s)	Not applicable. This indicator is best measured by tracking and monitoring pertinent local tobacco laws, ordinances, or regulations.
Example survey question(s)	Not applicable
Comments	Note that in *Lorillard* v. *Reilly* (533 U.S. 525 [2001]), the U.S. Supreme Court held that most regulations regarding cigarette advertising are preempted by the Federal Cigarette Labeling and Advertising Act, which makes it difficult for states and localities to regulate the extent and amount of retail tobacco advertising and promotion. Evaluators may also choose to gather data on the size and demographics of the population affected by the relevant laws or ordinances.

Rating

Overall quality low ⟷ high	Resources needed	Strength of evaluation evidence	Utility	Face validity	Accepted practice
▮▮▮▮▯	$$$ †	◗	◗	●	●

←○ ◐ ◗ ● → better

† Denotes low agreement among reviewers: that is, fewer than 75% of the valid ratings for this indicator were within one point of each other (see Appendix B for an explanation).

References
1. Rogers T, Feighery EC, Tencati EM, Butler JL, Weiner L. Community mobilizations to reduce point-of-purchase advertising of tobacco products. *Health Economics Quarterly*. 1995;22(4);427–42.
2. Jason LA, Pokorny SB, Mikulski K, Schoeny ME. Assessing storefront tobacco advertising after the billboard ban. *Evaluation and the Health Professions*. 2004;27(1):22–33.

Indicator 1.9.5

Extent of Tobacco Industry Sponsorship of Public and Private Events

Goal area 1	Preventing initiation of tobacco use among young people
Outcome 9	Reduced tobacco industry influences
What to measure	The extent of tobacco industry sponsorship of public and private events (e.g., sports, recreation, music, family, or work-related events)
Why this indicator is useful	The tobacco industry spends considerable resources sponsoring visible public events.[1] This sponsorship increases exposure to advertisements for tobacco product advertising and buys legitimacy for the tobacco industry.[1,2]
Example data source(s)	Event sponsorship tracking system California Tobacco Industry Monitoring Evaluation: Project SMART Money Information available at: http://www.ttac.org/enews/mailer09-30-03full.html#LinkF
Population group(s)	Not applicable. This indicator is best measured by observation.
Example survey question(s)	Not applicable
Comments	Evaluators may want to assess the types of events that are being sponsored and the numbers of attendees.

Rating

Overall quality low ⟵⟶ high	Resources needed	Strength of evaluation evidence	Utility	Face validity	Accepted practice
▬▬▬	$$$$◊	●	●	●	●

◯ ◐ ● ● ⟶ better

◊ Denotes that the experts' rating was modified (see Appendix B for an explanation).

References
1. Rosenberg NJ, Siegel M. Use of corporate sponsorship as a tobacco marketing tool: a review of tobacco industry sponsorship in the USA, 1995–99. *Tobacco Control*. 2001;10(3):239–46.
2. Federal Trade Commission. *Cigarette report for 2002*. Washington, DC: Federal Trade Commission; 2004.

Indicator 1.9.6

Proportion of Jurisdictions with Policies That Regulate Tobacco Industry Sponsorship of Public Events

Goal area 1	Preventing initiation of tobacco use among young people
Outcome 9	Reduced tobacco industry influences
What to measure	The proportion of local jurisdictions with public policies that regulate tobacco industry sponsorship of public events
Why this indicator is useful	The tobacco industry spends considerable resources to sponsor highly publicized events.[1] This sponsorship increases exposure to tobacco-product advertising and buys legitimacy for the tobacco industry.[1,2]
Example data source(s)	Policy tracking system
Population group(s)	Not applicable. This indicator is best measured by tracking and monitoring pertinent local tobacco laws, ordinances, or regulations.
Example survey question(s)	Not applicable
Comments	Evaluators may also choose to gather data on the size and demographics of the population affected by the relevant laws or ordinances.

Rating

Overall quality low ◄──► high	Resources needed	Strength of evaluation evidence	Utility	Face validity	Accepted practice
▇▇▇▇	$$$[†]	●	●	●	●

◄─ ○ ◐ ● ● ─► better

[†] Denotes low agreement among reviewers: that is, fewer than 75% of the valid ratings for this indicator were within one point of each other (see Appendix B for an explanation).

References
1. Rosenberg NJ, Siegel M. Use of corporate sponsorship as a tobacco marketing tool: a review of tobacco industry sponsorship in the USA, 1995–99. *Tobacco Control.* 2001;10(3):239–46.
2. Federal Trade Commission. *Cigarette report for 2002.* Washington, DC: Federal Trade Commission; 2004.

Indicator 1.9.7

Extent of Tobacco Advertising on School Property, at School Events, and Near Schools

Goal area 1	Preventing initiation of tobacco use among young people
Outcome 9	Reduced tobacco industry influences
What to measure	The extent of tobacco advertising on school property, at school events off campus, and within a designated distance from schools
Why this indicator is useful	Findings from a California study of retail tobacco advertising showed that stores near schools (within 1,000 feet) had significantly more tobacco advertising and promotional materials overall and more advertising on their exteriors than stores not near schools.[1] Stores near schools also had a significantly higher probability of having tobacco advertising or promotions near candy and low to the ground (at the eye level of children) than stores not near schools.[1]
Example data source(s)	CDC School Health Profiles: School Principal Questionnaire (Profiles), 2002 Environmental scan of tobacco advertising and promotional practices in retail outlets Operation Storefront: Youth Against Tobacco Advertising and Promotion Initiative Information available at: http://www.dhs.ca.gov/tobacco/html/Evaluation_Resources.htm
Population group(s)	School principals
Example survey question(s)	**From Profiles** Is tobacco advertising prohibited in each of the following locations? (Mark yes or no for each location.) Yes No • In the school building • On school grounds, including on the outside of the building, on playing fields, or other areas of the campus • On school buses or other vehicles used to transport students • In school publications (e.g., newsletters, newspapers, websites, in other school publications) Is tobacco advertising through sponsorship of school events prohibited? ☐ Yes ☐ No
Comments	None
Rating	Overall quality: high / Resources needed: $$$ / Strength of evaluation evidence: not available / Utility: medium-high / Face validity: high / Accepted practice: high

Reference

1. Roeseler A, Rogers T, Feighery E, Gehrman J. *Operation storefront: youth against tobacco advertising and promotion.* Sacramento, CA: California Department of Health Services; 2003. pp. 1–4.

Indicator 1.9.8

Extent of Tobacco Advertising in Print Media

Goal area 1	Preventing initiation of tobacco use among young people
Outcome 9	Reduced tobacco industry influences
What to measure	The extent of tobacco advertisement in print media (e.g., magazines or newspapers)
Why this indicator is useful	The Master Settlement Agreement (MSA) regulated aspects of tobacco advertising in print media. However, one study found that after the MSA, the combined advertising expenditures of the four major tobacco companies increased in 19 magazines that have a youth focus.[1] Another study found that 54% of teenagers' favorite magazines had cigarette advertisements.[2]
Example data source(s)	▸ Media Tracking Service (e.g., clipping service) ▸ TNS Media Intelligence Competitive Media Reporting (CMR) Information available at: http://www.tnsmi-cmr.com/products/index.html
Population group(s)	Not applicable. This indicator is best measured by tracking tobacco advertisements in print media.
Example survey question(s)	Not applicable
Comments	Evaluators may want to assess tobacco advertising by type of print media (e.g., magazines targeted to adults or magazines targeted to adolescents). Quantitative studies involve counting articles, measuring column-inches, or noting article placement. Qualitative studies require detailed content analyses to detect article themes.[3,4] More information on how to collect data on this indicator is in reference 5 below.

Rating

Overall quality low ◄——► high	Resources needed	Strength of evaluation evidence	Utility	Face validity	Accepted practice
(high)	$$$	●	●	◐	●

◄—○ ○ ◐ ● —► better

References
1. Hamilton WL, Turner-Bowker DM, Celebucki CC, Connolly GN. Cigarette advertising in magazines: the tobacco industry response to the Master Settlement Agreement and to public pressure. *Tobacco Control.* 2002;11(Suppl 2):ii54–8.
2. Schooler C, Feighery E, Flora JA. Seventh graders' self-reported exposure to cigarette marketing and its relationship to their smoking behavior. *American Journal of Public Health.* 1996;86(9):1216–21.
3. Lima JC, Siegel M. The tobacco settlement: an analysis of newspaper coverage of a national policy debate, 1997–98. *Tobacco Control.* 1999;8(3):247–53.
4. Menashe CL, Siegel M. The power of a frame: an analysis of newspaper coverage of tobacco issues—United States, 1985–1996. *Journal of Health Communication.* 1998;3(4):307–25.
5. Stillman F, Cronin K, Evans W, Ulasevich A. Can media advocacy influence newspaper coverage of tobacco: measuring the effectiveness of the American Stop Smoking Intervention Study's (ASSIST) media advocacy strategies. *Tobacco Control.* 2001;10(2):137–44.

Indicator 1.9.9

Amount and Quality of News Media Stories About Tobacco Industry Practices and Political Lobbying

Goal area 1	Preventing initiation of tobacco use among young people
Outcome 9	Reduced tobacco industry influences
What to measure	Media coverage of tobacco industry practices and political lobbying
Why this indicator is useful	Demonstrating the negative aspects of tobacco industry practices may influence young people's behavior.[1-3] For example, being aware that the tobacco industry is trying to manipulate behavior may reduce young people's susceptibility to tobacco marketing and increase overall support for anti-tobacco policies, laws, or regulations.[4]
Example data source(s)	Media Tracking Service (e.g., clipping service)
Population group(s)	Not applicable. This indicator is best measured by monitoring and tracking pertinent media coverage of tobacco industry practices.
Example survey question(s)	Not applicable
Comments	Quantitative studies involve counting articles, measuring column-inches, or noting article placement. Qualitative studies require detailed content analyses to detect article themes.[2,3] More information on how to collect data on this indicator is in reference 5 below.

Rating

Overall quality low ←——→ high	Resources needed	Strength of evaluation evidence	Utility	Face validity	Accepted practice
▬▬▬	$$$	⊘	●	●	●

←○◔●●→ better

⊘ Denotes no data.

References
1. Caburnay CA, Kreuter MW, Luke DA, Logan RA, Jacobsen HA, Reddy VC, Vempaty AR, Zayed HR. The news on health behavior: coverage of diet, activity, and tobacco in local newspapers. *Health Education & Behavior.* 2003;30(6):709–722.
2. Lima JC, Siegel M. The tobacco settlement: an analysis of newspaper coverage of a national policy debate, 1997–98. *Tobacco Control.* 1999;8(3):247–53.
3. Menashe CL, Siegel M. The power of a frame: an analysis of newspaper coverage of tobacco issues—United States, 1985–1996. *Journal of Health Communication.* 1998;3(4):307–25.
4. Hicks JJ. Crispin, Porter & Bogusky. The strategy behind Florida's truth campaign. Miami, FL: Truth Campaign; 2001. Online publication. Available from: http://www.tobaccofreedom.org/msa/articles/truth_review.html.
5. Stillman F, Cronin K, Evans W, Ulasevich A. Can media advocacy influence newspaper coverage of tobacco: measuring the effectiveness of the American Stop Smoking Intervention Study's (ASSIST) media advocacy strategies. *Tobacco Control.* 2001;10(2):137–44.

Indicator 1.9.10

Number and Type of Master Settlement Agreement Violations by Tobacco Companies

Goal area 1	Preventing initiation of tobacco use among young people
Outcome 9	Reduced tobacco industry influences
What to measure	The number and type of Master Settlement Agreement (MSA) violations by tobacco companies
Why this indicator is useful	In 2000, all of the major tobacco manufacturers failed to comply with the MSA, which bans the tobacco companies from targeting young people through magazine advertisements. The companies are selectively increasing their magazine advertisements targeted to young people.[1] Tracking these and other violations of the MSA will aid in the MSA's enforcement.[2,3]
Example data source(s)	▹ Tobacco industry monitoring system ▹ California Tobacco Industry Monitoring Evaluation: Project SMART Money Information available at: http://www.ttac.org/enews/mailer09-30-03full.html#LinkF
Population group(s)	Not applicable. This indicator is best measured by monitoring and tracking tobacco industry practices.
Example survey question(s)	Not applicable
Comments	None

Rating

Overall quality low ⟵⟶ high	Resources needed	Strength of evaluation evidence	Utility	Face validity	Accepted practice
▬▬▬ †	$$$$ ◊	○	◐	●	●

⟵ ○ ◔ ◐ ● ⟶ better

† Denotes low agreement among reviewers: that is, fewer than 75% of the valid ratings for this indicator were within one point of each other (see Appendix B for an explanation).
◊ Denotes that the experts' rating was modified (see Appendix B for an explanation).

References
1. Chung PJ, Garfield CF, Rathouz PJ, Lauderdale DS, Best D, Lantos J. Youth targeting by tobacco manufacturers since the Master Settlement Agreement: the first study to document violations of the youth-targeting ban in magazine ads by the three top U.S. tobacco companies. *Health Affairs.* 2002;21(2):254–63.
2. Hamilton WL, Turner-Bowker DM, Celebucki CC, Connolly GN. Cigarette advertising in magazines: the tobacco industry response to the Master Settlement Agreement and to public pressure. *Tobacco Control.* 2002; 11(Suppl 2):ii54–8.
3. Celebucki CC, Diskin K. A longitudinal study of externally visible cigarette advertising on retail storefronts in Massachusetts before and after the Master Settlement Agreement. *Tobacco Control.* 2002;11(Suppl 2):ii47–53.

Indicator 1.9.11

Extent of Tobacco Industry Contributions to Institutions and Groups

Goal area 1	Preventing initiation of tobacco use among young people
Outcome 9	Reduced tobacco industry influences
What to measure	The amount of funds contributed by the tobacco industry to institutions and groups (e.g., the hospitality industry, movie industry, sports organizations, and civic groups)
Why this indicator is useful	Studies show that the tobacco industry has a history of collaborating with businesses and community organizations. The amount of the tobacco industry's influence on these groups is directly related to the amount it contributes.[1-4] Tracking this indicator will help to understand tobacco industry influence.
Example data source(s)	• Public records of political contributions Information available from the Office of the State Secretary or equivalent in each state • Center for Responsive Politics (CRP) Information available at: http://www.opensecrets.org • Tobacco industry fiscal reports
Population group(s)	Not applicable. This indicator is best measured by reviewing public and tobacco industry records.
Example survey question(s)	Not applicable
Comments	Evaluators may want to categorize their findings by type of business or organization (e.g., the hospitality industry, movie industry, sports organizations, or civic groups) that received funds from the tobacco industry. More information on how to collect data on this indicator is in reference 5 below.

Rating

Overall quality low ←——→ high	Resources needed	Strength of evaluation evidence	Utility	Face validity	Accepted practice
▬▬▬▬▬	$◊	⊘	◐	●[†]	●

←○◔◑●→ better

† Denotes low agreement among reviewers: that is, fewer than 75% of the valid ratings for this indicator were within one point of each other (see Appendix B for an explanation).
◊ Denotes that the experts' rating was modified (see Appendix B for an explanation).
⊘ Denotes no data.

References
1. Ritch WA, Begay ME. Strange bedfellows: the history of collaboration between the Massachusetts Restaurant Association and the tobacco industry. *American Journal of Public Health.* 2001;91(4):598–603.
2. Rosenberg NJ, Siegel M. Use of corporate sponsorship as a tobacco marketing tool: a review of tobacco industry sponsorship in the USA, 1995–99. *Tobacco Control.* 2001;10(3):239–46.
3. Dearlove JV, Bialous SA, Glantz SA. Tobacco industry manipulation of the hospitality industry to maintain smoking in public places. *Tobacco Control.* 2002;11(2):94–104.
4. Mekemson C, Glantz SA. How the tobacco industry built its relationship with Hollywood. *Tobacco Control.* 2002;11 (Suppl 1):i81–91.
5. Rosenberg NJ, Siegel M. Use of corporate sponsorship as a tobacco marketing tool: a review of tobacco industry sponsorship in the USA, 1995–99. *Tobacco Control.* 2001;10(3):239–46.

Indicator 1.9.12

Amount of Tobacco Industry Campaign Contributions to Local and State Politicians

Goal area 1	Preventing initiation of tobacco use among young people
Outcome 9	Reduced tobacco industry influences
What to measure	The amount of funds contributed to local and state politicians by the tobacco industry
Why this indicator is useful	Studies show an association between political contributions from the tobacco industry and pro-tobacco legislation.[1-3] Tobacco industry contributions are a significant predictor of the industry's political influence, including its influence on votes for tobacco-related legislation.[1,2] Tracking this indicator may help states counter the influence of the tobacco industry.
Example data source(s)	▹ Public records of political contributions Information available from the Office of the State Secretary or equivalent in each state ▹ Federal Election Commission (FEC) Searchable database available at: http://www.fec.gov ▹ Center for Responsive Politics (CRP) Information available at: http://www.opensecrets.org
Population group(s)	Not applicable. This indicator is best measured by reviewing public records.
Example survey question(s)	Not applicable
Comments	More information on how to collect data on this indicator is in references 4 and 5 below.

Rating

Overall quality low ←→ high	Resources needed	Strength of evaluation evidence	Utility	Face validity	Accepted practice
▬▬▬▬▬†	$ ◊	⊘	●	●	●

←○◐●●→ better

† Denotes low agreement among reviewers: that is, fewer than 75% of the valid ratings for this indicator were within one point of each other (see Appendix B for an explanation).
◊ Denotes that the experts' rating was modified (see Appendix B for an explanation).
⊘ Denotes no data.

References
1. Glantz SA, Begay ME. Tobacco industry campaign contributions are affecting tobacco control policymaking in California. *Journal of the American Medical Association.* 1994;272(15):1176–82.
2. Monardi F, Glantz SA. Are tobacco industry campaign contributions influencing state legislative behavior? *American Journal of Public Health.* 1998;88(6):918–23.
3. Luke DA, Krauss M. Where there's smoking there's money: tobacco industry campaign contributions and U.S. Congressional voting. *American Journal of Preventive Medicine.* 2004;27(5):363–72.
4. Givel MS, Glantz SA. Tobacco lobby political influence on U.S. state legislatures in the 1990s. *Tobacco Control.* 2001;10(2):124–34.
5. Morley CP, Cummings KM, Hyland A, Giovino GA, Horan JK. Tobacco Institute lobbying at the state and local levels of government in the 1990s. *Tobacco Control.* 2002;11:102–9.

Outcome 10

Reduced Susceptibility to Experimentation with Tobacco Products

Susceptibility to smoking is defined as the intention to smoke or the absence of a strong intention not to smoke.[1] Studies show that susceptibility to experimentation is a valid and reliable predictor of future smoking behavior.[1] Studies also show that susceptible young people (those who have not made a firm decision not to smoke) are more likely than other young people to experiment with smoking.[1] Furthermore, recent evidence suggests that even low levels of smoking experimentation (two to four cigarettes smoked by age 10 years) substantially increase the likelihood of daily smoking in late adolescence.[2] To reduce the percentage of young people who take up smoking, it is therefore necessary to prevent young people from becoming susceptible to experimenting with tobacco.[3] In addition to tobacco industry influences, tobacco use by peers is strongly associated with early tobacco experimentation among children.[4] Parental involvement in young people's decision making about tobacco use is also an important contributor to reduced susceptibility to tobacco use.[5-7]

Listed below are the indicators associated with this outcome:

- **1.10.1** Proportion of young people who think that smoking is cool and helps them fit in
- **1.10.2** Proportion of young people who think that young people who smoke have more friends
- **1.10.3** Proportion of young people who report that their parents have discussed not smoking with them
- **1.10.4** Proportion of parents who report that they have discussed not smoking with their children
- **1.10.5** Proportion of young people who are susceptible never-smokers

References

1. Pierce JP, Choi WS, Gilpin EA, Farkas AJ, Merritt RK. Validation of susceptibility as a predictor of which adolescents take up smoking in the United States. *Health Psychology.* 1996;15(5):355–361.

2. Jackson C, Dickinson D. Cigarette consumption during childhood and persistence of smoking through adolescence. *Archives of Pediatrics & Adolescent Medicine.* 2004;158:1050–1056.

3. U.S. Department of Health and Human Services. *Preventing tobacco use among young people: a report of the Surgeon General.* Atlanta, GA: Centers for Disease Control and Prevention; 1994.

4. Jackson C. Initial and experimental stages of tobacco and alcohol use during late childhood: relation to peer, parent, and personal risk factors. *Addictive Behaviors.* 1997;22(5):685–98.

5. Distefan JM, Gilpin EA, Choi WS, Pierce JP. Parental influences predict adolescent smoking in the United States, 1989–1993. *Journal of Adolescent Health*. 1998;22(6):466–74.

6. Jackson C, Henriksen L. Do as I say: parent smoking, antismoking socialization, and smoking onset among children. *Addictive Behaviors*. 1997;22(1):107–14.

7. Sargent JD, Dalton M. Does parental disapproval of smoking prevent adolescents from becoming established smokers? *Pediatrics*. 2001;108(6):1256–62.

For Further Reading

Bidell MP, Furlong MJ, Dunn DM, Koegler JE. Case study of attempts to enact self-service tobacco display ordinances: a tale of three communities. *Tobacco Control*. 2000;9(1):71–7.

Centers for Disease Control and Prevention. Estimates of retailers willing to sell tobacco to minors: California, August–September 1995 and June–July 1996. *Morbidity and Mortality Weekly Report*. 1996;45(50):1095–9.

Feighery E, Altman DG, Shaffer G. The effects of combining education and enforcement to reduce tobacco sales to minors: a study of four northern California communities. *Journal of the American Medical Association*. 1991;266(22):3168–71.

Forster JL, Murray DM, Wolfson M, Blaine TM, Wagenaar AC, Hennrikus DJ. The effects of community policies to reduce youth access to tobacco. *American Journal of Public Health*. 1998;88(8):1193–8.

Howard KA, Ribisl KM, Howard-Pitney B, Norman GJ, Rohrbach LA. What factors are associated with local enforcement of laws banning illegal tobacco sales to minors? A study of 182 law enforcement agencies in California. *Preventive Medicine*. 2001 Aug;33(2 Pt 1):63–70.

Jason L, Billows W, Schnopp-Wyatt D, King C. Reducing the illegal sales of cigarettes to minors: analysis of alternative enforcement schedules. *Journal of Applied Behavior Analysis*. 1996;29(3):333–44.

Jason LA, Pokorny SB, Schoeny ME. Evaluating the effects of enforcements and fines on youth smoking. *Critical Public Health*. 2003;13(1):33–45.

Jason LA, Berk M, Schnopp-Wyatt DL, Talbot B. Effects of enforcement of youth access laws on smoking prevalence. *American Journal of Community Psychology*. 1999;27(2):143–61.

Jason LA, Ji PY, Anes MD, Birkhead SH. Active enforcement of cigarette control laws in the prevention of cigarette sales to minors. *Journal of the American Medical Association*. 1991;266(22):3159–61.

Luke DA, Stamatakis KA, Brownson RC. State youth-access tobacco control policies and youth smoking behavior in the United States. *American Journal of Preventive Medicine.* 2000;19(3):180–7.

Ma GX, Shive S, Tracy M. The effects of licensing and inspection enforcement to reduce tobacco sales to minors in greater Philadelphia, 1994–1998. *Addictive Behaviors.* 2001;26(5):677–87.

Rigotti NA, DiFranza JR, Chang Y, Tisdale T, Kemp B, Singer DE. The effect of enforcing tobacco-sales laws on adolescents' access to tobacco and smoking behavior. *New England Journal of Medicine.* 1997;337:1044–51.

Siegel M, Biener L, Rigotti NA. The effect of local tobacco sales laws on adolescent smoking initiation. *Preventive Medicine.* 1999;29(5):334–42.

Stead LF, Lancaster T. A systematic review of interventions for preventing tobacco sales to minors. *Tobacco Control.* 2000;9(2):169–76.

Teall AM, Graham MC. Youth access to tobacco in two communities. *Journal of Nursing Scholarship.* 2001;33(2):175–8.

U.S. Department of Health and Human Services. *Preventing tobacco use among young people: a report of the Surgeon General.* Atlanta, GA: Centers for Disease Control and Prevention; 1994.

Outcome 10

Reduced Susceptibility to Experimentation with Tobacco Products

Indicator Rating
← ○ ◐ ● ● → better

Number	Indicator	Overall quality low ←——→ high	Resources needed	Strength of evaluation evidence	Utility	Face validity	Accepted practice
1.10.1	Proportion of young people who think that smoking is cool and helps them fit in	▬▬▬▬▬	$$†	●	●	●	●
1.10.2	Proportion of young people who think that young people who smoke have more friends	▬▬▬▬	$$	●	○	●	●
1.10.3	Proportion of young people who report that their parents have discussed not smoking with them	▬▬▬▬	$$	●	●	●	●
1.10.4	Proportion of parents who report that they have discussed not smoking with their children	▬▬▬▬	$$$	⊘	●	●	●
1.10.5	Proportion of young people who are susceptible never-smokers	▬▬▬▬▬	$$†	●	●	●	●

† Denotes low agreement among reviewers: that is, fewer than 75% of the valid ratings for this indicator were within one point of each other (see Appendix B for an explanation).
⊘ Denotes no data.

Indicator 1.10.1

Proportion of Young People Who Think That Smoking Is Cool and Helps Them Fit In

Goal area 1	Preventing initiation of tobacco use among young people
Outcome 10	Reduced susceptibility to experimentation with tobacco products
What to measure	Proportion of young people who believe that smoking cigarettes will improve their social standing
Why this indicator is useful	Data indicate that adolescent cigarette smokers are significantly more likely to believe that smokers are more socially adept than nonsmokers.[1-5] These data can be used to estimate norms regarding the social desirability of smoking.
Example data source(s)	Youth Tobacco Survey (YTS): CDC Recommended Questions: Core, 2004
Population group(s)	Young people aged less than 18 years
Example survey question(s)	**From YTS** Do you think smoking cigarettes makes young people look cool or fit in? ☐ Definitely yes ☐ Probably yes ☐ Probably not ☐ Definitely not
Comments	None

Rating

Overall quality low ◄──► high	Resources needed	Strength of evaluation evidence	Utility	Face validity	Accepted practice
▬▬▬▬	$$†	◐	◐	◐	●

◄─ ○ ◔ ◐ ● ─► better

† Denotes low agreement among reviewers: that is, fewer than 75% of the valid ratings for this indicator were within one point of each other (see Appendix B for an explanation).

References
1. U.S. Department of Health and Human Services. *Preventing tobacco use among young people: a report of the Surgeon General.* Atlanta, GA: Centers for Disease Control and Prevention; 1994.
2. Unger JB, Rohrbach LA, Howard-Pitney B, Ritt-Olson A, Mouttapa M. Peer influences and susceptibility to smoking among California adolescents. *Substance Use and Misuse.* 2001;36(5):551–71.
3. Wang MQ. Social environmental influences on adolescents' smoking progression. *American Journal of Health Behavior.* 2001;25(4):418–25.
4. Distefan JM, Gilpin EA, Sargent JD, Pierce JP. Do movie stars encourage adolescents to start smoking? Evidence from California. *Preventive Medicine.* 1999;28(1):1–11.
5. Tickle JJ, Sargent JD, Dalton MA, Beach ML, Heatherton TF. Favorite movie stars, their tobacco use in contemporary movies, and its association with adolescent smoking. *Tobacco Control.* 2001;10(1):16–22.

Indicator 1.10.2

Proportion of Young People Who Think That Young People Who Smoke Have More Friends

Goal area 1	Preventing initiation of tobacco use among young people
Outcome 10	Reduced susceptibility to experimentation with tobacco products
What to measure	Proportion of young people who believe that those who smoke have more friends than those who do not smoke
Why this indicator is useful	Data indicate that cigarette smokers are significantly more likely to believe that those who smoke have more friends than those who do not smoke.[1-5] These data can be used as an estimate of norms concerning the social desirability of smoking.
Example data source(s)	Youth Tobacco Survey (YTS): CDC Recommended Questions: Core, 2004
Population group(s)	Young people aged less than 18 years
Example survey question(s)	**From YTS** Do you think young people who smoke cigarettes have more friends? ☐ Definitely yes ☐ Probably yes ☐ Probably not ☐ Definitely not
Comments	None

Rating

Overall quality low ← → high	Resources needed	Strength of evaluation evidence	Utility	Face validity	Accepted practice
▬▬▬	$$	◕	○	●	●

← ○ ◔ ◕ ● → better

References
1. U.S. Department of Health and Human Services. *Preventing tobacco use among young people: a report of the Surgeon General.* Atlanta, GA: Centers for Disease Control and Prevention; 1994.
2. Unger JB, Rohrbach LA, Howard-Pitney B, Ritt-Olson A, Mouttapa M. Peer influences and susceptibility to smoking among California adolescents. *Substance Use and Misuse.* 2001;36(5):551–71.
3. Wang MQ. Social environmental influences on adolescents' smoking progression. *American Journal of Health Behavior.* 2001;25(4):418–25.
4. Distefan JM, Gilpin EA, Sargent JD, Pierce JP. Do movie stars encourage adolescents to start smoking? Evidence from California. *Preventive Medicine.* 1999;28(1):1–11.
5. Tickle JJ, Sargent JD, Dalton MA, Beach ML, Heatherton TF. Favorite movie stars, their tobacco use in contemporary movies, and its association with adolescent smoking. *Tobacco Control.* 2001;10(1):16–22.

Indicator 1.10.3

Proportion of Young People Who Report That Their Parents Have Discussed Not Smoking with Them

Goal area 1	Preventing initiation of tobacco use among young people
Outcome 10	Reduced susceptibility to experimentation with tobacco products
What to measure	Proportion of young people who report that their parents have discussed the dangers of tobacco use with them in the past 12 months
Why this indicator is useful	Parental involvement in their children's smoking decisions is a predictor of whether their children take up smoking.[1-3] Teenagers who report that their parents are unconcerned about smoking or do not talk to them about it are more likely than other teenagers to take up smoking and to become regular smokers.[1-4]
Example data source(s)	Youth Tobacco Survey (YTS): CDC Recommended Questions: Core, 2004
Population group(s)	Young people aged less than 18 years
Example survey question(s)	**From YTS** In the past 12 months, how often have your parents or guardians discussed the dangers of tobacco use with you? ☐ Never ☐ Rarely ☐ Sometimes ☐ Often ☐ Very often
Comments	Evaluators may want to ask young people questions about parental rules about smoking and the perceived consequences of being caught smoking. Evaluators may also want to ask young people if their parents have discussed the dangers of tobacco use (not just smoking) with them.
Rating	Overall quality: low ←——→ high (high) Resources needed: $$ Strength of evaluation evidence: ● Utility: ● Face validity: ● Accepted practice: ● ←○◐●●→ better

References
1. Distefan JM, Gilpin EA, Choi WS, Pierce JP. Parental influences predict adolescent smoking in the United States, 1989–1993. *Journal of Adolescent Health*. 1998;22(6):466–74.
2. Jackson C, Henriksen L. Do as I say: parent smoking, antismoking socialization, and smoking onset among children. *Addictive Behaviors*. 1997;22(1):107–14.
3. Sargent JD, Dalton M. Does parental disapproval of smoking prevent adolescents from becoming established smokers? *Pediatrics*. 2001;108(6):1256–62.
4. Pierce JP, Distefan JM, Jackson C, White MM, Gilpin EA. Does tobacco marketing undermine the influence of recommended parenting in discouraging adolescents from smoking? *American Journal of Preventive Medicine*. 2002;23(2):73–81.

Indicator 1.10.4

Proportion of Parents Who Report That They Have Discussed Not Smoking with Their Children

Goal area 1	Preventing initiation of tobacco use among young people
Outcome 10	Reduced susceptibility to experimentation with tobacco products
What to measure	Proportion of parents who report that they talked to their children at least once in the previous 6 months about what their children may or may not do regarding tobacco use
Why this indicator is useful	Parental involvement in their children's smoking decisions is a predictor of whether their children take up smoking.[1-3] In addition, asking parents about their children and smoking sensitizes parents to the importance of discussing tobacco use with their children.[1-4]
Example data source(s)	Adult Tobacco Survey (ATS): CDC Recommended Questions: Supplemental Section G: Parental Involvement, 2003
Population group(s)	Parents of children aged less than 18 years
Example survey question(s)	**From ATS** During the last 6 months, how many times have you talked to your child about what he/she can or cannot do when it comes to tobacco? ☐ Never ☐ Once ☐ Twice ☐ Three or more times ☐ Don't know/Not sure ☐ Refused During the last 6 months, how many times have you told your child he/she cannot use tobacco? ☐ Never ☐ Once ☐ Twice ☐ Three or more times ☐ Don't know/Not sure ☐ Refused
Comments	None

Rating

Overall quality low ⟷ high	Resources needed	Strength of evaluation evidence	Utility	Face validity	Accepted practice
■■■	$$$	⊘	●	●	●

← ○ ◐ ● ● → better

⊘ Denotes no data.

References
1. Distefan JM, Gilpin EA, Choi WS, Pierce JP. Parental influences predict adolescent smoking in the United States, 1989–1993. *Journal of Adolescent Health.* 1998;22(6):466–74.
2. Jackson C, Henriksen L. Do as I say: parent smoking, antismoking socialization, and smoking onset among children. *Addictive Behaviors.* 1997;22(1):107–14.
3. Sargent JD, Dalton M. Does parental disapproval of smoking prevent adolescents from becoming established smokers? *Pediatrics.* 2001;108(6):1256–62.
4. Pierce JP, Distefan JM, Jackson C, White MM, Gilpin EA. Does tobacco marketing undermine the influence of recommended parenting in discouraging adolescents from smoking? *American Journal of Preventive Medicine.* 2002;23(2):73–81.

Indicator 1.10.5

Proportion of Young People Who Are Susceptible Never-smokers

Goal area 1	Preventing initiation of tobacco use among young people
Outcome 10	Reduced susceptibility to experimentation with tobacco products
What to measure	Proportion of young people who have never tried a cigarette but have not made a firm decision not to smoke
Why this indicator is useful	Studies show that susceptible young people (those who have not made a firm decision not to smoke) are more likely than other young people to experiment with smoking.[1]
Example data source(s)	Youth Tobacco Survey (YTS): CDC Recommended Questions: Core, 2004
Population group(s)	Young people aged less than 18 years
Example survey question(s)	**From YTS** Have you ever tried cigarette smoking, even one or two puffs? ☐ Yes ☐ No Do you think that you will try a cigarette soon? ☐ I have already tried smoking cigarettes ☐ Yes ☐ No Do you think you will smoke a cigarette at any time during the next year? ☐ Definitely yes ☐ Probably yes ☐ Probably not ☐ Definitely not If one of your best friends offered you a cigarette, would you smoke it? ☐ Definitely yes ☐ Probably yes ☐ Probably not ☐ Definitely not
Comments	Evaluators should ask all four example questions to create a susceptibility index.[1]

Rating

Overall quality low ⟵⟶ high	Resources needed	Strength of evaluation evidence	Utility	Face validity	Accepted practice
	$$†	◐	●	◐	●

⟵ ○ ◔ ◐ ● ⟶ better

† Denotes low agreement among reviewers: that is, fewer than 75% of the valid ratings for this indicator were within one point of each other (see Appendix B for an explanation).

Reference
1. Pierce JP, Choi WS, Gilpin EA, Farkas AJ, Merritt RK. Validation of susceptibility as a predictor of which adolescents take up smoking in the United States. *Health Psychology.* 1996;15(5):355–61.

Outcome 11

Decreased Access to Tobacco Products

As noted in the discussion of logic model component 8 (increased restriction and increased enforcement of restrictions on tobacco sales to minors), adopting and enforcing strong laws that restrict young people's access to tobacco can reduce the proportion of retailers that illegally sell tobacco products to minors. As also noted in that discussion, reductions in illegal sales to minors may not automatically translate into reductions in minors' self-reported access to tobacco products through commercial sources. In addition, reductions in illegal sales to young people would not be expected to affect minors' access to tobacco products through noncommercial (social) sources. More importantly, it is unclear whether reductions in retail tobacco sales to minors result in reductions in the actual rate of tobacco use by young people. Although some studies indicate that this is the case, other studies fail to support such a link.[1-3] The data suggest that to be successful in reducing young people's tobacco use, efforts to reduce commercial access must achieve high levels of retailer compliance (perhaps as high as 90% or more).[2] In practice, these levels may not always be attainable.

According to the *Guide to Community Preventive Services*, the most effective approach to preventing young people from gaining access to tobacco (as measured by minors' self-reported tobacco purchase or use behaviors) includes a combination of strong local and state laws, vigorous and sustained enforcement of these laws, retailer education, and—most importantly—community mobilization to generate community support for efforts to reduce youth access to tobacco products.[4] The *Guide to Community Preventive Services* notes that none of these interventions has been shown to be effective when implemented in isolation, in particular when implemented without a strong link to community mobilization initiatives.[4,5]

The *Guide to Community Preventive Services* and *Reducing Tobacco Use: A Report of the Surgeon General* also underscore the importance of taking a comprehensive approach to reducing tobacco use among young people.[4,5] Such an approach includes interventions to reduce the appeal of, and demand for, tobacco products among young people, as well as to restrict their access to these products. In addition, because young people are influenced by the social norms and environmental cues that they observe in adult society, efforts to reduce their tobacco use should be integrated into the broader framework of a comprehensive tobacco control program that also addresses tobacco use by adults.

Listed below are the indicators associated with this outcome:

- **1.11.1** Proportion of successful attempts to purchase tobacco products by young people
- **1.11.2** Proportion of young people reporting that they have been sold tobacco products by a retailer
- **1.11.3** Proportion of young people reporting that they have been unsuccessful in purchasing tobacco products from a retailer
- **1.11.4** Proportion of young people reporting that they have received tobacco products from a social source

1.11.5 Proportion of young people reporting that they purchased cigarettes from a vending machine

1.11.6[NR] Proportion of young people who believe that it is easy to obtain tobacco products

References

1. Rigotti NA, DiFranza JR, Chang Y, Tisdale T, Kemp B, Singer DE. The effect of enforcing tobacco-sales laws on adolescents' access to tobacco and smoking behavior. *New England Journal of Medicine.* 1997;337:1044–51.

2. National Cancer Institute. Smoking and Tobacco Control Monograph, No. 14. *Changing adolescent smoking prevalence: where it is and why.* Bethesda, MD: National Cancer Institute; 2001. NIH Publication No. 02–5086.

3. Fichtenberg CM, Glantz SA. Youth access interventions do not affect youth smoking. *Pediatrics.* 2002;109(6):1088–92.

4. U.S. Department of Health and Human Services. *Reducing tobacco use: a report of the Surgeon General.* 2000.

5. Fielding JE, Briss PA, Carande-Kulis VG, Hopkins DP, Husten CG, Pechacek TF, et al. Tobacco. In: Briss PA, Zaza S, Harris KW, editors. *The guide to community preventive services.* New York: Oxford University Press: [In press] 2005.

For Further Reading

Alexander C, Piazza M, Mekos D, Valente T. Peers, schools, and adolescent cigarette smoking. *Journal of Adolescent Health.* 2001;29(1):22–30.

Altman DG, Levine DW, Coeytaux R, Slade J, Jaffe R. Tobacco promotion and susceptibility to tobacco use among adolescents aged 12 through 17 years in a nationally representative sample. *American Journal of Public Health.* 1996;86(11):1590–3.

Biener L, Siegel M. Tobacco marketing and adolescent smoking: more support for a causal inference. *American Journal of Public Health.* 2000;90(3):407–11.

Castrucci BC, Gerlach KK, Kaufman NJ, Orleans CT. The association among adolescents' tobacco use, their beliefs and attitudes, and friends' and parents' opinions of smoking. *Maternal and Child Health Journal.* 2002;6(3):159–67.

Centers for Disease Control and Prevention. Youth tobacco surveillance: United States, 2000. *Morbidity and Mortality Weekly Report CDC Surveillance Summaries.* 2001;50(SS-4):1–84.

Distefan JM, Gilpin EA, Choi WS, Pierce JP. Parental influences predict adolescent smoking in the United States, 1989–1993. *Journal of Adolescent Health.* 1998; 22(6):466–74.

Forster JL, Murray DM, Wolfson M, Blaine TM, Wagenaar AC, Hennrikus DJ. The effects of community policies to reduce youth access to tobacco. *American Journal of Public Health.* 1998;88(8):1193–8.

Gilpin EA, Pierce JP, Rosbrook B. Are adolescents receptive to current sales promotion practices of the tobacco industry? *Preventive Medicine*. 1997;26(1):14–21.

Jackson C, Henriksen L. Do as I say: parent smoking, antismoking socialization, and smoking onset among children. *Addictive Behaviors*. 1997;22(1):107–14.

Jason LA, Berk M, Schnopp-Wyatt DL, Talbot B. Effects of enforcement of youth access laws on smoking prevalence. *American Journal of Community Psychology*. 1999;27(2):143–61.

Jason LA, Ji PY, Anes MD, Birkhead SH. Active enforcement of cigarette control laws in the prevention of cigarette sales to minors. *Journal of the American Medical Association*. 1991;266(22):3159–61.

Jason LA, Pokorny SB, Schoeny M.E. Evaluating the effects of enforcements and fines on youth smoking. *Critical Public Health*. 2003;13(1):33–45.

Luke DA, Stamatakis KA, Brownson RC. State youth-access tobacco control policies and youth smoking behavior in the United States. *American Journal of Preventive Medicine*. 2000;19(3):180–7.

Pierce JP, Distefan JM, Jackson C, White MM, Gilpin EA. Does tobacco marketing undermine the influence of recommended parenting in discouraging adolescents from smoking? *American Journal of Preventive Medicine*. 2002;23(2):73–81.

Sargent JD, Dalton M, Beach M, Bernhardt A, Heatherton T, Stevens M. Effect of cigarette promotions on smoking uptake among adolescents. *Preventive Medicine*. 2000;30(4):320–7.

Sargent JD, Dalton M. Does parental disapproval of smoking prevent adolescents from becoming established smokers? *Pediatrics*. 2001;108(6):1256–62.

Schooler C, Feighery E, Flora JA. Seventh graders' self-reported exposure to cigarette marketing and its relationship to their smoking behavior. *American Journal of Public Health*. 1996;86(9):1216–21.

Simons-Morton B, Haynie DL, Crump AD, Eitel SP, Saylor KE. Peer and parent influences on smoking and drinking among early adolescents. *Health Education & Behavior*. 2001;28(1):95–107.

U.S. Department of Health and Human Services. *Preventing tobacco use among young people: a report of the Surgeon General*. Atlanta, GA: Centers for Disease Control and Prevention; 1994.

Unger JB, Chen X. The role of social networks and media receptivity in predicting age of smoking initiation: a proportional hazards model of risk and protective factors. *Addictive Behaviors*. 1999;24(3):371–81.

Wang MQ. Social environmental influences on adolescents' smoking progression. *American Journal of Health Behavior*. 2001;25(4):418–25.

Outcome 11

Decreased Access to Tobacco Products

Indicator Rating

←○ ◐ ● ●→ better

Number	Indicator	Overall quality (low → high)	Resources needed	Strength of evaluation evidence	Utility	Face validity	Accepted practice
1.11.1	Proportion of successful attempts to purchase tobacco products by young people	†	$$$†	●	●	●	●†
1.11.2	Proportion of young people reporting that they have been sold tobacco products by a retailer		$$	●	●	●	●
1.11.3	Proportion of young people reporting that they have been unsuccessful in purchasing tobacco products from a retailer	†	$$	⊘	●†	●	●
1.11.4	Proportion of young people reporting that they have received tobacco products from a social source		$$	●	●	●	●
1.11.5	Proportion of young people reporting that they purchased cigarettes from a vending machine		$$	⊘	○	○	●
1.11.6[NR]	Proportion of young people who believe that it is easy to obtain tobacco products		⊘	⊘	⊘	⊘	⊘

† Denotes low agreement among reviewers: that is, fewer than 75% of the valid ratings for this indicator were within one point of each other (see Appendix B for an explanation).
⊘ Denotes no data.
[NR] Denotes an indicator that is not rated (see Appendix B for an explanation).

Indicator 1.11.1

Proportion of Successful Attempts to Purchase Tobacco Products by Young People

Goal area 1	Preventing initiation of tobacco use among young people
Outcome 11	Decreased access to tobacco products
What to measure	The proportion of retailers not in compliance with policies prohibiting the sale of tobacco products to minors
Why this indicator is useful	Decreasing the rate at which young people are successful in purchasing tobacco may contribute to a reduction in tobacco use by young people.[1]
Example data source(s)	Substance Abuse and Mental Health Services Administration (SAMHSA) Compliance Checks Information available at: http://prevention.samhsa.gov/tobacco/guidance.asp
Population group(s)	Tobacco retailers
Example survey question(s)	Not applicable
Comments	Evaluators must consider a number of factors when determining the proportion of successful purchase attempts, including (1) variations in the sampling frame (e.g., number, type, and location of stores), (2) number of successful and unsuccessful purchase attempts per store, and (3) real and apparent ages of minors attempting to purchase tobacco.[2]

Rating

Overall quality low ◄――► high	Resources needed	Strength of evaluation evidence	Utility	Face validity	Accepted practice
▬▬▬▬[†]	$$$[†]	◐	◐	●	●[†]

◄ ○ ◯ ◐ ● ► better

† Denotes low agreement among reviewers: that is, fewer than 75% of the valid ratings for this indicator were within one point of each other (see Appendix B for an explanation).

References
1. Rigotti NA, DiFranza JR, Chang Y, Tisdale T, Kemp B, Singer DE. The effect of enforcing tobacco-sales laws on adolescents' access to tobacco and smoking behavior. *New England Journal of Medicine.* 1997;337:1044–51.
2. DiFranza JR. Are the federal and state governments complying with the Synar Amendment? *Archives of Pediatrics & Adolescent Medicine.* 1999;153(10):1089–97.

GOAL AREA 1
Outcome 11

Indicator 1.11.2

Proportion of Young People Reporting That They Have Been Sold Tobacco Products by a Retailer

Goal area 1	Preventing initiation of tobacco use among young people
Outcome 11	Decreased access to tobacco products
What to measure	The proportion of young people who report having been sold tobacco products by a retailer in the previous 30 days
Why this indicator is useful	Even if most retailers in a community comply with laws prohibiting the sale of tobacco to young people and only a few continue to sell tobacco products to minors, young people's access to tobacco products through retail stores may remain unacceptably high. Young smokers will seek out the retailers that are willing to sell to them. Measuring this indicator helps determine the extent to which illegal sales of tobacco to young people are occurring.[1]
Example data source(s)	• Youth Tobacco Survey (YTS): CDC Recommended Questions: Core, 2004 • CDC Youth Risk Behavior Surveillance System (YRBSS), 2003
Population group(s)	Young people aged less than 18 years
Example survey question(s)	**From YTS** During the past 30 days, where did you buy the last pack of cigarettes you bought? ☐ I did not buy a pack of cigarettes during the past 30 days ☐ A gas station ☐ A convenience store ☐ A grocery store ☐ A drugstore ☐ A vending machine ☐ I bought them over the Internet ☐ Other _____ **From YTS and YRBSS** During the past 30 days, how did you usually get your own cigarettes? ☐ I did not smoke cigarettes during the past 30 days ☐ I bought them in a store such as a convenience store, supermarket, discount store, or gas station ☐ I bought them from a vending machine ☐ I borrowed (or bummed) them from someone else ☐ A person 18 years or older gave them to me ☐ I took them from a store or family member ☐ I got them some other way ☐ I gave someone else money to buy them for me
Comments	None
Rating	Overall quality: mid-range; Resources needed: $$; Strength of evaluation evidence: ●; Utility: ●; Face validity: ●; Accepted practice: ● ← ○ ◐ ● ● → better

Reference

1. Rigotti NA, DiFranza JR, Chang Y, Tisdale T, Kemp B, Singer DE. The effect of enforcing tobacco-sales laws on adolescents' access to tobacco and smoking behavior. *New England Journal of Medicine*. 1997;337:1044–51.

Indicator 1.11.3

Proportion of Young People Reporting That They Have Been Unsuccessful in Purchasing Tobacco Products from a Retailer

Goal area 1	Preventing initiation of tobacco use among young people
Outcome 11	Decreased access to tobacco products
What to measure	Proportion of young people who report that they were refused sale of cigarettes because of their age during the previous 30 days
Why this indicator is useful	Measuring this indicator helps determine the extent to which local and state policies and enforcement activities are reducing young people's access to tobacco products.[1]
Example data source(s)	Youth Tobacco Survey (YTS): CDC Recommended Questions: Core, 2004
Population group(s)	Young people aged less than 18 years
Example survey question(s)	**From YTS** During the past 30 days, did anyone ever refuse to sell you cigarettes because of your age? ☐ I did not try to buy cigarettes in a store during the past 30 days ☐ Yes, someone refused to sell me cigarettes because of my age ☐ No, no one refused to sell me cigarettes because of my age
Comments	Evaluators may also want to assess the type of retailer (e.g., gas station, convenience store, or grocery store) that sold tobacco to a minor.

Rating

Overall quality low ⟷ high	Resources needed	Strength of evaluation evidence	Utility	Face validity	Accepted practice
▬▬▬▬[†]	$$	⊘	●[†]	●	●

⬅ ○ ◔ ◕ ● ➡ better

† Denotes low agreement among reviewers: that is, fewer than 75% of the valid ratings for this indicator were within one point of each other (see Appendix B for an explanation).
⊘ Denotes no data.

Reference
1. Jones SE, Sharp DJ, Husten CG, Crossett LS. Cigarette acquisition and proof of age among US high school students who smoke. *Tobacco Control.* 2002;11:20–5.

Indicator 1.11.4

Proportion of Young People Reporting That They Have Received Tobacco Products from a Social Source

Goal area 1	Preventing initiation of tobacco use among young people
Outcome 11	Decreased access to tobacco products
What to measure	Proportion of young people who report getting their cigarettes from a social source such as a friend, family member, or schoolmate during the previous 30 days
Why this indicator is useful	Although increasing enforcement of laws prohibiting the sale of tobacco to minors reduces illegal sales, studies also suggest that more than half of high-school-aged smokers report obtaining cigarettes from social sources.[1]
Example data source(s)	Youth Tobacco Survey (YTS): CDC Recommended Questions: Core, 2004 CDC Youth Risk Behavior Surveillance System (YRBSS), 2003
Population group(s)	Young people aged less than 18 years
Example survey question(s)	**From YTS and YRBSS** During the past 30 days, how did you usually get your own cigarettes? ☐ I did not smoke cigarettes during the past 30 days ☐ I bought them in a store such as a convenience store, supermarket, discount store, or gas station ☐ I bought them from a vending machine ☐ I gave someone else money to buy them for me ☐ I borrowed (or bummed) them from someone else ☐ A person 18 years old or older gave them to me ☐ I took them from a store or family member ☐ I got them some other way
Comments	None

Rating	Overall quality low ←→ high	Resources needed	Strength of evaluation evidence	Utility	Face validity	Accepted practice
	■■■■■■■	$$	◐	●	●	●

← ○ ◔ ◐ ● → better

Reference
1. Centers for Disease Control and Prevention. Tobacco use and usual source of cigarettes among high school students– United States. *Morbidity and Mortality Weekly Report*. 1996;45(20);413–8.

Indicator 1.11.5

Proportion of Young People Reporting That They Purchased Cigarettes from a Vending Machine

Goal area 1	Preventing initiation of tobacco use among young people
Outcome 11	Decreased access to tobacco products
What to measure	The proportion of young people who usually purchased their cigarettes from a vending machine during the previous 30 days
Why this indicator is useful	Accessible vending machines provide virtually unrestricted access to cigarettes and can be used by even the youngest children. As of 2004, 46 states and the District of Columbia restricted minors' access to tobacco through vending machines, and 30 states and the District of Columbia banned vending machines in locations that are accessible to young people.[1]
Example data source(s)	▸ Youth Tobacco Survey (YTS): CDC Recommended Questions: Core, 2004 ▸ CDC Youth Risk Behavior Surveillance System (YRBSS), 2003
Population group(s)	Young people aged less than 18 years
Example survey question(s)	**From YTS** During the past 30 days, where did you buy the last pack of cigarettes you bought? ☐ I did not buy a pack of cigarettes during the past 30 days ☐ A gas station ☐ A convenience store ☐ A grocery store ☐ A drugstore ☐ A vending machine ☐ I bought them over the Internet **From YTS and YRBSS** During the past 30 days, how did you usually get your own cigarettes? ☐ I did not smoke cigarettes during the past 30 days ☐ I bought them in a store such as a convenience store, supermarket, discount store, or gas station ☐ I bought them from a vending machine ☐ I borrowed (or bummed) them from someone else ☐ A person 18 years or older gave them to me ☐ I took them from a store or family member ☐ I got them some other way ☐ I gave someone else money to buy them for me
Comments	None

Rating

Overall quality low ◄──► high	Resources needed	Strength of evaluation evidence	Utility	Face validity	Accepted practice
▬▬▬▬▬▬	$$	⊘	◐	◐	●

◄ ○ ◔ ◐ ● ► better

⊘ Denotes no data.

Reference
1. Centers for Disease Control and Prevention. *State Tobacco Activities Tracking and Evaluation (STATE) system.* Atlanta, GA: Centers for Disease Control and Prevention. Online database. Available from: http://www.cdc.gov/tobacco/statesystem. Accessed February 2005.

Indicator 1.11.6[NR]

Proportion of Young People Who Believe That It Is Easy to Obtain Tobacco Products

Goal area 1	Preventing initiation of tobacco use among young people
Outcome 11	Decreased access to tobacco products
What to measure	The degree to which young people believe that it is easy or difficult to obtain tobacco products
Why this indicator is useful	Changing the social norms regarding tobacco use by young people requires changing the perception among young people that tobacco products are easily obtained. If young people perceive that obtaining tobacco products is difficult, they are less likely to try to obtain such products.[1]
Example data source(s)	California Youth Tobacco Survey (CA YTS), 1999 Information available at: http://www.dhs.ca.gov/ps/cdic/ccb/TCS/html/Evaluation_Resources.htm
Population group(s)	Young people aged less than 18 years
Example survey question(s)	**From CA YTS** Do you think it would be easy or hard for you to get cigarettes if you wanted some? ☐ Easy ☐ Hard ☐ Don't know/Not sure ☐ Refused
Comments	This indicator was not rated by the panel of experts and, therefore, no rating information is available. See Appendix B for an explanation.

Rating

Overall quality low ◄—► high	Resources needed	Strength of evaluation evidence	Utility	Face validity	Accepted practice
▬▬▬▬▬	⊘	⊘	⊘	⊘	⊘

◄—○ ◐ ● ●—► better

⊘ Denotes no data.

[NR] Denotes an indicator that is not rated (see Appendix B for an explanation).

Reference
1. Gilpin EA, Lee L, Pierce JP. Does adolescent perception of difficulty in getting cigarettes deter experimentation? *Preventive Medicine.* 2004;38(4):485–91.

Outcome 12

Increased Price of Tobacco Products

Studies show an inverse relationship between cigarette price and smoking prevalence by young people and adults. Increasing state or local excise taxes on cigarettes is an effective method of increasing the real price of cigarettes. However, maintaining higher real prices requires further tax increases to offset the effects of inflation and industry practices designed to control retail product prices.[1,2] Recent efforts to offset industry pricing practices have focused on supporting minimum retail pricing laws.[3] Econometric studies show price elasticity for tobacco use among adolescents of –0.76, which means that a 10% increase in price would result in a 7.6% decrease in tobacco use.[4] In addition, to directly motivate people to quit or not start tobacco use, price increases can indirectly reduce tobacco use if a portion of the excise tax revenue is dedicated to the state's tobacco control program.[4]

Although young people usually start using tobacco by first experimenting with cigarettes, some begin by experimenting with other tobacco products such as spit tobacco (smokeless), bidis, small cigars, and loose tobacco (roll-your-own). All tobacco products are taxed. To prevent tobacco users from shifting to cheaper tobacco products, increasing taxes on all tobacco products is important.[5] Tax increases on tobacco products increase the real price of tobacco products and thus reduce young people's demand for such products.

Listed below is the indicator associated with this outcome:

1.12.1 Amount of tobacco product excise tax

References

1. U.S. Department of Health and Human Services. *Preventing tobacco use among young people: a report of the Surgeon General.* Atlanta, GA: Centers for Disease Control and Prevention; 1994.

2. Feighery EC, Ribisl KM, Clark PI, Haladjian HH. How tobacco companies ensure prime placement of their advertising and products in stores: interviews with retailers about tobacco company incentive programmes. *Tobacco Control.* 2003;12:184–8.

3. Bloom PN. Role of slotting fees and trade promotions in shaping how tobacco is marketed in retail stores. *Tobacco Control.* 2001;10(4):340–4.

4. Task Force on Community Preventive Services. The guide to community preventive services: tobacco use prevention and control. *American Journal of Preventive Medicine.* 2001;20(Suppl 2):1–88.

5. U.S. Department of Health and Human Services. *Reducing tobacco use: a report of the Surgeon General.* Atlanta, GA: Centers for Disease Control and Prevention; 2000.

For Further Reading

Gratias EJ, Krowchuk DP, Lawless MR, Durant RH. Middle school students' sources of acquiring cigarettes and requests for proof of age. *Journal of Adolescent Health.* 1999;25(4):276–83.

Ringel J, Pacula RL, Wasserman J. *Youth access to cigarettes: results from the 1999 National Youth Tobacco Survey.* Legacy First Look Report 10. Washington, DC: American Legacy Foundation; 2000.

U.S. Centers for Disease Control and Prevention. Responses to cigarette prices by race/ethnicity, income, and age groups—United States, 1976–1993. *Morbidity and Mortality Weekly Report.* 1998;47(29):605–9.

Outcome 12

Increased Price of Tobacco Products

Indicator Rating

← ○ ◐ ● ● → better

Number	Indicator	Overall quality low ←——→ high	Resources needed	Strength of evaluation evidence	Utility	Face validity	Accepted practice
1.12.1	Amount of tobacco product excise tax	▬▬▬▬▬	$	●	●	●	●

Indicator 1.12.1

Amount of Tobacco Product Excise Tax

Goal area 1	Preventing initiation of tobacco use among young people
Outcome 12	Increased price of tobacco products
What to measure	(1) The state excise tax per pack of cigarettes and (2) the percentage of the total price of a pack of cigarettes that is attributable to tax
Why this indicator is useful	Increasing tax on tobacco products reduces tobacco consumption and prevalence, especially among the most price-sensitive populations (e.g., young people).[1,2] Increasing cigarette excise taxes is an effective method of increasing the real price of cigarettes, although maintaining high prices requires further tax increases to offset the effects of inflation.[1,2]
Example data source(s)	CDC State Tobacco Activities Tracking and Evaluation (STATE) system Data available at: http://www.cdc.gov/tobacco/STATEsystem. Select "economics" and "cigarette sales." Campaign For Tobacco-Free Kids (CTFK) Information available at: http://tobaccofreekids.org/research/factsheets State departments of revenue
Population group(s)	Not applicable. This indicator is best measured by tracking and monitoring state excise taxes on tobacco products.
Example survey question(s)	Not applicable
Comments	States can also independently track the price of tobacco products by collecting scanner data (obtained from product bar codes), which provide information on product price, brand, and promotions. However, the cost of this type of data collection can be prohibitive. To gather more complete data on tobacco price, evaluators can also collect data on other tobacco products such as spit tobacco (smokeless), bidis, small cigars, and loose tobacco (roll-your-own).

Rating

Overall quality low ⟷ high	Resources needed	Strength of evaluation evidence	Utility	Face validity	Accepted practice
▬▬▬▬▬	$	●	●	●	●

← ○ ◔ ● ● → better

References
1. U.S. Department of Health and Human Services. *Preventing tobacco use among young people: a report of the Surgeon General.* Atlanta, GA: Centers for Disease Control and Prevention; 1994.
2. Task Force on Community Preventive Services. The guide to community preventive services: tobacco use prevention and control. *American Journal of Preventive Medicine.* 2001;20(Suppl 2):1–88.

Outcome 13

Reduced Initiation of Tobacco Use by Young People

Tobacco use begins primarily during adolescence, decades earlier than when the death and disability associated with tobacco use are likely to occur. Few people begin to use tobacco as adults; almost 90% of adult smokers began by age 18 years.[1] The earlier young people begin using tobacco products, the more likely they are to use them as adults and the longer they are likely to be users.[1,2] Both the duration and amount of tobacco use are related to eventual chronic health problems, with duration posing the stronger risk.[3,4] The processes of nicotine addiction further ensure that many of today's adolescent smokers will use tobacco regularly when they are adults.[1]

Listed below are the indicators associated with this outcome:

- **1.13.1**   Average age at which young people first smoked a whole cigarette
- **1.13.2**   Proportion of young people who report never having tried a cigarette

References

1. U.S. Department of Health and Human Services. *Preventing tobacco use among young people: a report of the Surgeon General.* Atlanta, GA: Centers for Disease Control and Prevention; 1994.

2. Jackson C, Dickinson D. Cigarette consumption during childhood and persistence of smoking through adolescence. *Archives of Pediatrics & Adolescent Medicine.* 2004;158:1050–6.

3. Doll R, Peto R. Cigarette smoking and lung cancer: dose and time relationships among regular smokers and lifelong non-smokers. *Journal of Epidemiology and Community Health.* 1978;32(4):303–13.

4. Flanders DW, Lally CA, Ahu BP, Henley J, Thun MJ. Lung cancer mortality in relation to age, duration of smoking, and daily cigarette consumption: results from Cancer Prevention Study II. *Cancer Research.* 2003;63:6556–62.

Outcome 13

Reduced Initiation of Tobacco Use by Young People

Indicator Rating

← ○ ◐ ● ● → better

Number	Indicator	Overall quality low ←——→ high	Resources needed	Strength of evaluation evidence	Utility	Face validity	Accepted practice
1.13.1	Average age at which young people first smoked a whole cigarette	▬▬▬▬▬	$$	●	◐	◐	●
1.13.2	Proportion of young people who report never having tried a cigarette	▬▬▬▬▬	$$	●	●	●	●

Indicator 1.13.1

Average Age at Which Young People First Smoked a Whole Cigarette

Goal area 1	Preventing initiation of tobacco use among young people
Outcome 13	Reduced initiation of tobacco use by young people
What to measure	The average age at which young smokers first smoked a whole cigarette
Why this indicator is useful	The age at which someone first smokes a whole cigarette is significantly related to that person's long-term smoking habits. The younger people are when they start using tobacco, the more likely they are to use tobacco products as adults.[1]
Example data source(s)	▸ Youth Tobacco Survey (YTS): CDC Recommended Questions: Core, 2004 ▸ CDC Youth Risk Behavior Surveillance System (YRBSS), 2003
Population group(s)	Young people aged less than 18 years
Example survey question(s)	**From YTS and YRBSS** How old were you when you smoked a whole cigarette for the first time? ☐ I have never smoked cigarettes ☐ 8 years or younger ☐ 9 or 10 years ☐ 11 or 12 years ☐ 13 or 14 years ☐ 15 or 16 years ☐ 17 years or older
Comments	To gather more complete data on tobacco use, evaluators can also ask questions about the use of other tobacco products such as spit tobacco (smokeless), bidis, small cigars, and loose tobacco (roll-your-own).

Rating

Overall quality low ◄――► high	Resources needed	Strength of evaluation evidence	Utility	Face validity	Accepted practice
▬▬▬▬▬	$$	●	●	●	●

◄―○ ◐ ● ●―► better

Reference
1. U.S. Department of Health and Human Services. *Preventing tobacco use among young people: a report of the Surgeon General.* Atlanta, GA: Centers for Disease Control and Prevention; 1994.

Indicator 1.13.2

Proportion of Young People Who Report Never Having Tried a Cigarette

Goal area 1	Preventing initiation of tobacco use among young people
Outcome 13	Reduced initiation of tobacco use by young people
What to measure	Proportion of young people who have never tried a cigarette, not even one or two puffs
Why this indicator is useful	Reducing the number of minors who experiment with tobacco will decrease the number who become established smokers.[1]
Example data source(s)	Youth Tobacco Survey (YTS): CDC Recommended Questions: Core, 2004 CDC Youth Risk Behavior Surveillance System (YRBSS), 2003
Population group(s)	Young people aged less than 18 years
Example survey question(s)	**From YTS and YRBSS** Have you ever tried cigarette smoking, even one or two puffs? ☐ Yes ☐ No
Comments	To gather more complete data on tobacco use, evaluators can also ask questions about the use of other tobacco products such as spit tobacco (smokeless), bidis, small cigars, and loose tobacco (roll-your-own).

Rating

Overall quality low ◄——► high	Resources needed	Strength of evaluation evidence	Utility	Face validity	Accepted practice
▬▬▬▬▬	$$	●	●	●	●

◄ ○ ◐ ● ● ► better

Reference

1. U.S. Department of Health and Human Services. *Preventing tobacco use among young people: a report of the Surgeon General.* Atlanta, GA: Centers for Disease Control and Prevention; 1994.

Outcome 14

Reduced Tobacco-use Prevalence Among Young People

Smoking by young people is associated with serious health problems, such as reduced lung capacity and physical fitness.[1] Smoking by young people also increases the likelihood that they will continue to smoke through adulthood, increasing their risk of tobacco-related diseases such as lung and other cancers, heart disease, and emphysema.[2,3]

Because the number of years of cigarette smoking produces a greater risk of disease than the number of cigarettes smoked per day, it is critically important to work on both preventing young people from starting to smoke and increasing the number and percentage of young smokers who quit.[4,5]

Listed below are the indicators associated with this outcome:

- **1.14.1** Prevalence of tobacco use among young people
- **1.14.2** Proportion of established young smokers

References

1. U.S. Department of Health and Human Services. *Preventing tobacco use among young people: a report of the Surgeon General.* Atlanta, GA: Centers for Disease Control and Prevention; 1994.

2. Jackson C, Dickinson D. Cigarette consumption during childhood and persistence of smoking through adolescence. *Archives of Pediatrics & Adolescent Medicine.* 2004;158(11):1050–6.

3. U.S. Department of Health and Human Services. *The health consequences of smoking: a report of the Surgeon General.* Atlanta, GA: Centers for Disease Control and Prevention; 2004.

4. Doll R, Peto R. Cigarette smoking and lung cancer: dose and time relationships among regular smokers and lifelong non-smokers. *Journal of Epidemiology and Community Health.* 1978;32(4):303–13.

5. Flanders DW, Lally CA, Ahu BP, Henley J, Thun MJ. Lung cancer mortality in relation to age, duration of smoking, and daily cigarette consumption: results from Cancer Prevention Study II. *Cancer Research.* 2003;63(19):6556–62.

For Further Reading

Centers for Disease Control and Prevention. *Targeting tobacco use: the nation's leading cause of death, 2004* [At a Glance]. Atlanta, GA: Centers for Disease Control and Prevention, National Center for Chronic Disease Prevention and Health Promotion; 2004. Available from: http://www.cdc.gov/nccdphp/aag/aag_osh.htm. Accessed March 2005.

Centers for Disease Control and Prevention. Projected smoking-related deaths among youth—United States. *Morbidity and Mortality Weekly Report.* 1996;45(44):971–4.

U.S. Department of Health and Human Services. *Women and smoking: a report of the Surgeon General.* Rockville, MD: U.S. Department of Health and Human Services, Public Health Service, Office of the Surgeon General; 2001.

Outcome 14

Reduced Tobacco-use Prevalence Among Young People

Indicator Rating
← ○ ◐ ● ● → better

Number	Indicator	Overall quality low ←→ high	Resources needed	Strength of evaluation evidence	Utility	Face validity	Accepted practice
1.14.1	Prevalence of tobacco use among young people	▬▬▬▬▬	$$	●	●	●	●
1.14.2	Proportion of established young smokers	▬▬▬▬▬	$$	●	●	●	●

Indicator 1.14.1

Prevalence of Tobacco Use Among Young People

Goal area 1	Preventing initiation of tobacco use among young people
Outcome 14	Reduced tobacco-use prevalence among young people
What to measure	Proportion of young people who have smoked on at least 1 day during the previous 30 days[1]
Why this indicator is useful	Reducing tobacco use among young people decreases their chances of smoking as adults.[2]
Example data source(s)	Youth Tobacco Survey (YTS): CDC Recommended Questions: Core, 2004 CDC Youth Risk Behavior Surveillance System (YRBSS), 2003
Population group(s)	Young people aged less than 18 years
Example survey question(s)	**From YTS and YRBSS** During the past 30 days, on how many days did you smoke cigarettes? ☐ 0 days ☐ 1 or 2 days ☐ 3 to 5 days ☐ 6 to 9 days ☐ 10 to 19 days ☐ 20 to 29 days ☐ All 30 days
Comments	Evaluators may also want to collect data on young people who ever smoked a cigarette and young people who frequently smoke. To gather more complete data on tobacco use, evaluators can also ask questions about the use of other tobacco products such as spit tobacco (smokeless), bidis, small cigars, and loose tobacco (roll-your-own).

Rating

Overall quality low ⟵⟶ high	Resources needed	Strength of evaluation evidence	Utility	Face validity	Accepted practice
▬▬▬▬	$$	●	●	●	●

⟵ ○ ◌ ◐ ● ⟶ better

References
1. Centers for Disease Control and Prevention. Cigarette use among high school students—United States, 1991–2003. *Morbidity and Mortality Weekly Report.* 2004;53(23):499–502.
2. U.S. Department of Health and Human Services. *Preventing tobacco use among young people: a report of the Surgeon General.* Atlanta, GA: Centers for Disease Control and Prevention; 1994.

Indicator 1.14.2

Proportion of Established Young Smokers

Goal area 1	Preventing initiation of tobacco use among young people
Outcome 14	Reduced tobacco-use prevalence among young people
What to measure	Proportion of young people who smoked 100 cigarettes or more during their lifetimes[1]
Why this indicator is useful	Young people who are established smokers are at high risk of becoming addicted to cigarettes and continuing to smoke as adults.[2]
Example data source(s)	▸ Youth Tobacco Survey (YTS): CDC Recommended Questions: Core, 2004 ▸ CDC Youth Risk Behavior Surveillance System (YRBSS), 2003
Population group(s)	Young people aged less than 18 years
Example survey question(s)	**From YTS and YRBSS** During the past 30 days, on how many days did you smoke cigarettes? ☐ 0 days ☐ 10 to 19 days ☐ 1 or 2 days ☐ 20 to 29 days ☐ 3 to 5 days ☐ All 30 days ☐ 6 to 9 days During the past 30 days, what brand of cigarettes did you usually smoke? (CHOOSE ONLY ONE ANSWER) ☐ I did not smoke cigarettes during the past 30 days ☐ Newport ☐ Virginia Slims ☐ I do not have a usual brand ☐ GPC, Basic, or Doral ☐ Camel ☐ Some other brand ☐ Marlboro About how many cigarettes have you smoked in your entire life? ☐ None ☐ 1 or more puffs but never a whole cigarette ☐ 1 cigarette ☐ 2 to 5 cigarettes ☐ 6 to 15 cigarettes (about half a pack total) ☐ 16 to 25 cigarettes (about 1 pack total) ☐ 26 to 99 cigarettes (more than 1 pack, but less than 5 packs) ☐ 100 or more cigarettes (5 or more packs)
Comments	To gather more complete data on tobacco use, evaluators can also ask questions about the use of other tobacco products such as spit tobacco (smokeless), bidis, small cigars, and loose tobacco (roll-your-own).

Rating

Overall quality low ⟷ high	Resources needed	Strength of evaluation evidence	Utility	Face validity	Accepted practice
▬▬▬	$$	●	●	●	●

←○◐●●→ better

References
1. Centers for Disease Control and Prevention. Cigarette use among high school students—United States, 1991–2003. *Morbidity and Mortality Weekly Report.* 2004;53(23):499–502.
2. U.S. Department of Health and Human Services. *Preventing tobacco use among young people: a report of the Surgeon General.* Atlanta, GA: Centers for Disease Control and Prevention; 1994.

CHAPTER 3

Goal Area 2: Eliminating Nonsmokers' Exposure to Secondhand Smoke

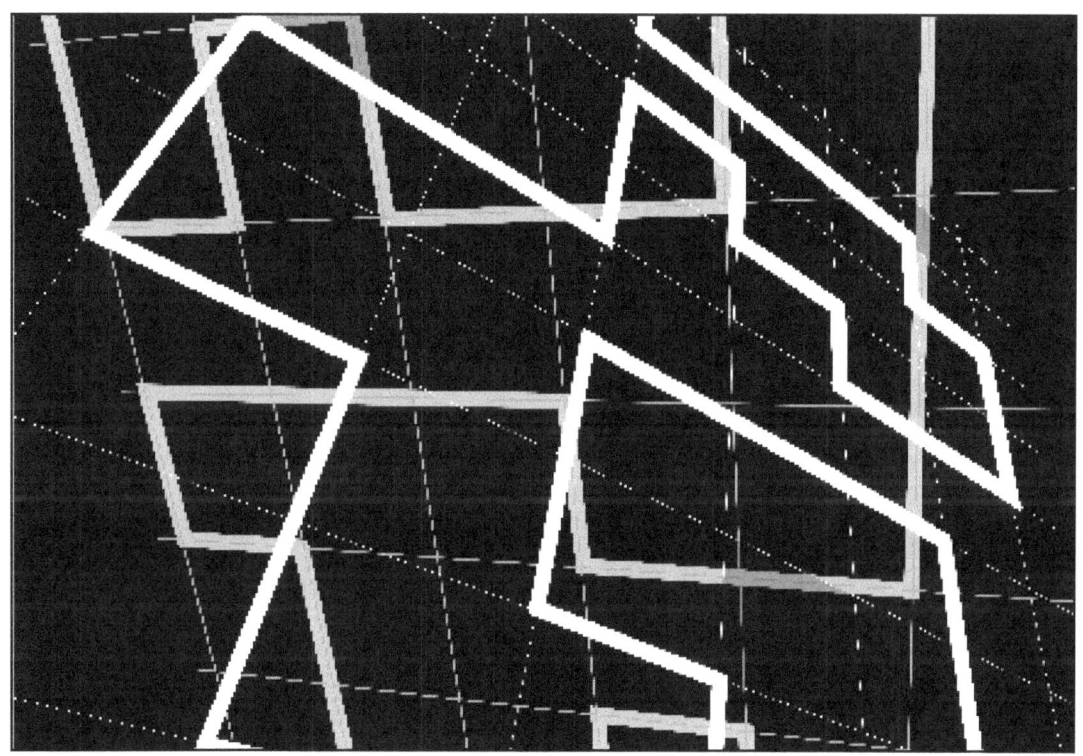

Goal Area 2

Eliminating Nonsmokers' Exposure to Secondhand Smoke

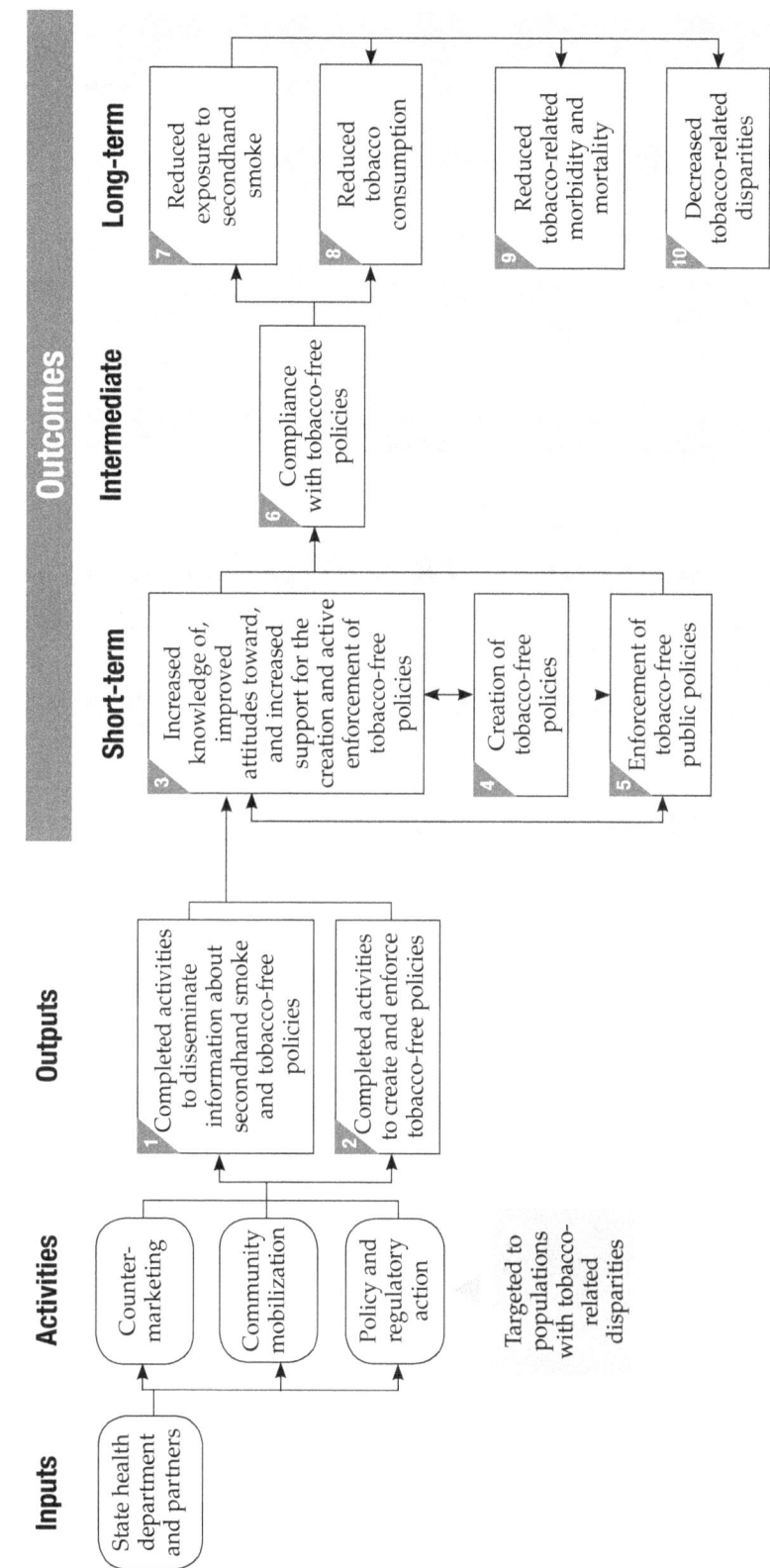

Goal Area 2

Eliminating Nonsmokers' Exposure to Secondhand Smoke

Short-term Outcomes

- **Outcome 3: Increased knowledge of, improved attitudes toward, and increased support for the creation and active enforcement of tobacco-free policies**

    - **2.3.1** Level of confirmed awareness of media messages on the dangers of secondhand smoke
    - **2.3.2** Level of receptivity to media messages about secondhand smoke
    - **2.3.3** Attitudes of smokers and nonsmokers about the acceptability of exposing others to secondhand smoke
    - **2.3.4** Proportion of the population willing to ask someone not to smoke in their presence
    - **2.3.5** Proportion of the population that thinks secondhand smoke is harmful
    - **2.3.6** Proportion of the population that thinks secondhand smoke is harmful to children and pregnant women
    - **2.3.7** Level of support for creating tobacco-free policies in public places and workplaces
    - **2.3.8** Level of support for adopting tobacco-free policies in homes and vehicles
    - **2.3.9** Level of support for active enforcement of tobacco-free public policies
    - **2.3.10**[NR] Level of support for creating tobacco-free policies in schools

- **Outcome 4: Creation of tobacco-free policies**

    - **2.4.1** Proportion of jurisdictions with public policies for tobacco-free workplaces and other indoor and outdoor public places
    - **2.4.2** Proportion of workplaces with voluntary tobacco-free policies
    - **2.4.3** Proportion of the population that works in environments with tobacco-free policies
    - **2.4.4** Proportion of the population reporting voluntary tobacco-free home or vehicle policies
    - **2.4.5** Proportion of schools or school districts reporting the implementation of 100% tobacco-free policies
    - **2.4.6** Changes in state tobacco control laws that preempt stronger local tobacco control laws

▪ **Outcome 5: Enforcement of tobacco-free public policies**

- 2.5.1 Number of compliance checks conducted by enforcement agencies
- 2.5.2 Number of enforcement agency responses to complaints regarding noncompliance with tobacco-free public policies
- 2.5.3 Number of warnings, citations, and fines issued for infractions of tobacco-free public policies

Intermediate Outcomes

▪ **Outcome 6: Compliance with tobacco-free policies**

- 2.6.1 Perceived compliance with tobacco-free policies in workplaces
- 2.6.2 Perceived compliance with tobacco-free policies in indoor and outdoor public places
- 2.6.3 Proportion of public places observed to be in compliance with tobacco-free policies
- 2.6.4 Perceived compliance with voluntary tobacco-free home or vehicle policies
- 2.6.5 Perceived compliance with tobacco-free policies in schools

Long-term Outcomes

▪ **Outcome 7: Reduced exposure to secondhand smoke**

- 2.7.1 Proportion of the population reporting exposure to secondhand smoke in the workplace
- 2.7.2 Proportion of the population reporting exposure to secondhand smoke in public places
- 2.7.3 Proportion of the population reporting exposure to secondhand smoke at home or in vehicles
- 2.7.4 Proportion of students reporting exposure to secondhand smoke in schools
- 2.7.5 Proportion of nonsmokers reporting overall exposure to secondhand smoke

▪ **Outcome 8: Reduced tobacco consumption**

- 2.8.1 Per capita consumption of tobacco products
- 2.8.2 Average number of cigarettes smoked per day by smokers
- 2.8.3 Smoking prevalence

Outcome 3

Increased Knowledge of, Improved Attitudes Toward, and Increased Support for the Creation and Active Enforcement of Tobacco-free Policies

The theory of change associated with eliminating nonsmokers' exposure to secondhand smoke starts with increasing people's knowledge of the dangers of exposure to secondhand smoke, changing their attitudes toward the acceptability of exposing nonsmokers to secondhand smoke, and increasing their support for passing and enforcing tobacco-free policies. Ideally, such changes should lead to increases in the number of environments with tobacco-free policies and increased compliance with those policies as people become more conscious of the importance of smoke-free air. In reality, passing tobacco-free policies is subject to many inhibiting and facilitating influences and factors. Moreover, adopting a policy does not ensure that the policy will be actively enforced or become self-enforcing.

Experience suggests that interventions intended to increase knowledge of and support for passing or enforcing tobacco-free policies can be effective.[1,2] In addition, experience and logic dictate that sufficient support for tobacco-free policies by either the public or decision makers will lead to the adoption of tobacco-free policies (including voluntary tobacco-free policies).[3]

Experience also shows that policy makers review data on public support for tobacco-free policies carefully before they decide whether to support such policies.[4-7] One study, for example, showed that support for a New York City law requiring that restaurants be tobacco free was associated with compliance with the law.[3] In addition, a study from California showed that exposure to a state media campaign promoting tobacco-free policies and laws was significantly associated with increases over time in reported smoking bans in homes.[8] Other studies show that increased knowledge of the adverse health effects of secondhand smoke is associated with increased efforts by individuals to minimize their exposure to secondhand smoke and with reductions in actual exposure to secondhand smoke.[9,10]

Listed below are the indicators associated with this outcome:

- **2.3.1** Level of confirmed awareness of media messages on the dangers of secondhand smoke
- **2.3.2** Level of receptivity to media messages about secondhand smoke
- **2.3.3** Attitudes of smokers and nonsmokers about the acceptability of exposing others to secondhand smoke
- **2.3.4** Proportion of the population willing to ask someone not to smoke in their presence
- **2.3.5** Proportion of the population that thinks secondhand smoke is harmful

- **2.3.6** Proportion of the population that thinks secondhand smoke is harmful to children and pregnant women
- **2.3.7** Level of support for creating tobacco-free policies in public places and workplaces
- **2.3.8** Level of support for adopting tobacco-free policies in homes and vehicles
- **2.3.9** Level of support for active enforcement of tobacco-free public policies
- **2.3.10**[NR] Level of support for creating tobacco-free policies in schools

References

1. Clarke H, Wilson MP, Cummings KM, Hyland A. The campaign to enact New York City's Smoke-Free Air Act. *Journal of Public Health Management and Practice.* 1999;5(1):1–13.

2. Magzamen S, Glantz SA. The new battleground: California's experience with smoke-free bars. *American Journal of Public Health.* 2001;91(2):245–52.

3. Hyland A, Cummings KM, Wilson MP. Compliance with the New York City Smoke-Free Air Act. *Journal of Public Health Management and Practice.* 1999; 5(1):43–52.

4. U.S. Department of Health and Human Services. *Reducing tobacco use: a report of the Surgeon General.* Atlanta, GA: Centers for Disease Control and Prevention; 2000.

5. U.S. Department of Health and Human Services. *Women and smoking: a report of the Surgeon General.* Rockville, MD: Office of the Surgeon General; Washington, DC: Government Printing Office; 2001.

6. Thomson GW, Wilson N. Public attitudes about tobacco smoke in workplaces: the importance of workers' rights in survey questions. *Tobacco Control.* 2004;13(2):206–7.

7. Howard KA, Rogers T, Howard-Pitney B, Flora JA, Norman GJ, Ribisl KM. Opinion leaders' support for tobacco control policies and participation in tobacco control activities. *American Journal of Public Health.* 2000;90(8):1283–7.

8. Rohrbach LA, Howard-Pitney B, Unger JB, Dent CW, Howard KA, Cruz TB, Ribisl KM, Norman GJ, Fishbein H, Johnson CA. Independent evaluation of the California Tobacco Control Program: relationships between program exposure and outcomes, 1996–1998. *American Journal of Public Health.* 2002;92(6):975–83.

9. Li C, Unger JB, Schuster D, Rohrbach LA, Howard-Pitney B, Norman G. Youths' exposure to environmental tobacco smoke (ETS): associations with health beliefs and social pressure. *Addictive Behaviors.* 2003;28(1):39–53.

10. Kurtz M, Kurtz JC, Johnson SM, Beverly EE. Exposure to environmental tobacco smoke: perceptions of African American children and adolescents. *Preventive Medicine.* 1996;25(3):286–92.

For Further Reading

Ashley M, Cohen J, Ferrence R, Bull S, Bondy S, Poland B, Pederson L. Smoking in the home: changing attitudes and current practices. *American Journal of Public Health* 1998;88(5):797–800.

Brenner H. Smoking behavior and attitude toward smoking regulations and passive smoking in the workplace. A study among 974 employees in the German metal industry. *Preventive Medicine.* 1997;26(1):138–43.

Crone MR, Reijneveld SA, Burgmeijer RJ, Hirasing RA. Factors that influence passive smoking in infancy: a study among mothers of newborn babies in The Netherlands. *Preventive Medicine.* 2001;32(3):209–17.

Fichtenberg CM, Glantz SA. Effect of smoke-free workplaces on smoking behaviour: systematic review. *British Medical Journal.* 2002;325(7357):188.

Gilpin EA, Emery SL, Farkas AJ, Distefan JM, White MM, Pierce JP. *The California Tobacco Control Program: a decade of progress. Results from the California Tobacco Surveys, 1990–1998.* La Jolla, CA: University of California, San Diego; 2001. Available from: http://repositories.cdlib.org/tc/surveys/. Accessed February 2005.

Gilpin EA, Pierce JP. The California Tobacco Control Program and potential harm reduction through reduced cigarette consumption in continuing smokers. *Nicotine and Tobacco Research.* 2002;4(Suppl 2):S157–66.

Glantz SA, Jamieson P. Attitudes toward secondhand smoke, smoking, and quitting among young people. *Pediatrics.* 2000;106(6):E82.

Hopper JA, Craig KA. Environmental tobacco smoke exposure among urban children. *Pediatrics.* 2000;106(4):E47.

Kegler M, Malcoe LH. Smoking restrictions in the home and car among rural Native American and white families with young children. *Preventive Medicine.* 2002;35(4):334–42.

Kurtz ME, Kurtz JC, Johnson SM, Beverly EE. Exposure to environmental tobacco smoke: perceptions of African American children and adolescents. *Preventive Medicine.* 1996;25(3):286–92.

Li C, Unger JB, Schuster D, Rohrbach LA, Howard-Pitney B, Norman G. Youths' exposure to environmental tobacco smoke (ETS): associations with health beliefs and social pressure. *Addictive Behaviors.* 2003;28(1):39–53.

Philpot SJ, Ryan SA, Torre LE, Wilcox HM, Jalleh G, Jamrozik Y. Effect of smoke-free policies on the behaviour of social smokers. *Tobacco Control.* 1999;8(3):278–81.

Pikora T, Phang J, Karro J, Corti B, Clarkson J, Donovan R, Frizzell S, Wilkinson A. Are smoke-free policies implemented and adhered to at sporting venues? *Australian and New Zealand Journal of Public Health.* 1999;23(4):407–9.

Popham WJ, Potter LD, Bal DG, Johnson MD, Duerr JM, Quinn V. Do anti-smoking media campaigns help smokers quit? *Public Health Reports.* 1993;108(4):510–3.

Outcome 3

Increased Knowledge of, Improved Attitudes Toward, and Increased Support for the Creation and Active Enforcement of Tobacco-free Policies

Indicator Rating
← ○ ◐ ◉ ● → better

Number	Indicator	Overall quality (low ←→ high)	Resources needed	Strength of evaluation evidence	Utility	Face validity	Accepted practice
2.3.1	Level of confirmed awareness of media messages on the dangers of secondhand smoke	▬▬▬	$$	◉	◉	◉	◉
2.3.2	Level of receptivity to media messages about secondhand smoke	▬▬▬†	$$†	◐	◉	◐	◉*
2.3.3	Attitudes of smokers and nonsmokers about the acceptability of exposing others to secondhand smoke	▬▬▬†	$$$†	◉	◉	◉	◉*
2.3.4	Proportion of the population willing to ask someone not to smoke in their presence	▬▬▬	$$†	◉	◉	◉†	◉*
2.3.5	Proportion of the population that thinks secondhand smoke is harmful	▬▬▬†	$$†	◉	◉	◉	◉
2.3.6	Proportion of the population that thinks secondhand smoke is harmful to children and pregnant women	▬▬▬	$$†	◉	◉	◉	◉
2.3.7	Level of support for creating tobacco-free policies in public places and workplaces	▬▬▬	$$†	◉	◉	◉	◉
2.3.8	Level of support for adopting tobacco-free policies in homes and vehicles	▬▬▬†	$$$	⊘	◉	◉	◉
2.3.9	Level of support for active enforcement of tobacco-free public policies	▬▬▬	$$$†	⊘	◉	◉	◉
2.3.10[NR]	Level of support for creating tobacco-free policies in schools	▬▬▬	⊘	⊘	⊘	⊘	⊘

* Denotes low reviewer response: that is, greater than 75% of the experts either did not rate the indicator, or gave the criterion an invalid rating (see Appendix B for an explanation).
† Denotes low agreement among reviewers: that is, fewer than 75% of the valid ratings for this indicator were within one point of each other (see Appendix B for an explanation).
⊘ Denotes no data.
[NR] Denotes an indicator that is not rated (see Appendix B for an explanation).

Indicator 2.3.1

Level of Confirmed Awareness of Media Messages on the Dangers of Secondhand Smoke

Goal area 2	Eliminating nonsmokers' exposure to secondhand smoke
Outcome 3	Increased knowledge of, improved attitudes toward, and increased support for the creation and active enforcement of tobacco-free policies
What to measure	Proportion of the target population that can accurately recall a media message about the dangers of exposure to secondhand smoke
Why this indicator is useful	Evaluators should measure exposure to media messages to confirm awareness of these messages by asking respondents to provide specific information about the message.[1] As people increase their knowledge about the health effects of secondhand smoke, the number of their actions to reduce exposure to secondhand smoke should also increase.[2]
Example data source(s)	Legacy Media Tracking Survey (LMTS), 2003 Information available at: http://tobacco.rti.org/data/lmts.cfm
Population group(s)	Young people aged less than 18 years
Example survey question(s)	**From LMTS** Have you recently seen an anti-smoking or anti-tobacco ad on TV that shows _____? ☐ Yes ☐ Maybe, not sure ☐ No ☐ Refused to answer What happens in this advertisement? (DO NOT READ RESPONSE CATEGORIES) _____ What do you think the main message of this ad was? (DO NOT READ RESPONSE CATEGORIES) _____
Comments	The example survey questions could be asked of adults. Evaluators may want to categorize awareness of the medium (e.g., billboard, television, print) through which respondents learned of the anti-tobacco media message. Programs may want to evaluate confirmed awareness of an advertisement by respondents' smoking status (current, former, or never) and addiction level (e.g., light, moderate, or heavy) because awareness levels may differ significantly among groups with different levels of addiction. Evaluators should work closely with countermarketing campaign managers to (1) develop a separate series of questions for each main media message and (2) coordinate data collection with the timing of the media campaign.

Rating	Overall quality low ←——→ high	Resources needed	Strength of evaluation evidence	Utility	Face validity	Accepted practice
	▬▬▬▬▬▬	$$	●	●	●	●

←○ ◔ ● ●→ better

References
1. Sly DF, Heald GR, Ray S. The Florida "truth" antitobacco media evaluation: design, first year results, and implications for planning future state media evaluations. *Tobacco Control.* 2001;10(1):9–15.
2. Task Force on Community Preventive Services. The guide to community preventive services: tobacco use prevention and control. *American Journal of Preventive Medicine.* 2001;20(Suppl 2):1–88.

Indicator 2.3.2

Level of Receptivity to Media Messages About Secondhand Smoke

Goal area 2	Eliminating nonsmokers' exposure to secondhand smoke
Outcome 3	Increased knowledge of, improved attitudes toward, and increased support for the creation and active enforcement of tobacco-free policies
What to measure	The level of receptivity to media messages by the intended audience. Receptivity is generally defined as the extent to which people are willing to listen to a persuasive message. In tobacco control evaluation, however, the definition is narrower; receptivity is the extent to which people believe that the message was convincing, made them think about their behavior, and stimulated discussion with others.[1]
Why this indicator is useful	Message awareness is necessary but not sufficient to change the knowledge of and attitudes toward tobacco-free policies, as well as for increasing support for creating and enforcing such policies. Media campaigns are effective only if their messages reach and resonate with the intended audience. A well-received message helps to ensure campaign effectiveness.[2-5]
Example data source(s)	Legacy Media Tracking Survey (LMTS), 2003 Information available at: http://tobacco.rti.org/data/lmts.cfm
Population group(s)	Young people aged less than 18 years
Example survey question(s)	**From LMTS** Tell me how much you agree or disagree with the following statement: This ad is convincing. Would you say you: ☐ Strongly agree ☐ Agree ☐ Disagree ☐ Strongly disagree ☐ Have no opinion ☐ Don't know Would you say the ad gave you good reasons not to smoke? ☐ Yes ☐ No ☐ Don't know Did you talk to your friends about this ad? ☐ Yes ☐ No ☐ Don't know
Comments	The example questions could be asked of adults. Evaluators may want to assess receptivity by the medium through which respondents learned of the media message (e.g., television, print, or radio). Evaluators should work closely with countermarketing campaign managers to (1) develop a separate series of questions for each main media message and (2) coordinate data collection with the timing of the media campaign.

Rating

Overall quality low ⟷ high	Resources needed	Strength of evaluation evidence	Utility	Face validity	Accepted practice
▰▰▰▰†	$$†	◐	●	◐	●*

←○◔●●→ better

* Denotes low reviewer response: that is, greater than 75% of the experts either did not rate the indicator, or gave the criterion an invalid rating (see Appendix B for an explanation).
† Denotes low agreement among reviewers: that is, fewer than 75% of the valid ratings for this indicator were within one point of each other (see Appendix B for an explanation).

References
1. Sly DF, Heald GR, Ray S. The Florida "truth" anti-tobacco media evaluation: design, first year results, and implications for planning future state media evaluations. *Tobacco Control.* 2001;10(1):9–15.
2. McGuire WJ. Public communication as a strategy for inducing health-promoting behavioral change. *Preventive Medicine.* 1984;13(3):299–319.
3. Kotler P, Armstrong G. *Principles of marketing,* 9th ed. Upper Saddle River, NJ: Prentice-Hall; 2001.
4. Carter WB. Health behavior as a rational process: theory of reasoned action and multiattribute utility theory. In: Glanz K, Lewis FM, Rimer BK, editors. *Health behavior and health education: theory, research, and practice.* San Francisco, CA: Jossey-Bass; 1990. pp. 63–91.
5. Maibach E, Parrott RL, editors. *Designing health messages: approaches from communication theory and public health practice.* Thousand Oaks, CA: Sage; 1995.

Indicator 2.3.3

Attitudes of Smokers and Nonsmokers About the Acceptability of Exposing Others to Secondhand Smoke

Goal area 2	Eliminating nonsmokers' exposure to secondhand smoke
Outcome 3	Increased knowledge of, improved attitudes toward, and increased support for the creation and active enforcement of tobacco-free policies
What to measure	The attitudes of smokers and nonsmokers concerning exposing others to secondhand smoke
Why this indicator is useful	Attitudes about the acceptability of exposing others to secondhand smoke are leading indicators of social norms with regard to smoking. Even in places without formal secondhand smoke regulations, changes in attitudes can increase (1) self-regulating behavior by smokers (i.e., they refrain from smoking in places where nonsmokers would be exposed to secondhand smoke) and (2) personal advocacy behavior by nonsmokers (i.e., they ask smokers not to smoke around them).[1,2]
Example data source(s)	National Social Climate Survey of Tobacco Control, 2001 Information available at: http://www.ssrc.msstate.edu/socialclimate
Population group(s)	Adults aged 18 years or older
Example survey question(s)	Smoking should not be allowed in any public place. Do you: ☐ Strongly agree ☐ Agree ☐ Disagree ☐ Strongly disagree **From National Social Climate Survey of Tobacco Control** It is acceptable for parents to smoke in front of children. Do you: ☐ Strongly agree ☐ Agree ☐ Disagree ☐ Strongly disagree
Comments	The authors created the first example question. It is not in any commonly used data source. The example survey questions could be asked of young people.
Rating	Overall quality: low → high [†]; Resources needed: $$$[†]; Strength of evaluation evidence: ●; Utility: ●; Face validity: ●; Accepted practice: ●[*] ← ○ ◐ ● ● → better

* Denotes low reviewer response: that is, greater than 75% of the experts either did not rate the indicator, or gave the criterion an invalid rating (see Appendix B for an explanation).
† Denotes low agreement among reviewers: that is, fewer than 75% of the valid ratings for this indicator were within one point of each other (see Appendix B for an explanation).

References
1. U.S. Department of Health and Human Services. *Reducing tobacco use: a report of the Surgeon General.* Atlanta, GA: Centers for Disease Control and Prevention; 2000.
2. McMillen RC, Winickoff JP, Klein JD, Weitzman M. U.S. adult attitudes and practices regarding smoking restrictions and child exposure to environmental tobacco smoke: changes in the social climate from 2000–2001. *Pediatrics.* 2003;112(1 Pt 1): E55–60.

Indicator 2.3.4

Proportion of the Population Willing to Ask Someone Not to Smoke in Their Presence

Goal area 2	Eliminating nonsmokers' exposure to secondhand smoke
Outcome 3	Increased knowledge of, improved attitudes toward, and increased support for the creation and active enforcement of tobacco-free policies
What to measure	Proportion of the population who report that they have asked or would ask someone not to smoke in their presence (including in homes, vehicles, and public places)
Why this indicator is useful	Compliance with tobacco-free policies and changes in smokers' behavior in places without policies require that nonsmokers be willing to ask smokers to refrain from smoking in their presence.[1,2] Experience in California suggests that nonsmokers' willingness to ask someone not to smoke increases over time and that smokers' responses are usually positive.[3]
Example data source(s)	Adult Tobacco Survey (ATS): CDC Recommended Questions: Supplemental Section D: Environmental Tobacco Smoke, 2003 California Adult Tobacco Survey (CATS), 1999 Information available at: http://www.dhs.ca.gov/ps/cdic/ccb/TCS/html/Evaluation_Resources.htm
Population group(s)	Adults aged 18 years or older
Example survey question(s)	**From ATS** If someone were smoking near you in the nonsmoking area of a restaurant, would you ask them to stop? ☐ Yes ☐ No ☐ Maybe ☐ Don't know/Not sure ☐ Refused In the past 12 months, have you ever asked a stranger not to smoke around you so you wouldn't have to avoid their tobacco smoke? ☐ Yes ☐ No ☐ Don't know/Not sure ☐ Refused **From CATS** In the past 12 months, have you ever asked someone not to smoke? ☐ Yes ☐ No ☐ Don't know/Not sure ☐ Refused *If the answer is "yes," ask the following:* On that same occasion, what was the primary reason you asked that person not to smoke? ☐ Smoke was annoying to you ☐ Concerned about long-term health effects of secondhand smoke ☐ Smoking was illegal ☐ Concerned about the smoker's health ☐ Concerned about your own health (respondent's health) ☐ Other (specify)_____ ☐ Don't know/Not sure ☐ Refused to answer
Comments	The example survey questions could be asked of young people.

Rating	Overall quality low ⟵⟶ high	Resources needed	Strength of evaluation evidence	Utility	Face validity	Accepted practice
	▬▬▬▬▬▬	$$ †	●	●	●†	●*

⟵ ○ ◐ ● ●⟶ better

* Denotes low reviewer response: that is, greater than 75% of the experts either did not rate the indicator, or gave the criterion an invalid rating (see Appendix B for an explanation).
† Denotes low agreement among reviewers: that is, fewer than 75% of the valid ratings for this indicator were within one point of each other (see Appendix B for an explanation).

References
1. Cains T, Cannata S, Poulos R, Ferson MJ, Stewart BW. Designated "no smoking" areas provide from partial to no protection from environmental tobacco smoke. *Tobacco Control.* 2004;13(1):17–22.
2. Repace J. *An air quality survey of respirable particles and particulate carcinogens in Delaware hospitality venues before and after a smoking ban.* Bowie, MD: Repace Associates; 2003. Available from: http://www.tobaccoscam.ucsf.edu/pdf/RepaceDelaware.pdf. Accessed December 2004.
3. Independent Evaluation Consortium. Final report. *Independent evaluation of the California Tobacco Control Prevention and Education Program: waves 1, 2, and 3 (1996–2000).* Rockville, MD: The Gallup Organization; 2002. Available from: http://www.dhs.ca.gov/tobacco/documents/WavesComplete.pdf. Accessed December 2004.

Indicator 2.3.5

Proportion of the Population That Thinks Secondhand Smoke Is Harmful

Goal area 2	Eliminating nonsmokers' exposure to secondhand smoke
Outcome 3	Increased knowledge of, improved attitudes toward, and increased support for the creation and active enforcement of tobacco-free policies
What to measure	Proportion of the population that believes exposure to secondhand smoke is harmful to one's health
Why this indicator is useful	Several studies found that increased knowledge of the adverse health effects of secondhand smoke was associated with (1) an increased number of actions to reduce exposure to secondhand smoke, (2) reduced exposure to secondhand smoke, and (3) increased intention to quit and higher quit rates among smokers.[1-3] Changes in attitudes and behaviors concerning secondhand smoke are often preceded by an understanding of its ill effects.
Example data source(s)	Adult Tobacco Survey (ATS): CDC Recommended Questions: Core, 2003 Youth Tobacco Survey (YTS): CDC Recommended Questions: Core, 2004
Population group(s)	Adults aged 18 years or older Young people aged less than 18 years
Example survey question(s)	**From ATS** Do you think that breathing smoke from other people's cigarettes is: ☐ Very harmful to one's health ☐ Not very harmful to one's health ☐ Somewhat harmful to one's health ☐ Not harmful at all to one's health Would you say that breathing smoke from other people's cigarettes causes: ☐ Lung cancer in adults ☐ Respiratory problems in children ☐ Heart disease in adults ☐ Sudden infant death syndrome ☐ Colon cancer in adults **From YTS** Do you think the smoke from other people's cigarettes is harmful to you? ☐ Definitely yes ☐ Probably yes ☐ Probably not ☐ Definitely not
Comments	The example questions could be asked of decision makers or opinion leaders.

Rating

Overall quality low ⟵⟶ high	Resources needed	Strength of evaluation evidence	Utility	Face validity	Accepted practice
▬▬▬†	$$†	◐	●	◐	●

⟵ ○ ◐ ● ● ⟶ better

† Denotes low agreement among reviewers: that is, fewer than 75% of the valid ratings for this indicator were within one point of each other (see Appendix B for an explanation).

References
1. Kurtz ME, Kurtz JE, Johnson SM, Beverly EE. Exposure to environmental tobacco smoke: perceptions of African American children and adolescents. *Preventive Medicine*. 1996;25(3):286–92.
2. Li C, Unger JB, Schuster D, Rohrbach LA, Howard-Pitney B, Norman G. Youths' exposure to environmental tobacco smoke (ETS): associations with health beliefs and social pressure. *Addictive Behaviors*. 2003;28(1):39–53.
3. Glantz SA, Jamieson P. Attitudes toward secondhand smoke, smoking, and quitting among young people. *Pediatrics*. 2000;106(6):E82.

Indicator 2.3.6

Proportion of the Population That Thinks Secondhand Smoke Is Harmful to Children and Pregnant Women

Goal area 2	Eliminating nonsmokers' exposure to secondhand smoke
Outcome 3	Increased knowledge of, improved attitudes toward, and increased support for the creation and active enforcement of tobacco-free policies
What to measure	Proportion of the population that believes exposure to secondhand smoke is harmful to children and pregnant women
Why this indicator is useful	Exposure to secondhand smoke is especially harmful to children and pregnant women.[1] Increased public awareness of this danger reduces exposure of children and pregnant women to secondhand smoke.[2]
Example data source(s)	Adult Tobacco Survey (ATS): CDC Recommended Questions: Core, 2003
Population group(s)	Adults aged 18 years or older
Example survey question(s)	**From ATS** Would you say that breathing smoke from other people's cigarettes causes: ☐ Lung cancer in adults ☐ Respiratory problems in children ☐ Heart disease in adults ☐ Sudden infant death syndrome ☐ Colon cancer in adults Do you agree or disagree with the following statement: Smoke from other people's cigarettes is harmful to children? ☐ Strongly agree ☐ Somewhat agree ☐ Neither agree nor disagree ☐ Somewhat disagree ☐ Strongly disagree ☐ Don't know/Not sure ☐ Refused to answer
Comments	The example survey questions could be asked of pregnant women and young people.

Rating

Overall quality low ⟷ high	Resources needed	Strength of evaluation evidence	Utility	Face validity	Accepted practice
▬▬▬	$$[†]	●	●	●	●

← ○ ◔ ● ● → better

[†] Denotes low agreement among reviewers: that is, fewer than 75% of the valid ratings for this indicator were within one point of each other (see Appendix B for an explanation).

References
1. U.S. Department of Health and Human Services. *Women and smoking: a report of the Surgeon General.* Rockville, MD: U.S. Department of Health and Human Services, Public Health Service, Office of the Surgeon General; 2001.
2. McMillen RC, Winickoff JP, Klein JD, Weitzman M. U.S. adult attitudes and practices regarding smoking restrictions and child exposure to environmental tobacco smoke: changes in the social climate from 2000–2001. *Pediatrics.* 2003;11(1 Pt 1): E55–60.

Indicator 2.3.7

Level of Support for Creating Tobacco-free Policies in Public Places and Workplaces

Goal area 2	Eliminating nonsmokers' exposure to secondhand smoke
Outcome 3	Increased knowledge of, improved attitudes toward, and increased support for the creation and active enforcement of tobacco-free policies
What to measure	Proportion of adults who support the creation of policies that restrict smoking in public places and workplaces
Why this indicator is useful	Tobacco-free policies are unlikely to be adopted without support among business owners, policy makers, and the general public.[1-4]
Example data source(s)	Adult Tobacco Survey (ATS): CDC Recommended Questions: Core, 2003 Adult Tobacco Survey (ATS): CDC Recommended Questions: Supplemental Section D: Environmental Tobacco Smoke, 2003 Behavioral Risk Factor Surveillance System (BRFSS): Tobacco Use Prevention Module, 2000
Population group(s)	Adults aged 18 years or older

Example survey question(s)

From ATS: Core

In indoor work areas, do you think that smoking should be allowed in all areas, some areas, or not at all?
☐ Allowed in all areas ☐ Allowed in some areas ☐ Not allowed at all
☐ Don't know/Not sure ☐ Refused

From ATS: Supplemental Section D

In _____, *(Fill blank with each of the following: public buildings, bars and cocktail lounges, day care centers, indoor sporting events)* do you think smoking should be allowed in all areas, some areas, or not allowed at all?
☐ Allowed in all areas ☐ Allowed in some areas ☐ Not allowed at all
☐ Don't know/Not sure ☐ Refused

Would you prefer a stronger workplace smoking policy, a weaker workplace smoking policy, or no change?
☐ Prefer stronger policy ☐ Prefer weaker policy ☐ Prefer no change
☐ Don't know/Not sure ☐ Refused

From BRFSS

In the following locations do you think that smoking should be allowed in all areas, some areas, or not allowed at all?

	Allowed in all areas	Some areas	Not allowed at all	Don't know Not sure	Refused to answer
Restaurants	☐	☐	☐	☐	☐
Schools	☐	☐	☐	☐	☐
Day Care Centers	☐	☐	☐	☐	☐
Indoor Work Areas	☐	☐	☐	☐	☐

Comments	Evaluators may want to analyze the level of support for creating tobacco-free policies according to (1) the smoking status of the responder and (2) the place where the smoking restrictions would or do apply.					
	These example questions could be asked of decision makers, employers, opinion leaders, or young people.					
Rating	Overall quality low ◄───► high	Resources needed	Strength of evaluation evidence	Utility	Face validity	Accepted practice
	▬▬▬▬▬	$$†	◐	●	●	●

◄─ ○ ◔ ◐ ● ─► better

† Denotes low agreement among reviewers: that is, fewer than 75% of the valid ratings for this indicator were within one point of each other (see Appendix B for an explanation).

References

1. U.S. Department of Health and Human Services. *Reducing tobacco use: a report of the Surgeon General.* Atlanta, GA: Centers for Disease Control and Prevention; 2000.
2. U.S. Department of Health and Human Services. *Women and smoking: a report of the Surgeon General.* Rockville, MD: U.S. Department of Health and Human Services, Public Health Service, Office of the Surgeon General; 2001.
3. Thomson GW, Wilson N. Public attitudes about tobacco smoke in workplaces: the importance of workers' rights in survey questions [letter]. *Tobacco Control.* 2004;13(2):206–7.
4. Howard KA, Rogers T, Howard-Pitney B, Flora JA, Norman GJ, Ribisl KM. Opinion leaders' support for tobacco control policies and participation in tobacco control activities. *American Journal of Public Health.* 2000;90(8):1283–7.

Indicator 2.3.8

Level of Support for Adopting Tobacco-free Policies in Homes and Vehicles

Goal area 2	Eliminating nonsmokers' exposure to secondhand smoke
Outcome 3	Increased knowledge of, improved attitudes toward, and increased support for the creation and active enforcement of tobacco-free policies
What to measure	Proportion of adults who support tobacco-free policies that restrict the use of tobacco products in homes and vehicles
Why this indicator is useful	Tobacco-free policies in private homes and vehicles are voluntary. To increase the number of homes and vehicles with these policies, it is necessary to increase the number of adults who support such policies.
Example data source(s)	University of California at San Diego, California Tobacco Survey (CTS): Adult Attitudes and Practices, 1996 Information available at: • http://ssdc.ucsd.edu/tobacco • http://www.dhs.ca.gov/ps/cdic/ccb/TCS/html/Evaluation_Resources.htm
Population group(s)	Adults aged 18 years or older
Example survey question(s)	**From CTS** I am going to read you some reasons why people have smoke-free homes. For each, please indicate whether it is very important, somewhat important, or not important to you for your household. The reasons are: ☐ To protect a household member who is sensitive to smoke ☐ To protect family from harmful health effects of environmental tobacco smoke ☐ To discourage young people from starting to smoke ☐ To encourage smokers to quit ☐ To avoid unpleasant odor of smoking ☐ Because it annoys others
Comments	Evaluators may want to modify the example question to address tobacco-free policies inside vehicles. Evaluators may want to analyze the level of support for creating tobacco-free policies in homes and vehicles based on the smoking status of the respondent. The example question could be asked of young people.

Rating

Overall quality low ◄——► high	Resources needed	Strength of evaluation evidence	Utility	Face validity	Accepted practice
▬▬▬▬▬▬†	$$$	⊘	●	●	●

◄ ○ ◐ ● ● ► better

† Denotes low agreement among reviewers: that is, fewer than 75% of the valid ratings for this indicator were within one point of each other (see Appendix B for an explanation).
⊘ Denotes no data.

Indicator 2.3.9

Level of Support for Active Enforcement of Tobacco-free Public Policies

Goal area 2	Eliminating nonsmokers' exposure to secondhand smoke
Outcome 3	Increased knowledge of, improved attitudes toward, and increased support for the creation and active enforcement of tobacco-free policies
What to measure	Proportion of adults who support active enforcement of tobacco-free policies. An example of active enforcement is issuing citations for establishments found not to be in compliance with tobacco-free laws.
Why this indicator is useful	Tobacco-free laws have a limited effect if they are not actively enforced. Policies are more likely to be actively enforced when business owners, decision makers, and the general public support them.[1-4]
Example data source(s)	California Independent Evaluation: Adult Survey, 1997 Information available at: http://www.dhs.ca.gov/ps/cdic/ccb/TCS/html/Evaluation_Resources.htm
Population group(s)	Adults aged 18 years or older
Example survey question(s)	**From California Independent Evaluation** Smoking bans in restaurants, cafeterias, and indoor work places should be strictly enforced. Do you: ☐ Strongly agree ☐ Agree ☐ Disagree ☐ Strongly disagree
Comments	This example question could be asked of decision makers or opinion leaders. More information about how to collect data on this indicator is in reference 5 below.

Rating

Overall quality low ⬅➡ high	Resources needed	Strength of evaluation evidence	Utility	Face validity	Accepted practice
▬▬▬▬▬	$$$†	⊘	●	●	●

⬅ ○ ◐ ● ● ➡ better

† Denotes low agreement among reviewers: that is, fewer than 75% of the valid ratings for this indicator were within one point of each other (see Appendix B for an explanation).
⊘ Denotes no data.

References
1. Howard KA, Rogers T, Howard-Pitney B, Flora JA, Norman GJ, Ribisl KM. Opinion leaders' support for tobacco control policies and participation in tobacco control activities. *American Journal of Public Health.* 2000;90(8):1283–7.
2. U.S. Department of Health and Human Services. *Reducing tobacco use: a report of the Surgeon General.* Atlanta, GA: Centers for Disease Control and Prevention; 2000.
3. U.S. Department of Health and Human Services. *Women and smoking: a report of the Surgeon General.* Rockville, MD: U.S. Department of Health and Human Services, Public Health Service, Office of the Surgeon General; 2001.
4. Thomson GW, Wilson N. Public attitudes about tobacco smoke in workplaces: the importance of workers' rights in survey questions [letter]. *Tobacco Control.* 2004;13(2):206–7.
5. California Independent Evaluation, Opinion Leader Survey [online]. 1997. Available from: http://www.dhs.ca.gov/ps/cdic/ccb/TCS/html/Evaluation_Resources.htm#os. Accessed December 2004.

Indicator 2.3.10[NR]

Level of Support for Creating Tobacco-free Policies in Schools

Goal area 2	Eliminating nonsmokers' exposure to secondhand smoke
Outcome 3	Increased knowledge of, improved attitudes toward, and increased support for the creation and active enforcement of tobacco-free policies
What to measure	Proportion of adults who support creating tobacco-free policies in schools
Why this indicator is useful	Young people's attitudes concerning the acceptability of smoking in general, and smoking around nonsmokers in particular, are influenced by what they see their peers and educators doing at school. Strong anti-tobacco school policies require the support of parents, teachers, principals, policy makers, and the general public.[1] High levels of compliance with tobacco-free school policies reduce students' exposure to secondhand smoke and reinforce anti-tobacco social norms.[2]
Example data source(s)	Adult Tobacco Survey (ATS): CDC Recommended Questions: Supplemental Section F: Policy Issues, 2003 University of California at San Diego, California Tobacco Survey (CTS): Adult Attitudes and Practices Instrument, 1996 Information available at: http://ssdc.ucsd.edu/tobacco Behavioral Risk Factor Surveillance System (BRFSS): Tobacco Use Prevention Module, 2000
Population group(s)	Adults aged 18 years or older
Example survey question(s)	**From ATS** How strongly do you agree or disagree with the following statement: Tobacco use by adults should not be allowed on school grounds or at any school events. ☐ Strongly agree ☐ Agree ☐ Disagree ☐ Strongly disagree ☐ Don't know/Not sure ☐ Refused **From CTS** Do you think schools should prohibit students from wearing clothing or bringing gear with tobacco brand logos to school? ☐ Yes ☐ No **From BRFSS** Do you think that smoking should be allowed in all areas of schools, restaurants, day care, and indoor work areas, some areas, or not allowed at all? ☐ All areas ☐ Some areas ☐ Not allowed ☐ Refused to answer
Comments	The example questions could also be asked of decision makers. Evaluators may want to analyze the level of support for creating tobacco-free policies in schools based on the smoking status of the respondent. This indicator was not rated by the panel of experts, and therefore no rating information is provided. See Appendix B for an explanation.

Rating	Overall quality low ←——→ high	Resources needed	Strength of evaluation evidence	Utility	Face validity	Accepted practice
	▬▬▬	⊘	⊘	⊘	⊘	⊘
				←○◔●●→ better		

⊘ Denotes no data.

NR Denotes an indicator that is not rated (see Appendix B for an explanation).

References
1. Task Force on Community Preventive Services Meeting, February 25, 2004. Meeting minutes available at: http://www.thecommunityguide.org.
2. Gilpin EA, White MM, White VM, Distefan JM, Trinidad DR, Lee L, Major J, Kealey S, Pierce JP. *Tobacco control successes in California: a focus on young people, results from the California Tobacco Surveys 1990–2002*. La Jolla, CA: University of California, San Diego; 2003. pp. 348–9. Available from: http://repositories.cdlib.org/tc/surveys/CTC1990–2002/. Accessed December 2004.

Outcome 4

Creation of Tobacco-free Policies

Creating tobacco-free policies in workplaces, other public places, and homes and vehicles not only protects nonsmokers from involuntary exposure to the toxins in tobacco smoke, but also may have the added benefit of reducing tobacco consumption by smokers and increasing the number of smokers who quit.[1-3] Smoking bans and restrictions are effective in reducing secondhand smoke exposure.[1,2]

Smoking bans may be implemented by governments (through legislation or regulation), oversight groups (e.g., the Joint Commission on Accreditation of Healthcare Organizations), individual employers or businesses, or private citizens (e.g., smoking bans in homes and vehicles). By approaching these groups or individuals and encouraging them to develop their own tobacco-free policies, tobacco control programs can protect the public from secondhand smoke. Where state law preempts stronger local laws, tobacco control programs retain the option of mobilizing the private sector to introduce voluntary smoking bans in workplaces and public places. In considering which channel to pursue, programs should take into account (1) the legal authority vested in various entities (e.g., counties, cities, local boards of health), (2) the level of support among relevant decision makers and their constituents, and (3) the feasibility of persuading these entities to implement tobacco-free policies. It is also worth remembering that despite the recent passage of a number of comprehensive state clean-indoor-air laws, comprehensive and strong laws can also be enacted at the local level, where such laws are easier to adopt and enforce.[4]

Experience shows that the education that occurs when a community debates whether it wants a local tobacco-free law—a debate that typically generates extensive media coverage—can greatly facilitate enforcement of the law, sometimes making it largely self-enforcing. Continued education of business proprietors, employers, and the public during the implementation process is also important in this regard. Preemptive laws prevent communities from engaging in the process of public education, mobilization, and debate that occurs when a local ordinance is under consideration, a process that can increase awareness and change social norms.[5] Such laws also pose a barrier to local enforcement because communities and local enforcement agencies may be less likely to enforce state laws that they were not directly involved in adopting than to enforce local ordinances.[5]

Regardless of which route is used to implement them, smoking bans are effective, cost-effective, feasible, and broadly supported by the public.[1,2,6] The dangers of secondhand smoke are well researched and well known, and the growth and spread of this knowledge has been accompanied by a radical reduction in the level of acceptability of smoking in public places and workplaces.[7,8]

Listed below are the indicators associated with this outcome:

- **2.4.1** Proportion of jurisdictions with public policies for tobacco-free workplaces and other indoor and outdoor public places
- **2.4.2** Proportion of workplaces with voluntary tobacco-free policies
- **2.4.3** Proportion of the population that works in environments with tobacco-free policies
- **2.4.4** Proportion of the population reporting voluntary tobacco-free home or vehicle policies
- **2.4.5** Proportion of schools or school districts reporting the implementation of 100% tobacco-free school policies
- **2.4.6** Changes in state tobacco control laws that preempt stronger local tobacco control laws

References

1. Task Force on Community Preventive Services. The guide to community preventive services: tobacco use prevention and control. *American Journal of Preventive Medicine.* 2001;20(Suppl 2):1–88.

2. U.S. Department of Health and Human Services. *Reducing tobacco use: a report of the Surgeon General.* Atlanta, GA: Centers for Disease Control and Prevention; 2000.

3. National Cancer Institute. Smoking and Tobacco Control Monograph No. 12. *Population-based smoking cessation: proceedings of a conference on What Works to Influence Cessation in the General Population.* Bethesda, MD: National Cancer Institute; 2000. NIH Publication No. 00-4892.

4. National Cancer Institute. Smoking and Tobacco Control Monograph No. 11. *State and local legislative action to reduce tobacco use.* Bethesda, MD: National Cancer Institute; 2000. NIH Publication No. 00-4804.

5. Centers for Disease Control and Prevention. Preemptive state tobacco-control laws—United States, 1982–1998. *Morbidity and Mortality Weekly Report.* 1999;47 (51 & 52):1112–4.

6. Gilpin EA, Lee L, and Pierce JP. Changes in population attitudes about where smoking should not be allowed: California versus the rest of the USA. *Tobacco Control.* 2004:13(1):38–44.

7. Brownson RC, Eriksen MP, Davis RM, Warner KE. Environmental tobacco smoke: health effects and policies to reduce exposure. *Annual Review of Public Health.* 1997;18:163–85.

8. Brownson RC, Hopkins DP, Wakefield MA. Effects of smoking restrictions in the workplace. *Annual Review of Public Health.* 2002;23:333–48.

For Further Reading

Gilpin EA, Pierce JP. The California Tobacco Control Program and potential harm reduction through reduced cigarette consumption in continuing smokers. *Nicotine and Tobacco Research.* 2002;4(Suppl 2):S157–66.

Hyland A, Cummings KM, Wilson MP. Compliance with the New York City Smoke-Free Air Act. *Journal of Public Health Management and Practice.* 1999;5(1):43–52.

Lakind J, Graves C, Ginevan M. Exposure to environmental tobacco smoke in the workplace and the impact of away-from-work exposure. *Risk Analysis.* 1999;19(3):349–58.

Moskowitz JM, Lin Z, Hudes ES. The impact of California's smoking ordinances on worksite smoking policy and exposure to environmental tobacco smoke. *American Journal of Health Promotion.* 1999;13(5):278–81, iii.

National Cancer Institute. Smoking and Tobacco Control Monograph No. 12. *Population-based smoking cessation: proceedings of a conference on What Works to Influence Cessation in the General Population.* Bethesda, MD: National Cancer Institute; 2000. NIH Publication No. 00-4892.

National Cancer Institute. Smoking and Tobacco Control Monograph No. 11. *State and local legislative action to reduce tobacco use.* Bethesda, MD: National Cancer Institute; 2000. NIH Publication No. 00-4804.

Rigotti NA, Stoto MA, Schelling TC. Do businesses comply with a no-smoking law? Assessing the self-enforcement approach. *Preventive Medicine.* 1994;23(2):223–9.

Sorensen G, Glasgow RE, Corbett K, Topor M. Compliance with worksite nonsmoking policies: baseline results from the COMMIT study of worksites. *American Journal of Health Promotion.* 1992;7(2):103–9.

Outcome 4

Creation of Tobacco-free Policies

Indicator Rating
← ○ ◐ ● ● → better

Number	Indicator	Overall quality (low → high)	Resources needed	Strength of evaluation evidence	Utility	Face validity	Accepted practice
2.4.1	Proportion of jurisdictions with public policies for tobacco-free workplaces and other indoor and outdoor public places	▬▬▬▬	$$$	◐	●	●	●
2.4.2	Proportion of workplaces with voluntary tobacco-free policies	▬▬▬▬	$$	●	◐	◐	●
2.4.3	Proportion of the population that works in environments with tobacco-free policies	▬▬▬▬	$$†	●	●	●	●
2.4.4	Proportion of the population reporting voluntary tobacco-free home or vehicle policies	▬▬▬▬	$$†	◐	●	◐	●
2.4.5	Proportion of schools or school districts reporting the implementation of 100% tobacco-free school policies	▬▬▬▬	$$	◐	●	◐	●
2.4.6	Changes in state tobacco control laws that preempt stronger local tobacco control laws	▬▬▬▬	$	⊘	●	◐	●

† Denotes low agreement among reviewers: that is, fewer than 75% of the valid ratings for this indicator were within one point of each other (see Appendix B for an explanation).
⊘ Denotes no data.

GOAL AREA 2
Outcome 4

Indicator 2.4.1

Proportion of Jurisdictions with Public Policies for Tobacco-free Workplaces and Other Indoor and Outdoor Public Places

Goal area 2	Eliminating nonsmokers' exposure to secondhand smoke
Outcome 4	Creation of tobacco-free policies
What to measure	Proportion of local jurisdictions that have public policies requiring tobacco-free workplaces, including restaurants, bars, and other indoor and outdoor public places
Why this indicator is useful	Evidence shows that workplace smoking restrictions reduce nonsmokers' exposure to secondhand smoke.[1,2] Policies that restrict smoking in workplaces are also linked to reduced tobacco use by smokers and possibly lower smoking prevalence.[2,3]
Example data source(s)	Policy tracking system Americans for Nonsmokers' Rights (ANR) Information available at: http://www.no-smoke.org
Population group(s)	Not applicable. This indicator is best measured by tracking and monitoring pertinent local tobacco laws, ordinances, and regulations.
Example survey question(s)	Not applicable
Comments	Evaluators may also choose to gather data on the size and demographics of the population affected by the relevant laws or ordinances.

Rating	Overall quality low ⬌ high	Resources needed	Strength of evaluation evidence	Utility	Face validity	Accepted practice
	▬▬▬▬▬▬	$$$	◑	●	●	●

← ○ ◐ ◑ ● → better

References
1. Task Force on Community Preventive Services. The guide to community preventive services: tobacco use prevention and control. *American Journal of Preventive Medicine.* 2001;20(Suppl 2):1–88.
2. U.S. Department of Health and Human Services. *Reducing tobacco use: a report of the Surgeon General.* Atlanta, GA: Centers for Disease Control and Prevention; 2000.
3. National Cancer Institute. Smoking and Tobacco Control Monograph No. 12. *Population-based smoking cessation: proceedings of a conference on What Works to Influence Cessation in the General Population.* Bethesda, MD: National Cancer Institute; 2000. NIH Publication No. 00-4892.

Indicator 2.4.2

Proportion of Workplaces with Voluntary Tobacco-free Policies

Goal area 2	Eliminating nonsmokers' exposure to secondhand smoke
Outcome 4	Creation of tobacco-free policies
What to measure	Proportion of workplaces (including restaurants and bars) with voluntary tobacco-free policies
Why this indicator is useful	Individual employers may opt to institute tobacco-free policies on their premises. These policies reduce nonsmokers' exposure to secondhand smoke.[1,2]
Example data source(s)	▸ Worksite Survey ▸ Adult Tobacco Survey (ATS): CDC Recommended Questions: Core, 2003 ▸ Current Population Survey: Tobacco Use Supplement (CPS TUS), 2003 ▸ Arizona Workplace Survey Information available at: http://www.tepp.org/evaluation
Population group(s)	Employers
Example survey question(s)	**From ATS** Which of the following best describes your place of work's official smoking policy for work areas? ☐ Not allowed in any work areas ☐ Allowed in some work areas ☐ Allowed in all work areas ☐ No official policy ☐ Don't know/Not sure ☐ Refused Which of these best describes your place of work's smoking policy for indoor public or common areas such as lobbies, restrooms, and lunch rooms? ☐ Not allowed in any public areas ☐ Allowed in some public areas ☐ Allowed in all public areas ☐ No official policy ☐ Don't know/Not sure ☐ Refused **From CPS TUS** Does your place of work have an official policy that restricts smoking in any way? ☐ Yes ☐ No **From Arizona Workplace Survey** According to the policy, are employees allowed to smoke in the following areas? ☐ Private offices ☐ Open work and production areas ☐ Reception areas ☐ Break areas and lounges ☐ Cafeterias ☐ Hallways and stairwells ☐ Restrooms ☐ Other areas inside the building ☐ Company vehicles ☐ Immediately outside entrances ☐ The rest of the grounds outside

GOAL AREA 2
Outcome 4

Comments	Few surveys have been conducted to assess the percentage of workplaces with tobacco-free policies.
	More information about how to collect data on this indicator is in reference 3 below.

Rating

Overall quality low ⟷ high	Resources needed	Strength of evaluation evidence	Utility	Face validity	Accepted practice
▬▬▬	$$	●	◐	◐	●

←○◔●●→ better

References
1. Task Force on Community Preventive Services. The guide to community preventive services: tobacco use prevention and control. *American Journal of Preventive Medicine.* 2001;20(Suppl 2):1–88.
2. U.S. Department of Health and Human Services. *Reducing tobacco use: a report of the Surgeon General.* Atlanta, GA: Centers for Disease Control and Prevention; 2000.
3. Eisenberg M, Ranger-Moore J, Taylor KA, Hall RA, Brown J, Lee H. Workplace tobacco policy: progress on a winding road. *Journal of Community Health.* 2001;26(1):23–37.

Indicator 2.4.3

Proportion of the Population That Works in Environments with Tobacco-free Policies

Goal area 2	Eliminating nonsmokers' exposure to secondhand smoke
Outcome 4	Creation of tobacco-free policies
What to measure	Proportion of adults employed outside the home whose place of work has a tobacco-free policy
Why this indicator is useful	Measuring this indicator shows the degree of protection provided to nonsmoking workers by policies that restrict smoking in the workplace.[1-4] Examples of such polices include a ban on using tobacco on the grounds, a ban on smoking indoors, or permitting smoking only in designated areas.
Example data source(s)	▸ Adult Tobacco Survey (ATS): CDC Recommended Questions: Core, 2003 ▸ Current Population Survey: Tobacco Use Supplement (CPS TUS), 2003
Population group(s)	Adults aged 18 years or older

Example survey question(s)

From ATS

Which of the following best describes your place of work's official smoking policy for work areas?
- ☐ Not allowed in any work areas   ☐ Allowed in some work areas
- ☐ Allowed in all work areas   ☐ No official policy
- ☐ Don't know/Not sure   ☐ Refused

Which of these best describes your place of work's smoking policy for indoor public or common areas such as lobbies, restrooms, and lunch rooms?
- ☐ Not allowed in any public areas   ☐ Allowed in some public areas
- ☐ Allowed in all public areas   ☐ No official policy
- ☐ Don't know/Not sure   ☐ Refused

From CPS TUS

Does your place of work have an official policy that restricts smoking in any way?
☐ Yes ☐ No

Comments	Evaluators may also want to categorize the data collected by occupation of the respondents.

Rating

Overall quality low ◀——▶ high	Resources needed	Strength of evaluation evidence	Utility	Face validity	Accepted practice
▰▰▰▰▱	$$[†]	◐	●	●	●

◀ ○ ◔ ◐ ● ▶ better

[†] Denotes low agreement among reviewers: that is, fewer than 75% of the valid ratings for this indicator were within one point of each other (see Appendix B for an explanation).

References

1. Shopland DR, Gerlach KK, Burns DM, Hartman AM, Gibson JT. State-specific trends in smoke-free workplace policy coverage: the current population survey tobacco use supplement, 1993 to 1999. *Journal of Occupational and Environmental Medicine.* 2001;43(8):680–6.
2. Gerlach KK, Shopland DR, Hartman AM, Gibson JT, Pechacek TF. Workplace smoking policies in the United States: results from a national survey of more than 100,000 workers. *Tobacco Control.* 1997;6(3):199–206.
3. Wortley PM, Caraballo RS, Pederson LL, Pechacek T. Exposure to secondhand smoke in the workplace: serum cotinine by occupation. *Journal of Occupational and Environmental Medicine.* 2002;44(6):503–9.
4. Shopland DR, Anderson CM, Burns DM, Gerlach KK. Disparities in smoke-free workplace policies among food service workers. *Journal of Occupational and Environmental Medicine.* 2004;46(4):347–56.

Indicator 2.4.4

Proportion of the Population Reporting Voluntary Tobacco-free Home or Vehicle Policies

Goal area 2	Eliminating nonsmokers' exposure to secondhand smoke
Outcome 4	Creation of tobacco-free policies
What to measure	Proportion of adults who report some form of voluntary tobacco-free policy in their homes or vehicles
Why this indicator is useful	Evidence shows that children living in households with smoking bans are exposed to substantially less secondhand smoke than children not protected by such policies.[1,2] This is especially true in households with at least one smoker.[1,2] Examples of such policies are (1) smoking not allowed anywhere in the home, (2) smoking restricted to some places in the home, or (3) smoking restricted to certain times in the home or vehicle.
Example data source(s)	Adult Tobacco Survey (ATS): CDC Recommended Questions: Core, 2003
Population group(s)	Adults aged 18 years or older
Example survey question(s)	**From ATS** Which statement best describes the rules about smoking inside your home? Do not include decks, garages, or porches. ☐ Smoking is not allowed anywhere inside the home ☐ Smoking is allowed in some places or at some times ☐ Smoking is allowed anywhere inside the home ☐ Don't know/Not sure ☐ Refused
Comments	Evaluators could modify the example question to address tobacco-free policies inside vehicles. The example question could be asked of young people.
Rating	Overall quality: low ⟵⟶ high (mid-range) Resources needed: $$[†] Strength of evaluation evidence: ◓ Utility: ● Face validity: ◓ Accepted practice: ● ⟵ ○ ◔ ◑ ● ⟶ better

[†] Denotes low agreement among reviewers: that is, fewer than 75% of the valid ratings for this indicator were within one point of each other (see Appendix B for an explanation).

References
1. Biener L, Cullen D, Di ZX, Hammond SK. Household smoking restrictions and adolescents' exposure to environmental tobacco smoke. *Preventive Medicine*. 1997;26(3):358–63.
2. Wakefield M, Banham D, Martin J, Ruffin R, McCaul K, Badcock N. Restrictions on smoking at home and urinary cotinine levels among children with asthma. *American Journal of Preventive Medicine*. 2000;19(3):188–92.

Indicator 2.4.5

Proportion of Schools or School Districts Reporting the Implementation of 100% Tobacco-free School Policies

Goal area 2	Eliminating nonsmokers' exposure to secondhand smoke
Outcome 4	Creation of tobacco-free policies
What to measure	Proportion of schools or school districts that report having a policy that prohibits anyone from using tobacco at all times on school grounds, at all school-sponsored functions, and in school vehicles
Why this indicator is useful	Young people spend much of their time in school. Their attitudes about the acceptability of smoking in general and smoking around nonsmokers in particular are influenced by the actions of their peers and educators at school.[1,2]
Example data source(s)	CDC School Health Profiles: School Principal Questionnaire (Profiles), 2002
Population group(s)	School principals
Example survey question(s)	**From Profiles** Has this school adopted a policy prohibiting tobacco use? ☐ Yes ☐ No Does the tobacco-free policy specifically prohibit use of each of these types of tobacco products for each for the following groups? Type of tobacco product — Students (Yes/No), Faculty/Staff (Yes/No), Visitors (Yes/No) • Cigarettes • Smokeless tobacco • Cigars • Pipes Does the school's tobacco-free policy specifically prohibit tobacco use during each of the following times for each for the following groups? Time — Students (Yes/No), Faculty/Staff (Yes/No), Visitors (Yes/No) • During school hours • During non-school hours Does the school's tobacco prevention policy specifically prohibit tobacco use in each of the following locations for each of the following groups? Location — Students (Yes/No), Faculty/Staff (Yes/No), Visitors (Yes/No) • In school buildings • On school grounds • In school buses or other vehicles used to transport students • At off-campus, school-sponsored events

GOAL AREA 2
Outcome 4

Comments	To measure this indicator fully, evaluators should use all four example questions, not just one or two.
	Evaluators may also want to collect information on school districts in order to measure the proportion of students in the district who are covered by anti-tobacco policies.
	This indicator can be used to measure progress toward achieving Recommendation 1 of CDC's "Guidelines for School Health Programs to Prevent Tobacco Use and Addiction."[1]

Rating	Overall quality low ⟵⟶ high	Resources needed	Strength of evaluation evidence	Utility	Face validity	Accepted practice
	▬▬▬▬	$$	◖	●	◖	●

⟵ ○ ◐ ◖ ● ⟶ better

References
1. Centers for Disease Control and Prevention. Guidelines for school health programs to prevent tobacco use and addiction. *Morbidity and Mortality Weekly Report Recommendations and Reports.* 1994;43(RR-2):1–18.
2. U.S. Department of Health and Human Services. *Preventing tobacco use among young people: a report of the Surgeon General.* Atlanta, GA: Centers for Disease Control and Prevention; 1994.

Indicator 2.4.6

Changes in State Tobacco Control Laws That Preempt Stronger Local Tobacco Control Laws

Goal area 2	Eliminating nonsmokers' exposure to secondhand smoke
Outcome 4	Creation of tobacco-free policies
What to measure	Any change in legislation that prevents local jurisdictions from enacting restrictions that are more stringent than the state's restrictions on smoke-free indoor air laws
Why this indicator is useful	Preemptive legislation is the tobacco industry's chief strategy for eradicating local tobacco control ordinances.[1] Because of the striking increase in the number of local tobacco control ordinances from the mid-1980s to the mid-1990s, the tobacco industry aggressively pushed for states to pass legislation that preempted local regulation of tobacco in various areas, including smoke-free indoor air, minors' access, and marketing.[2] As of December 31, 2004, a total of 19 states had at least one type of preemptive provision for smoke-free indoor air legislation.[2] As of December 31, 2004, only two states, Maine and Delaware, had successfully repealed preemption laws in their entirety in any area of tobacco control policy. Preemptive laws prevent communities from engaging in the process of public education, mobilization, and debate that occurs when a local ordinance is under consideration, a process that can increase awareness and change social norms. These laws also pose a barrier to local enforcement because communities may be less likely to enforce state laws that they were not directly involved in adopting.[2]
Example data source(s)	CDC State Tobacco Activities Tracking and Evaluation (STATE) system Data available at: http://www.cdc.gov/tobacco/STATEsystem
Population group(s)	Not applicable. This indicator is best measured by tracking and monitoring state tobacco control laws.
Example survey question(s)	Not applicable
Comments	None

Rating	Overall quality low ←→ high	Resources needed	Strength of evaluation evidence	Utility	Face validity	Accepted practice
	▨	$	⊘	●	●	●

←○◔●●→ better

⊘ Denotes no data.

References
1. National Cancer Institute. Smoking and Tobacco Control Monograph No. 11. *State and local legislative action to reduce tobacco use.* Bethesda, MD: National Cancer Institute; 2000. NIH Publication No. 00-4804.
2. Centers for Disease Control and Prevention. Preemptive state smoke-free indoor air laws—United States, 1999–2004. *Morbidity and Mortality Weekly Report.* 2005;54(10):250–3.

Outcome 5

Enforcement of Tobacco-free Public Policies

Experience shows that tobacco-free policies make a difference only when voluntary compliance is adequate or the policies are actively enforced. If the entities that are regulated (e.g., businesses, public agencies) do not experience any pressure to follow newly legislated policies, the policies will contribute little to reducing exposure to secondhand smoke. Although little research has been done on the effects of enforcing tobacco-free policies, research concerning other policies shows that policy enforcement is effective in improving compliance.[1] With the recent trend toward passing comprehensive smoke-free laws that cover bars, the need for active enforcement of those laws is likely to become greater.[2]

Listed below are the indicators associated with this outcome:

- **2.5.1** Number of compliance checks conducted by enforcement agencies
- **2.5.2** Number of enforcement agency responses to complaints regarding noncompliance with tobacco-free public policies
- **2.5.3** Number of warnings, citations, and fines issued for infractions of tobacco-free public policies

References

1. U.S. Department of Health and Human Services. *Preventing tobacco use among young people: a report of the Surgeon General.* Atlanta, GA: Centers for Disease Control and Prevention; 1994.

2. Weber MD, Bagwell DA, Fielding JE, Glantz SA. Long-term compliance with California's Smoke-Free Workplace Law among bars and restaurants in Los Angeles County. *Tobacco Control.* 2003;12(3):269–73.

For Further Reading

Biener L, Cullen D, Di ZX, Hammond SK. Household smoking restrictions and adolescents' exposure to environmental tobacco smoke. *Preventive Medicine.* 1997;26(3):358–63.

Farkas A, Gilpin EA, Distefan JM, Pierce JP. The effects of household and workplace smoking restrictions on quitting behaviours. *Tobacco Control.* 1999;8(3):261–5.

Farkas AJ, Gilpin EA, White MM, Pierce JP. Association between household and workplace smoking restrictions and adolescent smoking. *Journal of the American Medical Association.* 2000;284(6):717–22.

Gilpin EA, Pierce JP. The California Tobacco Control Program and potential harm reduction through reduced cigarette consumption in continuing smokers. *Nicotine and Tobacco Research.* 2002;4(Suppl 2):S157–66.

Gilpin EA, White MM, Farkas AJ, Pierce JP. Home smoking restrictions: which smokers have them and how they are associated with smoking behavior. *Nicotine and Tobacco Research.* 1999;1(2):153–62.

Hopper JA, Craig KA. Environmental tobacco smoke exposure among urban children. *Pediatrics.* 2000;106(4):E47.

Hyland A, Cummings KM, Wilson MP. Compliance with the New York City Smoke-Free Air Act. *Journal of Public Health Management and Practice.* 1999;5(1):43–52.

Jacobson PD, Wasserman J. The implementation and enforcement of tobacco control laws: policy implications for activists and the industry. *Journal of Health Politics, Policy and Law.* 1999;24(3):567–98.

Kegler M, Malcoe LH. Smoking restrictions in the home and car among rural Native American and white families with young children. *Preventive Medicine.* 2002;35(4):334–42.

Lynch BS, Bonnie RJ. *Growing up tobacco free: preventing nicotine addiction in children and youths.* Washington, DC: National Academy Press; 1994.

Pentz MA, Brannon BR, Charlin VL, Barrett EJ, MacKinnon DP, Flay BR. The power of policy: the relationship of smoking policy to adolescent smoking. *American Journal of Public Health.* 1989;79:857–62.

Task Force on Community Preventive Services. The guide to community preventive services: tobacco use prevention and control. *American Journal of Preventive Medicine.* 2001;20(Suppl 2):1–88.

Wakefield M, Banham D, Martin J, Ruffin R, McCaul K, Badcock N. Restrictions of smoking at home and urinary cotinine levels among children with asthma. *American Journal of Preventive Medicine.* 2000;19(3):188–92.

Outcome 5

Enforcement of Tobacco-free Public Policies

Indicator Rating

← ○ ◐ ● ● → better

Number	Indicator	Overall quality low ←→ high	Resources needed	Strength of evaluation evidence	Utility	Face validity	Accepted practice
2.5.1	Number of compliance checks conducted by enforcement agencies	▬▬▬▬	$$$	⊘	●	●	●
2.5.2	Number of enforcement agency responses to complaints regarding noncompliance with tobacco-free public policies	▬▬▬▬ †	$$$	⊘	●	●	●
2.5.3	Number of warnings, citations, and fines issued for infractions of tobacco-free public policies	▬▬▬▬	$$$	⊘	●	●	●

† Denotes low agreement among reviewers: that is, fewer than 75% of the valid ratings for this indicator were within one point of each other (see Appendix B for an explanation).
⊘ Denotes no data.

Indicator 2.5.1

Number of Compliance Checks Conducted by Enforcement Agencies

Goal area 2	Eliminating nonsmokers' exposure to secondhand smoke
Outcome 5	Enforcement of tobacco-free public policies
What to measure	The number of checks conducted by enforcement agencies (e.g., police, health department inspectors, and building inspectors) to assess the level of compliance with laws, regulations, and ordinances related to tobacco-free policies
Why this indicator is useful	An effective means of enforcing tobacco-free public policies is to conduct regular compliance checks. Such checks convey the message that policy makers and the public care about tobacco-free policies and are serious about enforcing them.[1,2]
Example data source(s)	▸ Enforcement Agency Survey ▸ California Independent Evaluation: Policy Enforcement Survey: Exposure to Environmental Tobacco Smoke, 2000 Information available at: http://www.dhs.ca.gov/ps/cdic/ccb/TCS/html/Evaluation_Resources.htm
Population group(s)	Agency representatives responsible for enforcement
Example survey question(s)	**From California Independent Evaluation** In the last year, how often has your agency conducted any of the following types of enforcement activities related to clean indoor air laws? 1–7, where 1 = never and 7 = very often; Don't know / Not applicable • Responded to inquiries 1 2 3 4 5 6 7 ☐ • Responded to complaints 1 2 3 4 5 6 7 ☐ • Issued warnings 1 2 3 4 5 6 7 ☐ • Issued citations 1 2 3 4 5 6 7 ☐ • Issued fines 1 2 3 4 5 6 7 ☐ • Conducted compliance checks 1 2 3 4 5 6 7 ☐ • Educated business owners about the law 1 2 3 4 5 6 7 ☐ • Educated others about the law 1 2 3 4 5 6 7 ☐
Comments	Survey respondents may not have access to all requested information.

Rating

Overall quality low ⟷ high	Resources needed	Strength of evaluation evidence	Utility	Face validity	Accepted practice
■■■■■	$$$	⊘	●	●	●

⬅ ○ ◐ ● ● ➡ better

⊘ Denotes no data.

References
1. Kiser D, Boschert T. Eliminating smoking in bars, restaurants, and gaming clubs in California: BREATH, the California Smoke-Free Bar Program. *Journal of Public Health Policy.* 2001;22(1):81–7.
2. Weber MD, Bagwell DA, Fielding JE, Glantz SA. Long-term compliance with California's Smoke-Free Workplace Law among bars and restaurants in Los Angeles County. *Tobacco Control.* 2003;12(3):269–73.

GOAL AREA 2
Outcome 5

Indicator 2.5.2

Number of Enforcement Agency Responses to Complaints Regarding Noncompliance with Tobacco-free Public Policies

Goal area 2	Eliminating nonsmokers' exposure to secondhand smoke
Outcome 5	Enforcement of tobacco-free public policies
What to measure	The number of checks (prompted by outside complaints) by enforcement agencies (e.g., police, health department inspectors, and building inspectors) to assess the level of compliance with tobacco-free public policies
Why this indicator is useful	Recording complaints of noncompliance with tobacco-free public policies is one way of identifying noncompliance with such policies. Such checks convey the message that policy makers and the public care about tobacco-free policies and are serious about enforcing them.[1,2] Following up on these complaints is an easy way of targeting noncompliance. The number of complaints received by enforcement agencies also provides a sense of the public's attitude toward tobacco-free policies.
Example data source(s)	Enforcement Agency Survey California Independent Evaluation: Policy Enforcement Survey: Exposure to Environmental Tobacco Smoke, 2000 Information available at: http://www.dhs.ca.gov/ps/cdic/ccb/TCS/html/Evaluation_Resources.htm
Population group(s)	Agency representatives responsible for enforcement
Example survey question(s)	**From California Independent Evaluation** In the last year, how often has your agency conducted any of the following types of enforcement activities related to clean indoor air laws? 1–7, where 1 = never and 7 = very often; Don't know / Not applicable • Responded to inquiries 1 2 3 4 5 6 7 ☐ • Responded to complaints 1 2 3 4 5 6 7 ☐ • Issued warnings 1 2 3 4 5 6 7 ☐ • Issued citations 1 2 3 4 5 6 7 ☐ • Issued fines 1 2 3 4 5 6 7 ☐ • Conducted compliance checks 1 2 3 4 5 6 7 ☐ • Educated business owners about the law 1 2 3 4 5 6 7 ☐ • Educated others about the law 1 2 3 4 5 6 7 ☐
Comments	Survey respondents may not have access to all the requested information.
Rating	Overall quality: low ←→ high † Resources needed: $$$ Strength of evaluation evidence: no data Utility: ● Face validity: ● Accepted practice: ● ← ○ ◐ ● ● → better † Denotes low agreement among reviewers: that is, fewer than 75% of the valid ratings for this indicator were within one point of each other (see Appendix B for an explanation). ⊘ Denotes no data.

References
1. Kiser D, Boschert T. Eliminating smoking in bars, restaurants, and gaming clubs in California: BREATH, the California Smoke-Free Bar Program. *Journal of Public Health Policy*. 2001;22(1):81–7.
2. Weber MD, Bagwell DA, Fielding JE, Glantz SA. Long-term compliance with California's Smoke-Free Workplace Law among bars and restaurants in Los Angeles County. *Tobacco Control*. 2003;12(3):269–73.

Indicator 2.5.3

Number of Warnings, Citations, and Fines Issued for Infractions of Tobacco-free Public Policies

Goal area 2	Eliminating nonsmokers' exposure to secondhand smoke
Outcome 5	Enforcement of tobacco-free public policies
What to measure	The number of the warnings, citations, and fines issued to retailers for infractions of tobacco-free public policies
Why this indicator is useful	Compliance with tobacco-free public policies improves when noncompliance has repercussions.[1,2] Issuing warnings or citations sets an example and shows that noncompliance with tobacco-free policies has adverse consequences.
Example data source(s)	▹ Enforcement Agency Survey ▹ California Independent Evaluation: Policy Enforcement Survey: Exposure to Environmental Tobacco Smoke, 2000 Information available at: http://www.dhs.ca.gov/ps/cdic/ccb/TCS/html/Evaluation_Resources.htm
Population group(s)	Agency representatives responsible for enforcement
Example survey question(s)	**From California Independent Evaluation** In the last six months, please estimate how many citations for violation of clean indoor air laws were • Issued in your jurisdiction? ____(# of citations issued) • Prosecuted in your jurisdiction? ____(# of citations prosecuted)
Comments	The example survey question does not measure warnings given for noncompliance. Evaluators may also want to assess the effects that different penalties (e.g., graduated fines) have on compliance with tobacco-free public policies. Data must be interpreted in context. For example, a low number of citations may indicate either high compliance or low enforcement.

Rating

Overall quality low ⟵⟶ high	Resources needed	Strength of evaluation evidence	Utility	Face validity	Accepted practice
▬▬▬▬▬	$$$	⊘	●	◐	●

⟵ ○ ◐ ● ● ⟶ better

⊘ Denotes no data.

References
1. Centers for Disease Control and Prevention. *Best practices for comprehensive tobacco control programs*. Atlanta, GA: Centers for Disease Control and Prevention; 1999.
2. Task Force on Community Preventive Services. The guide to community preventive services: tobacco use prevention and control. *American Journal of Preventive Medicine*. 2001;20(Suppl 2):1–88.

Outcome 6

Compliance with Tobacco-free Policies

The evidence is clear that exposure to secondhand smoke is harmful and that increasing the number of tobacco-free environments can save lives.[1] Compliance with voluntary tobacco-free policies in homes and vehicles is an important marker of social normative changes that have an effect on the health of children and on tobacco use among young people.[2] Although the need for compliance with tobacco-free policies is apparent, little research has been done specifically on whether increased compliance leads to decreased exposure to secondhand smoke (perhaps because the connection has face validity). Perceived compliance can be measured as that reported by members of a community responding to questionnaires and interviews. Actual compliance can be measured by observation. Observational measures capture a point in time, while population-based surveys capture the perceptions of individuals regarding compliance over a prior period.

Listed below are the indicators associated with this outcome:

- 2.6.1 Perceived compliance with tobacco-free policies in workplaces
- 2.6.2 Perceived compliance with tobacco-free policies in indoor and outdoor public places
- 2.6.3 Proportion of public places observed to be in compliance with tobacco-free policies
- 2.6.4 Perceived compliance with voluntary tobacco-free home or vehicle policies
- 2.6.5 Perceived compliance with tobacco-free policies in schools

References

1. U.S. Department of Health and Human Services. *The health consequences of smoking: a report of the Surgeon General.* Atlanta, GA: Centers for Disease Control and Prevention; 2004.
2. Wakefield M, Chaloupka F, Kaufman N, Orleans C, Barker D, Ruel E. Effect of restrictions at home, at school, and in public places on teenage smoking: cross sectional study. *British Medical Journal.* 2000;321(7257):333–7. Erratum in: *British Medical Journal.* 2000;321(7261):623.

For Further Reading

Lynch BS, Bonnie RJ. *Growing up tobacco free: preventing nicotine addiction in children and youths.* Washington, DC: National Academy Press; 1994.

Pentz MA, Brannon BR, Charlin VL, Barrett EJ, MacKinnon DP, Flay BR. The power of policy: the relationship of smoking policy to adolescent smoking. *American Journal of Public Health.* 1989;79(7):857–862.

U.S. Department of Health and Human Services. *Preventing tobacco use among young people: a report of the Surgeon General.* Atlanta, GA: Centers for Disease Control and Prevention; 1994.

Outcome 6

Compliance with Tobacco-free Policies

Indicator Rating

← ○ ◔ ◐ ● → better

Number	Indicator	Overall quality low ←→ high	Resources needed	Strength of evaluation evidence	Utility	Face validity	Accepted practice
2.6.1	Perceived compliance with tobacco-free policies in workplaces	├─┼─┼─┤ │	$$†	⊘	◐	◐	●
2.6.2	Perceived compliance with tobacco-free policies in indoor and outdoor public places	▬▬▬▬	$$$†	⊘	◐	◐	●
2.6.3	Proportion of public places observed to be in compliance with tobacco-free policies	▬▬▬▬	$$$$†	⊘	◐	◐	●
2.6.4	Perceived compliance with voluntary tobacco-free home or vehicle policies	▬▬▬▬	$$†	◐	◐	◐	●
2.6.5	Perceived compliance with tobacco-free policies in schools	▬▬▬▬	$$	◔	◐	◐	●

† Denotes low agreement among reviewers: that is, fewer than 75% of the valid ratings for this indicator were within one point of each other (see Appendix B for an explanation).
⊘ Denotes no data.

Indicator 2.6.1

Perceived Compliance with Tobacco-free Policies in Workplaces

Goal area 2	Eliminating nonsmokers' exposure to secondhand smoke
Outcome 6	Compliance with tobacco-free policies
What to measure	Proportion of adults employed outside the home reporting employee compliance with their workplace's tobacco-free policies
Why this indicator is useful	Perceived compliance with tobacco-free policies is one measure of actual compliance with these policies.[1,2] If tobacco-free policies are not followed, they are unlikely to protect nonsmokers from the harmful effects of secondhand smoke or change social norms.[1]
Example data source(s)	Adult Tobacco Survey (ATS): CDC Recommended Questions: Core, 2003
Population group(s)	Adults aged 18 years or older
Example survey question(s)	**From ATS** As far as you know, in the past 7 days, that is since [fill in date], has anyone smoked in your work area? ☐ Yes ☐ No ☐ Don't know/Not sure ☐ Refused
Comments	Evaluators may also want to gather each company's demographic data (e.g., on the company's size or type of business). Evaluators should determine the scope of the tobacco-free policies before evaluating perceived compliance with them. The example questions could also be asked of employers.

Rating

Overall quality low ←→ high	Resources needed	Strength of evaluation evidence	Utility	Face validity	Accepted practice
▬▬▬▬▬	$$†	⊘	◐	◐	●

←○ ◔ ◐ ● → better

† Denotes low agreement among reviewers: that is, fewer than 75% of the valid ratings for this indicator were within one point of each other (see Appendix B for an explanation).
⊘ Denotes no data.

References
1. Shopland DR, Anderson CM, Burns DM, Gerlach KK. Disparities in smoke-free workplace policies among food service workers. *Journal of Occupational and Environmental Medicine.* 2004;46(4):347–56.
2. Weber MD, Bagwell DA, Fielding JE, Glantz SA. Long-term compliance with California's smoke-free workplace law among bars and restaurants in Los Angeles County. *Tobacco Control.* 2003;12(3):269–73.

GOAL AREA 2
Outcome 6

Indicator 2.6.2

Perceived Compliance with Tobacco-free Policies in Indoor and Outdoor Public Places

Goal area 2	Eliminating nonsmokers' exposure to secondhand smoke
Outcome 6	Compliance with tobacco-free policies
What to measure	Proportion of adults and young people who report compliance with tobacco-free policies in public places (e.g., bars, restaurants, and sporting arenas)
Why this indicator is useful	Perceived compliance with tobacco-free policies is one measure of actual compliance with these policies.[1,2] If tobacco-free policies are not followed, they are not likely to protect nonsmokers from the harmful effects of secondhand smoke or change social norms.[1]
Example data source(s)	No commonly used data sources were found
Population group(s)	Adults aged 18 years or older Young people aged less than 18 years
Example survey question(s)	In your community, how many people break the policy that bans smoking in: Response options: None, A few, Some, Most, All of them, Don't know/Not sure, Not applicable, Refused to answer • Bars • Restaurants • Indoor public places • Outdoor public places
Comments	The authors created this example question. It is not in any commonly used data source. Evaluators should determine the scope of tobacco-free policies before evaluating perceived compliance with them.
Rating	Overall quality: low ←——→ high Resources needed: $$$† Strength of evaluation evidence: no data Utility: ● Face validity: ● Accepted practice: ● ←○○●●→ better

† Denotes low agreement among reviewers: that is, fewer than 75% of the valid ratings for this indicator were within one point of each other (see Appendix B for an explanation).
⊘ Denotes no data.

References
1. Shopland DR, Anderson CM, Burns DM, Gerlach KK. Disparities in smoke-free workplace policies among food service workers. *Journal of Occupational and Environmental Medicine.* 2004;46(4):347–56.
2. Weber MD, Bagwell DA, Fielding JE, Glantz SA. Long-term compliance with California's smoke-free workplace law among bars and restaurants in Los Angeles County. *Tobacco Control.* 2003;12(3):269–73.

Indicator 2.6.3

Proportion of Public Places Observed to Be in Compliance with Tobacco-free Policies

Goal area 2	Eliminating nonsmokers' exposure to secondhand smoke
Outcome 6	Compliance with tobacco-free policies
What to measure	Proportion of indoor or outdoor places (e.g., bars, restaurants, and sporting arenas) in a community in which employees and patrons comply with tobacco-free policies
Why this indicator is useful	Observing whether people (employees and patrons) comply with tobacco-free policies is a systematic way to measure compliance at a given place and time.[1] If tobacco-free policies are not followed, they are not likely to protect nonsmokers from the harmful effects of secondhand smoke or change social norms.[2]
Example data source(s)	▸ Direct observation of employees' and patrons' behavior ▸ California's BREATH (Smoke-Free Bars, Workplaces, and Communities Program) Information available at: http://www.breath-ala.org
Population group(s)	Not applicable. This indicator is best measured by observation.
Example survey question(s)	Not applicable. This indicator is best measured by observation.
Comments	In addition to observing smoking-related behavior in public places, evaluators can measure the environmental tobacco smoke in these places by monitoring indoor air quality.[3-5]

Rating

Overall quality low ◄——► high	Resources needed	Strength of evaluation evidence	Utility	Face validity	Accepted practice
▬▬▬▬▬	$$$$[†]	⊘	◐	●	●

◄ ○ ◔ ◑ ● ► better

† Denotes low agreement among reviewers: that is, fewer than 75% of the valid ratings for this indicator were within one point of each other (see Appendix B for an explanation).
⊘ Denotes no data.

References
1. Weber MD, Bagwell DA, Fielding JE, Glantz SA. Long-term compliance with California's Smoke-Free Workplace Law among bars and restaurants in Los Angeles County. *Tobacco Control*. 2003;12(3):269–73.
2. Shopland DR, Anderson CM, Burns DM, Gerlach KK. Disparities in smoke-free workplace policies among food service workers. *Journal of Occupational and Environmental Medicine*. 2004;46(4):347–56.
3. Cains T, Cannata S, Poulos R, Ferson M, Stewart B. Designated "no smoking" areas provide from partial to no protection from environmental tobacco smoke. *Tobacco Control*. 2004;13(1):17–22.
4. Repace J. *An air quality survey of respirable particles and particulate carcinogens in Delaware hospitality venues before and after a smoking ban*. Bowie, MD: Repace Associates; 2003. Available from: http://www.tobaccoscam.ucsf.edu/pdf/RepaceDelaware.pdf. Accessed December 2004.
5. Kiser D, Boschert T. Eliminating smoking in bars, restaurants, and gaming clubs in California: BREATH, the California Smoke-Free Bar Program. *Journal of Public Health Policy*. 2001;22(1):81–7.

GOAL AREA 2
Outcome 6

Indicator 2.6.4

Perceived Compliance with Voluntary Tobacco-free Home or Vehicle Policies

Goal area 2	Eliminating nonsmokers' exposure to secondhand smoke
Outcome 6	Compliance with tobacco-free policies
What to measure	Proportion of adults and young people who report compliance with tobacco-free policies in their homes or vehicles
Why this indicator is useful	Perceived compliance with tobacco-free policies is one measure of actual compliance with these policies.[1,2] Self-reported data on people's exposure to secondhand smoke at home or in vehicles can be used to measure compliance with tobacco-free policies.[3,4] Compliance with home and vehicle tobacco-free policies is especially important for protecting the health of children and for supporting anti-tobacco social norms.[5,6]
Example data source(s)	Adult Tobacco Survey (ATS): CDC Recommended Questions: Core, 2003
Population group(s)	Adults aged 18 years or older
Example survey question(s)	**From ATS** *For respondents who report they have a smoke-free home policy* During the past 7 days (that is, since [fill in date]), how many days did anyone smoke cigarettes, cigars, or pipes anywhere inside your home? ☐ ___ days (0–7) ☐ Don't know/Not sure ☐ Refused
Comments	Evaluators may want to modify the example question to address tobacco-free policies inside vehicles. Evaluators should determine the scope of the tobacco-free policies before evaluating perceived compliance with them. The example survey question could be asked of young people. |️
Rating	Overall quality: low ←——→ high (high) Resources needed: $$[†] Strength of evaluation evidence: ● Utility: ● Face validity: ● Accepted practice: ● ←○◐●●→ better

[†] Denotes low agreement among reviewers: that is, fewer than 75% of the valid ratings for this indicator were within one point of each other (see Appendix B for an explanation).

References
1. Shopland DR, Anderson CM, Burns DM, Gerlach KK. Disparities in smoke-free workplace policies among food service workers. *Journal of Occupational and Environmental Medicine.* 2004;46(4):347–56.
2. Weber MD, Bagwell DA, Fielding JE, Glantz SA. Long-term compliance with California's smoke-free workplace law among bars and restaurants in Los Angeles County. *Tobacco Control.* 2003;12(3):269–73.
3. Biener L, Cullen D, Di ZX, Hammond SK. Household smoking restrictions and adolescents' exposure to environmental tobacco smoke. *Preventive Medicine.* 1997;26(3):358–63.
4. Wakefield M, Banham D, Martin J, Ruffin R, McCaul K, Badcock N. Restrictions on smoking at home and urinary cotinine levels among children with asthma. *American Journal of Preventive Medicine.* 2000;19(3):188–92.
5. U.S. Environmental Protection Agency. *Respiratory health effects of passive smoking: lung cancer and other disorders.* Washington, DC: EPA Office of Research and Development; 1992. Publication No. EPA/600/6-90/006F.
6. National Cancer Institute. Smoking and Tobacco Control Monograph No. 10. *Health effects of exposure to environmental tobacco smoke: the report of the California Environmental Protection Agency.* Bethesda, MD: National Cancer Institute; 1999. NIH Publication No. 99-4645.

Indicator 2.6.5

Perceived Compliance with Tobacco-free Policies in Schools

Goal area 2	Eliminating nonsmokers' exposure to secondhand smoke
Outcome 6	Compliance with tobacco-free policies
What to measure	Proportion of students who report that the school population is complying with the school's tobacco-free policies
Why this indicator is useful	Perceived compliance with tobacco-free policies is one measure of actual compliance with these policies.[1,2] Compliance with tobacco-free school policies reduces students' exposure to secondhand smoke and reinforces anti-tobacco social norms.[3]
Example data source(s)	▸ Youth Tobacco Survey (YTS): CDC Recommended Questions: Core, 2004 ▸ CDC Youth Risk Behavior Surveillance System (YRBSS), 2003 ▸ California Independent Evaluation: Youth Survey, 2000 Information available at: http://www.dhs.ca.gov/ps/cdic/ccb/TCS/html/Evaluation_Resources.htm
Population group(s)	Young people aged less than 18 years
Example survey question(s)	**From YTS and YRBSS** During the past 30 days, on how many days did you smoke cigarettes on school property? ☐ 0 days ☐ 1 or 2 days ☐ 3 to 5 days ☐ 6 to 9 days ☐ 10 to 19 days ☐ 20 to 29 days ☐ All 30 days During the past 30 days, on how many days did you use chewing tobacco, snuff, or dip on school property? ☐ 0 days ☐ 1 or 2 days ☐ 3 to 5 days ☐ 6 to 9 days ☐ 10 to 19 days ☐ 20 to 29 days ☐ All 30 days **From California Independent Evaluation** Is there a rule at your school that no one is allowed to smoke cigarettes in the school building or on the school yard? ☐ Yes ☐ No ☐ I don't know/I'm not sure Have you seen any students break that rule? ☐ Yes ☐ No ☐ My school does not have a no-smoking rule ☐ I don't know/I'm not sure How many students who are smokers break that rule? ☐ None ☐ A few ☐ Some ☐ Most ☐ All of them ☐ My school does not have a no-smoking rule ☐ I don't know/I'm not sure Have you seen adults break that rule? ☐ Yes ☐ No ☐ My school does not have a no-smoking rule ☐ I don't know/I'm not sure Is there a rule at your school that no one is allowed to use chewing tobacco or snuff in the school building or on the school yard? ☐ Yes ☐ No ☐ I don't know/I'm not sure

GOAL AREA 2
Outcome 6

Comments	If students report on the YTS or YRBSS instruments (1) the existence of a tobacco-free school policy and (2) having personally used tobacco products more than 1 day on school property, they are considered noncompliant.
	Evaluators may also want to categorize data by grade level and type of school (e.g., elementary, middle, high school, private, parochial, public).
	Evaluators should determine the scope of the tobacco-free policies before evaluating perceived compliance with them.
	The example survey questions could be asked of teachers and principals.

Rating	Overall quality low ◄——► high	Resources needed	Strength of evaluation evidence	Utility	Face validity	Accepted practice
	(mid-high)	$$	◐	●	●	●

◄ ○ ◔ ◐ ● ► better

References
1. Shopland DR, Anderson CM, Burns DM, Gerlach KK. Disparities in smoke-free workplace policies among food service workers. *Journal of Occupational and Environmental Medicine.* 2004;46(4):347–56.
2. Weber MD, Bagwell DA, Fielding JE, Glantz SA. Long-term compliance with California's smoke-free workplace law among bars and restaurants in Los Angeles County. *Tobacco Control.* 2003;12(3):269–73.
3. Gilpin EA, White MM, White VM, Distefan JM, Trinidad DR, Lee L, Major J, Kealey S, Pierce JP. *Tobacco control successes in California: a focus on young people, results from the California Tobacco Surveys 1990–2002.* La Jolla, CA: University of California, San Diego; 2003. pp. 348–9. Available from: http://repositories.cdlib.org/tc/surveys/CTC1990-2002. Accessed December 2004.

Outcome 7

Reduced Exposure to Secondhand Smoke

There is substantial evidence regarding the harm caused by exposure to secondhand smoke. Secondhand smoke can lead to lung cancer and heart disease in adults and to many serious health problems (e.g., lower respiratory infections, asthma, sudden infant death syndrome, ear infections) in children.[1-3] Evidence also indicates that tobacco smoke is especially harmful to pregnant women and to fetal development.[1,2] Reducing nonsmokers' exposure to secondhand smoke can prevent disease and save lives.[1-4] Median exposure levels and the percentage of nonsmokers in the United States who are exposed to secondhand smoke have decreased significantly.[5]

Listed below are the indicators associated with this outcome:

- **2.7.1**   Proportion of the population reporting exposure to secondhand smoke in the workplace
- **2.7.2**   Proportion of the population reporting exposure to secondhand smoke in public places
- **2.7.3**   Proportion of the population reporting exposure to secondhand smoke at home or in vehicles
- **2.7.4**   Proportion of students reporting exposure to secondhand smoke in schools
- **2.7.5**   Proportion of nonsmokers reporting overall exposure to secondhand smoke

References

1. U.S. Department of Health and Human Services. *The health consequences of smoking: a report of the Surgeon General.* Atlanta, GA: Centers for Disease Control and Prevention; 2004.

2. U.S. Department of Health and Human Services. *Women and smoking: a report of the Surgeon General.* Rockville, MD: Office of the Surgeon General; Washington, DC: Government Printing Office; 2001.

3. National Cancer Institute. Smoking and Tobacco Control Monograph No. 10. *Health effects of exposure to environmental tobacco smoke: the report of the California Environmental Protection Agency.* Bethesda, MD: National Cancer Institute; 1999. NIH Publication No. 99-4645.

4. U.S. Environmental Protection Agency. *Respiratory health effects of passive smoking: lung cancer and other disorders.* Washington, DC: EPA Office of Research and Development; 1992. Publication No. EPA/600/6-90/006F.

5. Changes in secondhand smoke exposure among nonsmokers from different racial/ethnic groups: United States, 1988–1994 and 1999–2000. Data from 1988–1994 NHANES III survey and 1999–2000 NHANES survey. Poster Presentation. 132nd Annual American Public Health Association Meeting, Washington, DC, November 6–10, 2004.

For Further Reading

Mannino DM, Caraballo R, Benowitz N, Repace J. Predictors of cotinine levels in U.S. children: data from the Third National Health and Nutrition Examination Survey. *Chest.* 2001;120(3):718–24.

Pizacani BA, Martin DP, Stark MJ, Koepsell TD, Thompson B, Diehr P. Household smoking bans: which households have them and do they work? *Preventive Medicine.* 2003;36(1):99–107.

Poulsen L. Exposure to teachers smoking and adolescent smoking behaviour: analysis of cross sectional data from Denmark. *Tobacco Control.* 2002;11(3):246–51.

Wakefield M, Banham D, Martin J, Ruffin R, McCaul K, Badcock N. Restrictions of smoking at home and urinary cotinine levels among children with asthma. *American Journal of Preventive Medicine.* 2000;19(3):188–92.

Outcome 7

Reduced Exposure to Secondhand Smoke

Indicator Rating

← ○ ◐ ● ● → better

Number	Indicator	Overall quality (low → high)	Resources needed	Strength of evaluation evidence	Utility	Face validity	Accepted practice
2.7.1	Proportion of the population reporting exposure to secondhand smoke in the workplace	▬▬▬▬▬	$$†	◐	●	●	●
2.7.2	Proportion of the population reporting exposure to secondhand smoke in public places	▬▬▬▬†	$$$	◐	◐	◐	●
2.7.3	Proportion of the population reporting exposure to secondhand smoke at home or in vehicles	▬▬▬▬	$$†	◐	◐	◐	●
2.7.4	Proportion of students reporting exposure to secondhand smoke in schools	▬▬▬▬	$$$	⊘	●	●	●
2.7.5	Proportion of nonsmokers reporting overall exposure to secondhand smoke	▬▬▬▬▬	$$	●	◐	◐	●

† Denotes low agreement among reviewers: that is, fewer than 75% of the valid ratings for this indicator were within one point of each other (see Appendix B for an explanation).
⊘ Denotes no data.

GOAL AREA 2
Outcome 7

Indicator 2.7.1

Proportion of the Population Reporting Exposure to Secondhand Smoke in the Workplace

Goal area 2	Eliminating nonsmokers' exposure to secondhand smoke
Outcome 7	Reduced exposure to secondhand smoke
What to measure	Proportion of adults who are employed outside the home and who report exposure to secondhand smoke in the workplace
Why this indicator is useful	Exposure to secondhand smoke is a major cause of death and disease.[1-4] For nonsmokers who are not exposed to secondhand smoke in their homes, the workplace is typically their greatest source of exposure. Studies show that after only 3 months of decreased workplace exposure to secondhand smoke, nonsmokers' lung function improves and their respiratory symptoms are reduced.[5]
Example data source(s)	California Adult Tobacco Survey (CATS), 1999 Information available at: http://www.dhs.ca.gov/ps/cdic/ccb/TCS/html/Evaluation_Resources.htm
Population group(s)	Adults aged 18 years or older
Example survey question(s)	**From CATS** During the past two weeks has anyone smoked in the area in which you work? ☐ Yes ☐ No ☐ Don't know/Not sure ☐ Refused
Comments	None

Rating

Overall quality low ⟷ high	Resources needed	Strength of evaluation evidence	Utility	Face validity	Accepted practice
▬▬▬▬▬	$$†	◐	●	●	●

←○◌◐●→ better

† Denotes low agreement among reviewers: that is, fewer than 75% of the valid ratings for this indicator were within one point of each other (see Appendix B for an explanation).

References

1. U.S. Department of Health and Human Services. *The health consequences of smoking: a report of the Surgeon General.* Atlanta, GA: Centers for Disease Control and Prevention; 2004.
2. U.S. Department of Health and Human Services. *Women and smoking: a report of the Surgeon General.* Rockville, MD: U.S. Department of Health and Human Services, Public Health Service, Office of the Surgeon General; 2001.
3. U.S. Environmental Protection Agency. *Respiratory health effects of passive smoking: lung cancer and other disorders.* Washington, DC: EPA Office of Research and Development; 1992. Publication No. EPA/600/6-90/006F.
4. National Cancer Institute. Smoking and Tobacco Control Monograph No. 10. *Health effects of exposure to environmental tobacco smoke: the report of the California Environmental Protection Agency.* Bethesda, MD: National Cancer Institute; 1999. NIH Publication No. 99-4645.
5. Eisner MD, Smith AK, Blanc PD. Bartenders' respiratory health after establishment of smoke-free bars and taverns. *Journal of the American Medical Association.* 1998;280(22);1909–14.

Indicator 2.7.2

Proportion of the Population Reporting Exposure to Secondhand Smoke in Public Places

Goal area 2	Eliminating nonsmokers' exposure to secondhand smoke
Outcome 7	Reduced exposure to secondhand smoke
What to measure	Proportion of the population reporting exposure to secondhand smoke in public places, including bars, restaurants, sporting arenas, and concert venues
Why this indicator is useful	Exposure to secondhand smoke is a major cause of death and disease.[1-4] Many studies show that exposure to secondhand smoke leads to lung cancer and heart disease in adults and to multiple health problems, such as severe asthma, lower respiratory tract infections, and ear infections in children.[1-4] The public is exposed to secondhand smoke in many public places. Measuring exposure in public settings is necessary for assessing overall exposure levels.[5]
Example data source(s)	California Adult Tobacco Survey (CATS), 1999 Information available at: http://www.dhs.ca.gov/ps/cdic/ccb/TCS/html/Evaluation_Resources.htm
Population group(s)	Adults aged 18 years or older
Example survey question(s)	**From CATS** During the past 7 days, when you were some place other than work or home, how many days were you exposed to other people's tobacco smoke?
Comments	The example survey question could be asked of young people.

Rating

Overall quality low ⟵⟶ high	Resources needed	Strength of evaluation evidence	Utility	Face validity	Accepted practice
▬▬▬▬▬ †	$$$	◐	◐	◐	●

⟵ ○ ◔ ◐ ● ⟶ better

† Denotes low agreement among reviewers: that is, fewer than 75% of the valid ratings for this indicator were within one point of each other (see Appendix B for an explanation).

References
1. U.S. Department of Health and Human Services. *The health consequences of smoking: a report of the Surgeon General.* Atlanta, GA: Centers for Disease Control and Prevention; 2004.
2. U.S. Department of Health and Human Services. *Women and smoking: a report of the Surgeon General.* Rockville, MD: U.S. Department of Health and Human Services, Public Health Service, Office of the Surgeon General; 2001.
3. U.S. Environmental Protection Agency. *Respiratory health effects of passive smoking: lung cancer and other disorders.* Washington, DC: EPA Office of Research and Development; 1992. Publication No. EPA/600/6-90/006F.
4. National Cancer Institute. Smoking and Tobacco Control Monograph No. 10. *Health effects of exposure to environmental tobacco smoke: the report of the California Environmental Protection Agency.* Bethesda, MD: National Cancer Institute; 1999. NIH Publication No. 99-4645.
5. Centers for Disease Control and Prevention. *Taking action against secondhand smoke.* Atlanta, GA: Centers for Disease Control and Prevention; 2004. Available from: http://www.cdc.gov/tobacco/ETS_Toolkit. Accessed March 2005.

Indicator 2.7.3

Proportion of the Population Reporting Exposure to Secondhand Smoke at Home or in Vehicles

Goal area 2	Eliminating nonsmokers' exposure to secondhand smoke
Outcome 7	Reduced exposure to secondhand smoke
What to measure	Proportion of the population reporting exposure to secondhand smoke at home or in vehicles
Why this indicator is useful	Exposure to secondhand smoke at home or in vehicles is a serious health hazard.[1-4] Many studies show that exposure to secondhand smoke leads to lung cancer and heart disease in adults and to multiple health problems, such as severe asthma, lower respiratory tract infections, and ear infections in children.[1-4]
Example data source(s)	Adult Tobacco Survey (ATS): CDC Recommended Questions: Core, 2003 Youth Tobacco Survey (YTS): CDC Recommended Questions: Core, 2004
Population group(s)	Adults aged 18 years or older Young people aged less than 18 years
Example survey question(s)	**From ATS** During the past 7 days (that is, since [fill in date]), how many days did anyone smoke cigarettes, cigars, or pipes anywhere inside your home? ☐ Less than 1 day per week ☐ Rarely ☐ None ☐ ___days (1–7) ☐ Don't know/Not sure ☐ Refused In the past 7 days (that is, since [fill in date]), have you been in a car with someone who was smoking? ☐ Yes ☐ No **From YTS** During the past 7 days, on how many days were you in the same room with someone who was smoking cigarettes? ☐ 0 days ☐ 1 or 2 days ☐ 3 or 4 days ☐ 5 or 6 days ☐ 7 days During the past 7 days, on how many days did you ride in a car with someone who was smoking cigarettes? ☐ 0 days ☐ 1 or 2 days ☐ 3 or 4 days ☐ 5 or 6 days ☐ 7 days
Comments	The ATS and YTS example survey questions can only be used to gather data on exposure to smoke during the previous 7 days and not to quantify exposure level.

Rating

Overall quality low ⟷ high	Resources needed	Strength of evaluation evidence	Utility	Face validity	Accepted practice
▬▬▬▬▬	$$†	●	●	●	●

← ○ ◔ ● ● → better

† Denotes low agreement among reviewers: that is, fewer than 75% of the valid ratings for this indicator were within one point of each other (see Appendix B for an explanation).

References
1. U.S. Department of Health and Human Services. *The health consequences of smoking: a report of the Surgeon General.* Atlanta, GA: Centers for Disease Control and Prevention; 2004.
2. U.S. Department of Health and Human Services. *Women and smoking: a report of the Surgeon General.* Rockville, MD: U.S. Department of Health and Human Services, Public Health Service, Office of the Surgeon General; 2001.
3. U.S. Environmental Protection Agency. *Respiratory health effects of passive smoking: lung cancer and other disorders.* Washington, DC: EPA Office of Research and Development; 1992. Publication No. EPA/600/6-90/006F.
4. National Cancer Institute. Smoking and Tobacco Control Monograph No. 10. *Health effects of exposure to environmental tobacco smoke: the report of the California Environmental Protection Agency.* Bethesda, MD: National Cancer Institute; 1999. NIH Publication No. 99-4645.

GOAL AREA 2
Outcome 7

Indicator 2.7.4

Proportion of Students Reporting Exposure to Secondhand Smoke in Schools

Goal area 2	Eliminating nonsmokers' exposure to secondhand smoke
Outcome 7	Reduced exposure to secondhand smoke
What to measure	Proportion of students reporting exposure to tobacco smoke while on school grounds, at school-sponsored functions, and in school vehicles (exposure can occur during or after regular school hours)
Why this indicator is useful	Exposure to secondhand smoke is a major cause of death and disease.[1-4] Young people spend many of their waking hours in school, where they might be exposed to second-hand smoke. Compliance with tobacco-free school policies reduces students' exposure to secondhand smoke and reinforces anti-tobacco social norms.[5]
Example data source(s)	No commonly used data sources were found
Population group(s)	Students
Example survey question(s)	When you are at school, are you exposed to smoke from other people's cigarettes, pipes, or cigars? ☐ Yes ☐ No
Comments	The authors created this example question. It is not in any commonly used data source. Evaluators might also want to measure secondhand smoke exposure on college campuses.

Rating

Overall quality low ◄────► high	Resources needed	Strength of evaluation evidence	Utility	Face validity	Accepted practice
▬▬▬▬▬▬	$$$	⊘	●	●	●

◄ ○ ◐ ● ● ► better

⊘ Denotes no data.

References
1. U.S. Department of Health and Human Services. *The health consequences of smoking: a report of the Surgeon General.* Atlanta, GA: Centers for Disease Control and Prevention; 2004.
2. U.S. Environmental Protection Agency. *Respiratory health effects of passive smoking: lung cancer and other disorders.* Washington, DC: EPA Office of Research and Development; 1992. Publication No. EPA/600/6-90/006F.
3. National Cancer Institute. Smoking and Tobacco Control Monograph No. 10. *Health effects of exposure to environmental tobacco smoke: the report of the California Environmental Protection Agency.* Bethesda, MD: National Cancer Institute; 1999. NIH Publication No. 99-4645.
4. U.S. Department of Health and Human Services. *Women and smoking: a report of the Surgeon General.* Rockville, MD: U.S. Department of Health and Human Services, Public Health Service, Office of the Surgeon General; 2001.
5. Gilpin EA, White MM, White VM, Distefan JM, Trinidad DR, Lee L, Major J, Kealey S, Pierce JP. *Tobacco control successes in California: a focus on young people, results from the California Tobacco Surveys 1990–2002.* La Jolla, CA: University of California, San Diego; 2003. pp. 348–349. Available from: http://repositories.cdlib.org/tc/surveys/CTC1990-2002/. Accessed December 2004.

Indicator 2.7.5

Proportion of Nonsmokers Reporting Overall Exposure to Secondhand Smoke

Goal area 2	Eliminating nonsmokers' exposure to secondhand smoke
Outcome 7	Reduced exposure to secondhand smoke
What to measure	Nonsmokers' level of exposure to secondhand smoke. Such exposure can be caused by family members, co-workers, or strangers in public places.
Why this indicator is useful	Exposure to secondhand smoke is a major cause of death and disease.[1-4] Trends in nonsmokers' overall level of exposure to secondhand smoke are an important gauge of the success of efforts to reduce this exposure.[5-7]
Example data source(s)	▸ Youth Tobacco Survey (YTS): CDC Recommended Questions: Core, 2004 ▸ California Independent Evaluation: Adult Survey, 2000 Information available at: http://www.dhs.ca.gov/ps/cdic/ccb/TCS/html/Evaluation_Resources.htm
Population group(s)	▸ Adults aged 18 years or older ▸ Young people aged less than 18 years
Example survey question(s)	**From YTS** During the past 7 days, on how many days were you in the same room with someone who was smoking cigarettes? ☐ 0 day ☐ 1 or 2 days ☐ 3 or 4 days ☐ 5 or 6 days ☐ 7 days During the past 7 days, on how many days did you ride in a car with someone who was smoking cigarettes? ☐ 0 day ☐ 1 or 2 days ☐ 3 or 4 days ☐ 5 or 6 days ☐ 7 days **From California Independent Evaluation** During the past 7 days, when you were at home, how many days were you exposed to other family members' or visitors' tobacco smoke? ☐ None ☐ 1 day ☐ 2 days ☐ 3 days ☐ 4 days ☐ 5 days ☐ 6 days ☐ 7 days ☐ Was not home in the past 7 days *Of those who were exposed on some days, ask the following:* On these days, about how many hours per day were you exposed to other people's smoke? Write the actual number of hours per day _____ During the past 7 days, when you were at work, how many days were you exposed to other people's tobacco smoke? ☐ None ☐ 1 day ☐ 2 days ☐ 3 days ☐ 4 days ☐ 5 days ☐ 6 days ☐ 7 days ☐ Was not at work in the past 7 days *Of those who were exposed on some days, ask the following:* On these days, about how many hours per day were you exposed to other people's smoke? Write the actual number of hours per day _____ During the past 7 days, when you were some place other than work or home, how many days were you exposed to other people's tobacco smoke? ☐ None ☐ 1 day ☐ 2 days ☐ 3 days ☐ 4 days ☐ 5 days ☐ 6 days ☐ 7 days

Example survey question(s) (cont.)

Of those who were exposed on some days, ask the following:
On these days, about how many hours per day were you exposed to other people's smoke?
Write the actual number of hours per day_____

Comments None

Rating

Overall quality low ⟷ high	Resources needed	Strength of evaluation evidence	Utility	Face validity	Accepted practice
▬▬▬▬▬	$$	◓	◓	◓	●

←○◔◑●→ better

References

1. U.S. Department of Health and Human Services. *The health consequences of smoking: a report of the Surgeon General.* Atlanta, GA: Centers for Disease Control and Prevention; 2004.
2. U.S. Environmental Protection Agency. *Respiratory health effects of passive smoking: lung cancer and other disorders.* Washington, DC: EPA Office of Research and Development; 1992. Publication No. EPA/600/6-90/006F.
3. National Cancer Institute. Smoking and Tobacco Control Monograph No. 10. *Health effects of exposure to environmental tobacco smoke: the report of the California Environmental Protection Agency.* Bethesda, MD: National Cancer Institute; 1999. NIH Publication No. 99-4645.
4. U.S. Department of Health and Human Services. *Women and smoking: a report of the Surgeon General.* Rockville, MD: U.S. Department of Health and Human Services, Public Health Service, Office of the Surgeon General; 2001.
5. U.S. Department of Health and Human Services. *Healthy people 2010.* 2nd ed. With *Understanding and improving health and objectives for improving health.* 2 vols. Washington, DC: Government Printing Office; 2000.
6. International Agency for Research on Cancer. Monographs on the Evaluation of Carcinogenic Risks to Humans, Volume 83. *Tobacco smoke and involuntary smoking: summary of data reported and evaluation.* Lyon, France: World Health Organization; 2002. Available from: http://monographs.iarc.fr/htdocs/indexes/vol83index.html. Accessed December 2004.
7. National Institutes of Health, National Toxicology Program. *10th report on carcinogens, 2000.* Research Triangle Park, NC: National Institute of Environmental Health Sciences; 2002. Available from: http://ehp.niehs.nih.gov/roc/toc10.html. Accessed December 2004.

Outcome 8

Reduced Tobacco Consumption

Although the main goal of activities to eliminate exposure to secondhand smoke is protecting nonsmokers, another possible outcome is the reduced cigarette use that may result from cessation by smokers or the decreased number of cigarettes smoked per day by continuing smokers. Research shows that smokers in workplaces with tobacco-free policies may reduce the number of cigarettes they smoke or quit smoking altogether.[1,2] In addition, young people who live in households with tobacco-free policies are less likely to smoke than those who live in households in which people smoke.[3]

Listed below are the indicators associated with this outcome:

2.8.1 Per capita consumption of tobacco products

2.8.2 Average number of cigarettes smoked per day by smokers

2.8.3 Smoking prevalence

References

1. Fichtenberg CM, Glantz SA. Effect of smoke-free workplaces on smoking behaviour: systematic review. *British Medical Journal.* 2002;325(7357):188.

2. Farrelly MC, Pechacek TF, Chaloupka FJ. The impact of tobacco control expenditures on aggregate cigarette sales: 1981–2000. *Journal of Health Economics.* 2003;22(5):843–59. Erratum in: *Journal of Health Economics.* 2004;23(2):419.

3. Farkas AJ, Gilpin EA, White MM, Pierce JP. Association between household and workplace smoking restrictions and adolescent smoking. *Journal of the American Medical Association.* 2000;284(6):717–22.

For Further Reading

Biener L, Cullen D, Di ZX, Hammond SK. Household smoking restrictions and adolescents' exposure to environmental tobacco smoke. *Preventive Medicine.* 1997;26(3):358–63.

National Cancer Institute. Smoking and Tobacco Control Monograph No. 11. *State and local legislative action to reduce tobacco use.* Bethesda, MD: National Cancer Institute; 2000. NIH Publication No. 00-4804.

Outcome 8

Reduced Tobacco Consumption

Indicator Rating

← ○ ◐ ● ● → better

Number	Indicator	Overall quality low ←→ high	Resources needed	Strength of evaluation evidence	Utility	Face validity	Accepted practice
2.8.1	Per capita consumption of tobacco products	▬▬▬▬	$	●	●	◐	●
2.8.2	Average number of cigarettes smoked per day by smokers	▬▬▬▬	$$†	●	●	◐	●
2.8.3	Smoking prevalence	▬▬▬▬	$$†	●	◐	●	●

† Denotes low agreement among reviewers: that is, fewer than 75% of the valid ratings for this indicator were within one point of each other (see Appendix B for an explanation).

Indicator 2.8.1

Per Capita Consumption of Tobacco Products

Goal area 2	Eliminating nonsmokers' exposure to secondhand smoke
Outcome 8	Reduced tobacco consumption
What to measure	The number of cigarette packs sold per adult aged 18 years or older in the state
Why this indicator is useful	In addition to decreasing nonsmokers' exposure to secondhand smoke, smoke-free policies decrease the number of cigarettes smoked.[1]
Example data source(s)	▸ CDC State Tobacco Activities Tracking and Evaluation (STATE) system Data available at: http://www.cdc.gov/tobacco/STATEsystem ▸ State departments of revenue
Population group(s)	Not applicable. This indicator is best measured by examining tax records to assess the state's sales of cigarettes.
Example survey question(s)	Not applicable
Comments	Evaluators need to measure statewide consumption of cigarettes, smokeless tobacco, and other tobacco products separately.

Rating	Overall quality low ◀——▶ high	Resources needed	Strength of evaluation evidence	Utility	Face validity	Accepted practice
	▬▬▬	$	●	●	◐	●

◀ ○ ◌ ◉ ● ▶ better

Reference
1. Fichtenberg CM, Glantz SA. Effect of smoke-free workplaces on smoking behaviour: systematic review. *British Medical Journal.* 2002;325(7357):188.

Indicator 2.8.2

Average Number of Cigarettes Smoked per Day by Smokers

Goal area 2	Eliminating nonsmokers' exposure to secondhand smoke
Outcome 8	Reduced tobacco consumption
What to measure	The average number of cigarettes smoked per day by adult and young smokers
Why this indicator is useful	Daily cigarette use by employees who smoke decreases when smoke-free policies are adopted in the workplace.[1] In addition, young people who live in households with tobacco-free policies are less likely to smoke than those who live in households in which people smoke.[2]
Example data source(s)	CDC State Tobacco Activities Tracking and Evaluation (STATE) system Data available at: http://www.cdc.gov/tobacco/STATEsystem Youth Tobacco Survey (YTS): CDC Recommended Questions: Core, 2004 CDC Youth Risk Behavior Surveillance System (YRBSS), 2003 Adult Tobacco Survey (ATS): CDC Recommended Questions: Core, 2003
Population group(s)	Smokers 18 years of age or older Smokers aged less than 18 years
Example survey question(s)	**From YTS and YRBSS** During the past 30 days, on the days you smoked, how many cigarettes did you smoke per day? ☐ I did not smoke cigarettes during the past 30 days ☐ Less than 1 cigarette per day ☐ 1 cigarette per day ☐ 2 to 5 cigarettes per day ☐ 6 to 10 cigarettes per day ☐ 11 to 20 cigarettes per day ☐ More than 20 cigarettes per day **From ATS** *For everyday smokers* On the average, about how many cigarettes a day do you now smoke? Number of cigarettes _____ *For some-day smokers* On the average, on days when you smoked during the past 30 days, about how many cigarettes did you smoke a day? Number of cigarettes _____
Comments	Calculating the average number of cigarettes smoked per day by adults requires combining data for everyday smokers and some-day smokers.

Rating	Overall quality low ←→ high	Resources needed	Strength of evaluation evidence	Utility	Face validity	Accepted practice
	▬▬▬▬▬	$$†	●	●	◐	●

←○◔●●→ better

† Denotes low agreement among reviewers: that is, fewer than 75% of the valid ratings for this indicator were within one point of each other (see Appendix B for an explanation).

References
1. Farrelly MC, Evans WN, Sfekas AE. The impact of workplace smoking bans: results from a national survey. *Tobacco Control*. 1999;8(3):272–7.
2. Farkas AJ, Gilpin EA, White MM, Pierce JP. Association between household and workplace smoking restrictions and adolescent smoking. *Journal of the American Medical Association*. 2000;284(6):717–22.

GOAL AREA 2
Outcome 8

Indicator 2.8.3

Smoking Prevalence

Goal area 2	Eliminating nonsmokers' exposure to secondhand smoke
Outcome 8	Reduced tobacco consumption
What to measure	Proportion of adults employed outside the home who have ever smoked at least 100 cigarettes in their lives and who smoke every day or some days[1] Proportion of young people who have smoked on at least 1 day during the previous 30 days[2]
Why this indicator is useful	Studies show that tobacco-free work policies lead to an increase in the number of employees who quit smoking.[3] In addition, smoke-free workplaces and homes are associated with significantly lower rates of adolescent smoking and an increased likelihood of adolescent smoking cessation.[4]
Example data source(s)	Adult Tobacco Survey (ATS): CDC Recommended Questions: Core, 2003 Behavioral Risk Factor Surveillance System (BRFSS), 2003 Youth Tobacco Survey (YTS): CDC Recommended Questions: Core, 2004 CDC Youth Risk Behavior Surveillance System (YRBSS), 2003
Population group(s)	Adults aged 18 years or older Young people less than 18 years of age
Example survey question(s)	**From ATS and BRFSS** Have you smoked at least 100 cigarettes in your entire life? ☐ Yes ☐ No ☐ Don't know/Not sure ☐ Refused Do you now smoke cigarettes every day, some days, or not at all? ☐ Every day ☐ Some days ☐ Not at all ☐ Refused **From YTS and YRBSS** During the past 30 days, on how many days did you smoke cigarettes? ☐ 0 days ☐ 1 or 2 days ☐ 3 to 5 days ☐ 6 to 9 days ☐ 10 to 19 days ☐ 20 to 29 days ☐ All 30 days
Comments	To gather more complete data on tobacco use, evaluators may also want to ask questions about the use of other tobacco products such as spit (smokeless) tobacco, bidis, small cigars, and loose (roll-your-own) tobacco.

Rating

Overall quality low ◄──► high	Resources needed	Strength of evaluation evidence	Utility	Face validity	Accepted practice
■■■■■■	$$[†]	●	◐	●	●

◄─○ ◐ ● ●─► better

[†] Denotes low agreement among reviewers: that is, fewer than 75% of the valid ratings for this indicator were within one point of each other (see Appendix B for an explanation).

References
1. Centers for Disease Control and Prevention. Prevalence of current cigarette smoking among adults and changes in prevalence of current and some day smoking—United States, 1996–2001. *Morbidity and Mortality Weekly Report.* 2003;52(14):303–7.
2. Centers for Disease Control and Prevention. Cigarette use among high school students—United States, 1991–2003. *Morbidity and Mortality Weekly Report.* 2004;53(23):499–502.
3. Farrelly MC, Evans WN, Sfekas AE. The impact of workplace smoking bans: results from a national survey. *Tobacco Control.* 1999;8(3):272–7.
4. Farkas AJ, Gilpin EA, White MM, Pierce JP. Association between household and workplace smoking restrictions and adolescent smoking. *Journal of the American Medical Association.* 2000;284(6):717–22.

CHAPTER 4

Goal Area 3: Promoting Quitting Among Adults and Young People

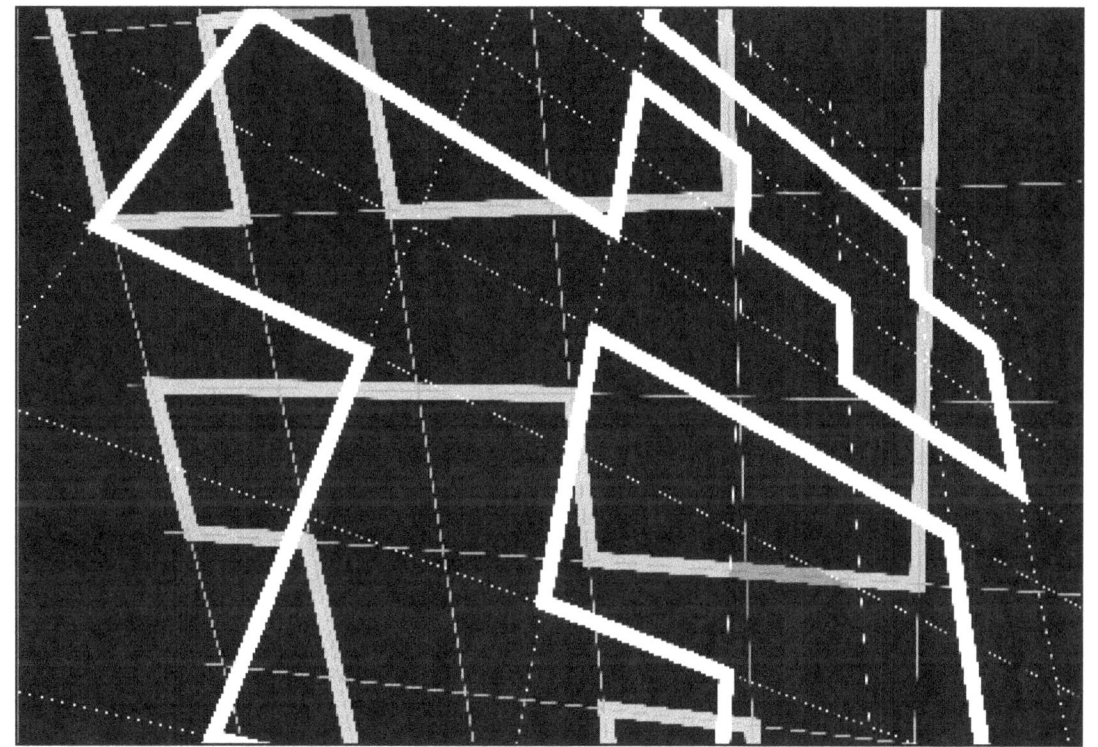

Goal Area 3

Promoting Quitting Among Adults and Young People

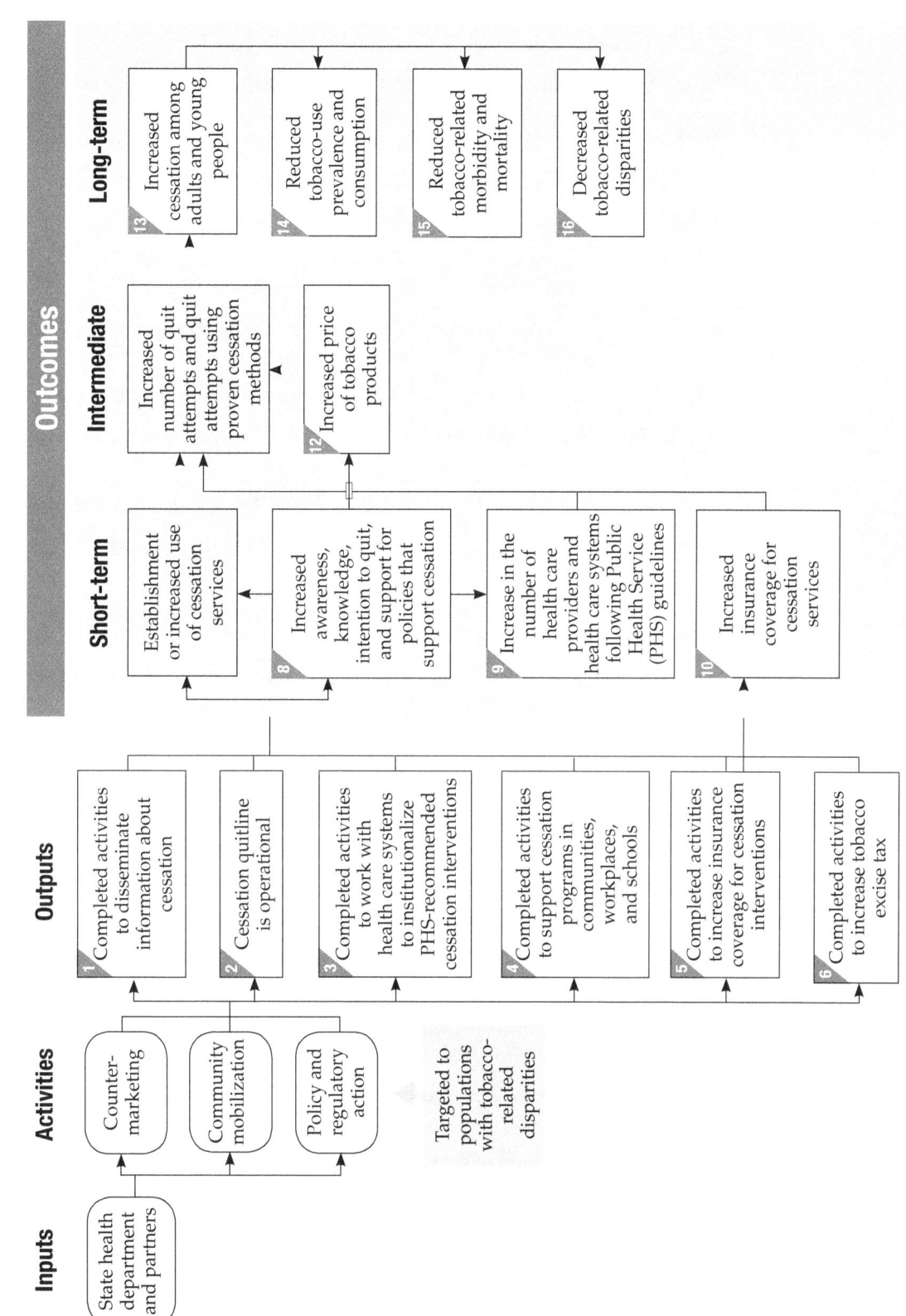

CHAPTER 4 ▸ Goal Area 3: Promoting Quitting Among Adults and Young People | 193

Goal Area 3

Promoting Quitting Among Adults and Young People

Short-term Outcomes

- Outcome 7: Establishment or increased use of cessation services
    - 3.7.1   Number of callers to telephone quitlines
    - 3.7.2^{NR} Number of calls to telephone quitlines from users who heard about the quitline through a media campaign
    - 3.7.3   Number of calls to telephone quitlines from users who heard about the quitline through a source other than a media campaign
    - 3.7.4   Proportion of smokers who have used group cessation programs
    - 3.7.5   Proportion of health care systems with telephone quitlines or contracts with state quitlines
    - 3.7.6   Proportion of worksites with a cessation program or a contract with a quitline

- Outcome 8: Increased awareness, knowledge, intention to quit, and support for policies that support cessation
    - 3.8.1   Level of confirmed awareness of media campaign messages on the dangers of smoking and the benefits of cessation
    - 3.8.2   Level of receptivity to anti-tobacco media messages on the dangers of smoking and the benefits of cessation
    - 3.8.3   Proportion of smokers who intend to quit
    - 3.8.4   Proportion of smokers who intend to quit smoking by using proven cessation methods
    - 3.8.5   Level of support for increasing excise tax on tobacco products
    - 3.8.6   Proportion of smokers who are aware of the cessation services available to them
    - 3.8.7   Proportion of smokers who are aware of their insurance coverage for cessation treatment
    - 3.8.8   Level of support for increasing insurance coverage for cessation treatment
    - 3.8.9^{NR} Proportion of employers who are aware of the benefits of providing coverage for cessation treatment

Outcome 9: Increase in the number of health care providers and health care systems following Public Health Service (PHS) guidelines

- 3.9.1 Proportion of health care providers and health care systems that have fully implemented the Public Health Service (PHS) guidelines
- 3.9.2 Proportion of adults who have been asked by a health care professional about smoking
- 3.9.3 Proportion of smokers who have been advised to quit smoking by a health care professional
- 3.9.4 Proportion of smokers who have been assessed regarding their willingness to make a quit attempt by a health care professional
- 3.9.5 Proportion of smokers who have been assisted in quitting smoking by a health care professional
- 3.9.6 Proportion of smokers for whom a health care professional has arranged for follow-up contact regarding a quit attempt
- 3.9.7 Proportion of pregnant women who report that a health care professional advised them to quit smoking during a prenatal visit
- 3.9.8 Proportion of health care systems that have provider-reminder systems in place

Outcome 10: Increased insurance coverage for cessation services

- 3.10.1 Proportion of insurance purchasers and payers that reimburse for tobacco cessation services

Intermediate Outcomes

Outcome 11: Increased number of quit attempts and quit attempts using proven cessation methods

- 3.11.1 Proportion of adult smokers who have made a quit attempt
- 3.11.2 Proportion of young smokers who have made a quit attempt
- 3.11.3 Proportion of adult and young smokers who have made a quit attempt using proven cessation methods

Outcome 12: Increased price of tobacco products

- 3.12.1 Amount of tobacco product excise tax

Long-term Outcomes

■ Outcome 13: Increased cessation among adults and young people

- **3.13.1** Proportion of smokers who have sustained abstinence from tobacco use
- **3.13.2**[NR] Proportion of recent successful quit attempts

■ Outcome 14: Reduced tobacco-use prevalence and consumption

- **3.14.1** Smoking prevalence
- **3.14.2** Prevalence of tobacco use during pregnancy
- **3.14.3** Prevalence of postpartum tobacco use
- **3.14.4** Per capita consumption of tobacco products

Outcome 7

Establishment or Increased Use of Cessation Services

Tobacco is highly addictive.[1] Although it is possible to quit without help, evidence shows that the chance of success is much higher with the use of support services.[2] State-supported telephone quitlines overcome many of the barriers to smoking cessation classes because they are free and available at smokers' convenience.[2] They also bring services to smokers in areas that have few resources. Group cessation programs and workplace cessation programs also improve the likelihood of success. Integrated services—which link quitlines, provider services, workplace cessation initiatives, and approved pharmacotherapies—offer smokers several help options and lead to greater use of cessation services and more success.[3]

Listed below are the indicators associated with this outcome:

- 3.7.1   Number of callers to telephone quitlines
- 3.7.2[NR]   Number of calls to telephone quitlines from users who heard about the quitline through a media campaign
- 3.7.3   Number of calls to telephone quitlines from users who heard about the quitline through a source other than a media campaign
- 3.7.4   Proportion of smokers who have used group cessation programs
- 3.7.5   Proportion of health care systems with telephone quitlines or contracts with state quitlines
- 3.7.6   Proportion of worksites with a cessation program or a contract with a quitline

References

1. U.S. Department of Health and Human Services. *Reducing tobacco use: a report of the Surgeon General.* Atlanta, GA: Centers for Disease Control and Prevention; 2000.

2. Task Force on Community Preventive Services. The guide to community preventive services: tobacco use prevention and control. *American Journal of Preventive Medicine.* 2001;20(Suppl 2):1–88.

3. Fiore MC, Bailey WC, Cohen SJ, Dorfman S, Goldstein M, Gritz E, Heyman RB, Jaén CR, Kottke TE, Lando HA, Mecklenburg RE, Mullen PD, Nett LM, Robinson L, Stitzer ML, Tommasello AC, Villejo L, Wewers ME. *Treating tobacco use and dependence: clinical practice guideline.* Rockville, MD: U.S. Department of Health and Human Services; 2000.

For Further Reading

Abt Associates. *Independent evaluation of the Massachusetts tobacco control program. 6th annual report.* Cambridge, MA: Abt Associates; 1994.

Campion P, Owen L, McNeill A, McGuire C. Evaluation of a mass media campaign on smoking and pregnancy. *Addiction.* 1994;89(10):1245–54.

Cummings KM, Sciandra R, Davis S, Rimer BK. Results of an antismoking media campaign utilizing the cancer information service. *Journal of the National Cancer Institute. Monographs.* 1993;(14):113–8.

Kozlowski LT, Goldberg ME, Sweeney CT, Palmer RF, Pillitteri JL, Yost BA, White EL, Stine MM. Smoker reactions to a "radio message" that Light cigarettes are as dangerous as Regular cigarettes. *Nicotine and Tobacco Research.* 1999;1(1):67–76.

Lichtenstein E, Glasgow RE, Lando HA, Ossip-Klein DJ, Boles SM. Telephone counseling for smoking cessation: rationales and meta-analytic review of evidence. *Health Education Research.* 1996;11(2):243–57.

National Cancer Institute. Changing adolescent smoking prevalence: where it is and why. *Smoking and Tobacco Control Monograph No. 14.* Bethesda, MD: National Cancer Institute; 2001. NIH Publication No. 02-5086.

National Cancer Institute. Population-based smoking cessation: proceedings of a conference on What Works to Influence Cessation in the General Population. *Smoking and Tobacco Control Monograph No. 12.* Bethesda, MD: National Cancer Institute; 2000. NIH Publication No. 00-4892.

Owen L. Impact of a telephone helpline for smokers who called during a mass media campaign. *Tobacco Control.* 2000;9(2):148–54.

Pierce JP, Anderson DM, Romano RM, Meissner HI, Odenkirchen JC. Promoting smoking cessation in the United States: effect of public service announcements on the Cancer Information Service telephone line. *Journal of the National Cancer Institute.* 1992;84(9):677–83.

Platt S, Tannahill A, Watson J, Fraser E. Effectiveness of antismoking telephone helpline: follow up survey. *British Medical Journal.* 1997;314(7091):1371–5.

Popham WJ, Potter LD, Bal DG, Johnson MD, Duerr JM, Quinn V. Do anti-smoking media campaigns help smokers quit? *Public Health Reports.* 1993;108(4):510–3.

Sly DF, Heald GR, Ray S. The Florida "truth" anti-tobacco media evaluation: design, first year results, and implications for planning future state media evaluations. *Tobacco Control.* 2001;10(1):9–15.

Wakefield M, Borland R. Saved by the bell: the role of telephone helpline services in the context of mass-media anti-smoking campaigns. *Tobacco Control.* 2000;9(2):117–9.

Warner KE. Effects of the antismoking campaign: an update. *American Journal of Public Health.* 1989;79(2):144–51.

Zhu S, Rosbrook B, Anderson CM, Gilpin E, Sadler GP. The demographics of help-seeking for smoking cessation in California and the role of the California Smoker's Helpline. *Tobacco Control.* 1995;4(1):9–15.

Zhu SH, Anderson CM, Johnson CE, Tedeschi G, Roeseler A. A centralised telephone service for tobacco cessation: the California experience. *Tobacco Control.* 2000;9(Suppl 2):ii48–55.

Zucker D, Hopkins RS, Sly DF, Urich J, Kershaw JM, Solari S. Florida's "truth" campaign: a counter-marketing, anti-tobacco media campaign. *Journal of Public Health Management and Practice.* 2000;6(3):1–6.

Outcome 7

Establishment or Increased Use of Cessation Services

Indicator Rating
← ○ ◐ ● ● → better

Number	Indicator	Overall quality low ←——→ high	Resources needed	Strength of evaluation evidence	Utility	Face validity	Accepted practice
3.7.1	Number of callers to telephone quitlines	▬▬▬▬▬	$$	●	●	●	●
3.7.2[NR]	Number of calls to telephone quitlines from users who heard about the quitline through a media campaign	▬▬▬▬▬	⊘	⊘	⊘	⊘	⊘
3.7.3	Number of calls to telephone quitlines from users who heard about the quitline through a source other than a media campaign	▬▬▬▬▬	$$	◐	◐	◐	◐
3.7.4	Proportion of smokers who have used group cessation programs	▬▬▬▬▬	$$	●	◐	◐	◐
3.7.5	Proportion of health care systems with telephone quitlines or contracts with state quitlines	▬▬▬▬▬†	$$$†	●	○	●	●
3.7.6	Proportion of worksites with a cessation program or a contract with a quitline	▬▬▬▬▬	$$$	⊘	●	●	●

† Denotes low agreement among reviewers: that is, fewer than 75% of the valid ratings for this indicator were within one point of each other (see Appendix B for an explanation).
⊘ Denotes no data.
[NR] Denotes an indicator that is not rated (see Appendix B for an explanation).

Indicator 3.7.1

Number of Callers to Telephone Quitlines

Goal area 3	Promoting quitting among adults and young people
Outcome 7	Establishment or increased use of cessation services
What to measure	The number of calls to telephone-based tobacco use cessation services
Why this indicator is useful	Evidence shows that telephone quitlines are an effective method of increasing tobacco cessation.[1-5] Quit rates among users of the California quitline were twice as high as among those who used self-help methods alone.[3] Quitlines can reach large numbers of smokers and services can be provided in multiple languages.[6]
Example data source(s)	Quitline call monitoring
Population group(s)	Quitline telephone callers
Example survey question(s)	Not applicable. This indicator is best measured by tracking calls to telephone quitlines.
Comments	Evaluators may also want to collect information about the proportion of smokers in the state who have received counseling from the quitline.
	Multiple types of information (e.g., caller demographics and location, call variability by month and time of day, and client satisfaction with quitline services) can be tracked through quitline monitoring.
	Additional information about quitline monitoring is available through the North American Quitline Consortium at: http://naquitline.org.
	For more information on how to collect data on this indicator, see references 7 and 8 below.

Rating

Overall quality low ⟵⟶ high	Resources needed	Strength of evaluation evidence	Utility	Face validity	Accepted practice
(high)	$$	●	●	●	●

⟵ ○ ◯ ● ● ⟶ better

References

1. Fiore MC, Bailey WC, Cohen SJ, Dorfman SF, Goldstein MG, Gritz EG, Heyman RB, Jaén CR, Kottke TE, Lando HA, Mecklenburg RE, Mullen PD, Nett LM, Robinson L, Stitzer ML, Tommasello AC, Villejo L, Wewers ME. *Treating tobacco use and dependence: clinical practice guideline.* Rockville, MD: U.S. Department of Health and Human Services; 2000.
2. Stead LF, Lancaster T, Perera R. Telephone counselling for smoking cessation. *Cochrane Database of Systematic Reviews.* 2003;(1):CD002850.
3. Zhu SH, Anderson CM, Tedeschi GJ, Rosbrook B, Johnson CE, Byrd M, Gutierrez-Terrell E. Evidence of real-world effectiveness of a telephone quitline for smokers. *New England Journal of Medicine.* 2002;347(14):1087–93.
4. Task Force on Community Preventive Services. The guide to community preventive services: tobacco use prevention and control. *American Journal of Preventive Medicine.* 2001;20(Suppl 2):1–88.

References (cont.)

5. National Cancer Institute. Population-based smoking cessation: proceedings of a conference on What Works to Influence Cessation in the General Population. *Smoking and Tobacco Control Monograph No. 12.* Bethesda, MD: National Cancer Institute; 2000. NIH Publication No. 00-4892.
6. Prout MN, Martinez O, Ballas J, Geller AC, Lash TL, Brooks D, Heeren T. Who uses the Smoker's Quitline in Massachusetts? *Tobacco Control.* 2002;11(Suppl 2):ii74–5.
7. Centers for Disease Control and Prevention. *Telephone quitlines: a resource for development, implementation, and evaluation.* Atlanta, GA: Centers for Disease Control and Prevention; 2004.
8. Miller CL, Wakefield M, Roberts L. Uptake and effectiveness of the Australian telephone quitline service in the context of a mass media campaign. *Tobacco Control.* 2003;12(Suppl 2):ii53–8.

GOAL AREA 3
Outcome 7

Indicator 3.7.2[NR]

Number of Calls to Telephone Quitlines from Users Who Heard About the Quitline Through a Media Campaign

Goal area 3	Promoting quitting among adults and young people
Outcome 7	Establishment or increased use of cessation services
What to measure	The number of calls to telephone-based tobacco use cessation services from people who heard about the service through a media campaign
Why this indicator is useful	Media programs are a cost efficient way to promote cessation services because media advertisements can promote a single telephone number and broadcast it across a wide area.[1,2] Quitline media campaigns can be a cost-effective method to promote both state and local cessation programs because quitlines can also refer callers to local programs as appropriate.[1,2]
Example data source(s)	Quitline call monitoring
Population group(s)	Quitline telephone callers
Example survey question(s)	Not applicable. This indicator is best measured by tracking calls to telephone quitlines.
Comments	Evaluators may also want to collect information about the proportion of smokers in the state who received counseling from the quitline.
	Multiple types of information (e.g., caller demographics and location, call variability by month and time of day, and client satisfaction with quitline services) can be tracked through quitline monitoring.
	Additional information on quitline monitoring is also available through the North American Quitline Consortium at: http://naquitline.org.

Rating

Overall quality low ◄——► high	Resources needed	Strength of evaluation evidence	Utility	Face validity	Accepted practice
▬▬▬▬▬	⊘	⊘	⊘	⊘	⊘

◄–○–◔–●–●–► better

⊘ Denotes no data.

[NR] Denotes an indicator that is not rated (see Appendix B for an explanation).

References
1. Centers for Disease Control and Prevention. *Telephone quitlines: a resource for development, implementation, and evaluation.* Atlanta, GA: Centers for Disease Control and Prevention; 2004.
2. The World Bank. *Tobacco quitlines: at a glance.* Washington, DC: The World Bank; 2002. Available from: http://wbln0018.worldbank.org/HDNet/hddocs.nsf/vtlw/7de69862c4402da485256ea1004e73b2 or http://www.cdc.gov/tobacco/quit/CRC/TobaccoQuitlineataGlance.pdf. Accessed March 2005.

Indicator 3.7.3

Number of Calls to Telephone Quitlines from Users Who Heard About the Quitline Through a Source Other Than a Media Campaign

Goal area 3	Promoting quitting among adults and young people
Outcome 7	Establishment or increased use of cessation services
What to measure	The number of calls to a telephone-based tobacco use cessation service from people who heard about the service through sources other than media campaigns, including workplaces, community programs, and health care providers
Why this indicator is useful	Integrating multiple cessation services is an important way of increasing the use of these services.[1,2] The use of telephone quitlines can be increased by promoting them through workplaces, mass media, public insurers (e.g., Medicaid), and health care providers.[2]
Example data source(s)	Quitline call monitoring
Population group(s)	Quitline telephone callers
Example survey question(s)	Not applicable. This indicator is best measured by tracking calls to telephone quitlines.
Comments	Evaluators may also want to collect information about the proportion of smokers in the state who received counseling from the quitline.
	Multiple types of information (e.g., caller demographics and location, call variability by month and time of day, and client satisfaction with quitline services) can be tracked through quitline monitoring.
	Additional information about quitline monitoring is available through the North American Quitline Consortium at: http://naquitline.org.
	For more information on how to collect data on this indicator, see references 2 and 3 below.

Rating

Overall quality low ← → high	Resources needed	Strength of evaluation evidence	Utility	Face validity	Accepted practice
▬▬▬▬▬	$$	●	●	●	●

← ○ ◐ ● ● → better

References
1. The Pacific Center on Health & Tobacco. *Linking a network: integrate quitlines with health care systems.* Portland, OR: The Pacific Center on Health & Tobacco; 2003. Available from: http://www.paccenter.org/pages/pub_reports.htm. Accessed March 2005.
2. Centers for Disease Control and Prevention. *Telephone quitlines: a resource for development, implementation, and evaluation.* Atlanta, GA: Centers for Disease Control and Prevention; 2004.
3. Miller CL, Wakefield M, Roberts L. Uptake and effectiveness of the Australian telephone quitline service in the context of a mass media campaign. *Tobacco Control.* 2003;12(Suppl 2):ii53–8.

GOAL AREA 3
Outcome 7

Indicator 3.7.4

Proportion of Smokers Who Have Used Group Cessation Programs

Goal area 3	Promoting quitting among adults and young people
Outcome 7	Establishment or increased use of cessation services
What to measure	Proportion of smokers who report using a group cessation service or program (e.g., stop-smoking classes or group counseling)
Why this indicator is useful	Evidence shows that group cessation programs are effective in increasing tobacco use cessation.[1] For example, studies have shown that the quit rates of people who attended group programs were significantly higher than the quit rates of control subjects who did not attend group programs.[2]
Example data source(s)	Adult Tobacco Survey (ATS): CDC Recommended Questions: Supplemental Section C: Cessation, 2003
Population group(s)	Smokers aged 18 years or older

Example survey question(s)

From ATS

The last time you tried to quit smoking, did you use any other assistance such as classes or counseling?
☐ Yes ☐ No ☐ Don't know/Not sure ☐ Refused

If respondent answers "yes," ask the following question for each option below:
Did you use:

	Yes	No	Don't know / Not sure	Refused
1. A stop-smoking clinic or class?	☐	☐	☐	☐
2. A telephone quitline?	☐	☐	☐	☐
3. One-on-one counseling from a doctor or nurse?	☐	☐	☐	☐
4. Self-help material, books, or videos?	☐	☐	☐	☐
5. Acupuncture?	☐	☐	☐	☐
6. Hypnosis?	☐	☐	☐	☐
7. Did you use anything else to help you quit?	☐	☐	☐	☐

Comments

The example survey questions could also be asked of young smokers.

Evaluators might want to collect information on the proportion of smokers in the state who have used group cessation programs.

Rating

Overall quality low ◄——► high	Resources needed	Strength of evaluation evidence	Utility	Face validity	Accepted practice
▬▬▬▬	$$	●	●	●	●

◄ ○ ◐ ● ● ► better

References
1. Fiore MC, Bailey WC, Cohen SJ, Dorfman SF, Goldstein MG, Gritz EG, Heyman RB, Jaén CR, Kottke TE, Lando HA, Mecklenburg RE, Mullen PD, Nett LM, Robinson L, Stitzer ML, Tommasello AC, Villejo L, Wewers ME. *Treating tobacco use and dependence: clinical practice guideline.* Rockville, MD: U.S. Department of Health and Human Services; 2000.
2. Stead LF, Lancaster T. Group behavior therapy programmes for smoking cessation. *Cochrane Database of Systematic Reviews.* 2002;(3):CD001007.

Indicator 3.7.5

Proportion of Health Care Systems with Telephone Quitlines or Contracts with State Quitlines

Goal area 3	Promoting quitting among adults and young people
Outcome 7	Establishment or increased use of cessation services
What to measure	Proportion of health care systems (e.g., managed care organizations) that include telephone quitlines in their tobacco cessation services
Why this indicator is useful	Not all states have statewide telephone quitlines, and in those that do, the quitlines are not always adequately funded to counsel all tobacco users in the state.[1-4] In these situations, health care systems can either contribute financially to the state quitline or develop a quitline for their own patients.
Example data source(s)	Addressing Tobacco in Managed Care (ATMC), Survey of Health Plans, 1997–1998
Population group(s)	Managed care or health care system administrators

Example survey question(s)

From ATMC

Which of the following cessation interventions are available in your plan, and which are included in your plan's formulary? [Mark all that apply.]

	Unavailable	Full coverage	Partial coverage	In formulary
1. Nicotine replacement therapy				
Over-the-counter	☐	☐	☐	☐
Prescription	☐	☐	☐	☐
Only with enrollment in cessation program	☐	☐	☐	☐
2. Buproprion (e.g., Zyban®)	☐	☐	☐	☐
3. Telephone counseling	☐	☐	☐	☐
4. Face-to-face counseling	☐	☐	☐	☐
5. Classes or group meeting	☐	☐	☐	☐
6. Self-help materials	☐	☐	☐	☐

Example questions

Does [your organization] operate a telephone quitline for smokers?
☐ Yes ☐ No ☐ Don't know

Does [your organization] inform beneficiaries about the state's telephone quitline?
☐ Yes ☐ No

Does [your organization] contribute to the financing of the state's telephone quitline?
☐ Yes ☐ No

Comments	For the second set of example questions, the authors modified questions from the State Medicaid Tobacco Dependence Treatment Survey, 2003. Information available from the Center for Health and Public Policy Studies, School of Public Health, University of California Berkeley.

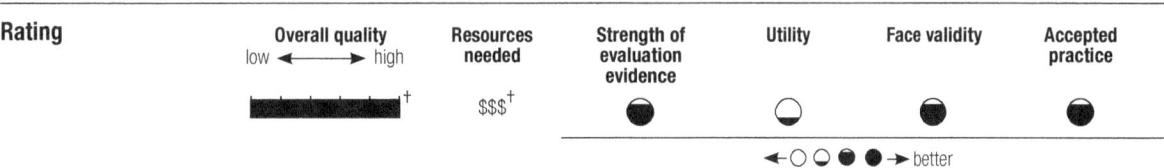

† Denotes low agreement among reviewers: that is, fewer than 75% of the valid ratings for this indicator were within one point of each other (see Appendix B for an explanation).

References
1. Centers for Disease Control and Prevention. *Telephone quitlines: a resource for development, implementation, and evaluation.* Atlanta, GA: Centers for Disease Control and Prevention; 2004.
2. The Pacific Center on Health & Tobacco. *Linking a network: integrate quitlines with health care systems.* Portland, OR: The Pacific Center on Health & Tobacco; 2003. Available from: http://www.paccenter.org/pages/pub_reports.htm. Accessed March 2005.
3. Task Force on Community Preventive Services. The guide to community preventive services: tobacco use prevention and control. *American Journal of Preventive Medicine.* 2001;20(Suppl 2):1–88.
4. Centers for Disease Control and Prevention. *Coverage for tobacco use cessation treatments.* Atlanta, GA: Centers for Disease Control and Prevention; 2004.

Indicator 3.7.6

Proportion of Worksites with a Cessation Program or a Contract with a Quitline

Goal area 3	Promoting quitting among adults and young people
Outcome 7	Establishment or increased use of cessation services
What to measure	Proportion of worksites that support a tobacco cessation program for employees
Why this indicator is useful	Like health care systems, employers can contribute financially to the state quitline in order to ensure access to these services for their employees.[1] Employers can also set up their own cessation programs, although the results to date from numerous worksite-based cessation projects suggest either no impact or a small net effect.[2]
Example data source(s)	Partnership for Prevention, Tobacco Survey: National Survey of Employer-sponsored Health Plans, 2002 Information available at: http://www.mercerhr.com
Population group(s)	Employers
Example survey question(s)	**From Partnership for Prevention, Tobacco Survey: National Survey of Employer-sponsored Health Plans** Which of the following tobacco/smoking cessation (tobacco/nicotine dependence) service(s) are offered at the worksite/outside of the health plan? *Check all that apply* ☐ Individual counseling (face-to-face) ☐ Group counseling (face-to-face) ☐ Telephone counseling (including referrals to quitlines) ☐ Self-help programs (such as brochures, videos, Internet support) ☐ Cessation treatment as part of prenatal care ☐ Prescription medications ☐ Over-the-counter medications ☐ Other (please specify)_____ ☐ No services covered ☐ Don't know
Comments	None

Rating

Overall quality low ←——→ high	Resources needed	Strength of evaluation evidence	Utility	Face validity	Accepted practice
▬▬▬▬▬	$$$	⊘	●	●	●

← ○ ◐ ● ● → better

⊘ Denotes no data.

References
1. The Pacific Center on Health & Tobacco. *Comprehensive statewide tobacco cessation.* Portland, OR: The Pacific Center on Health & Tobacco; 2003. Available from: http://www.paccenter.org/pages/pub_reports.htm. Accessed March 2005.
2. U.S. Department of Health and Human Services. *Reducing tobacco use: a report of the Surgeon General.* Atlanta, GA: Centers for Disease Control and Prevention; 2000.

Outcome 8

Increased Awareness, Knowledge, Intention to Quit, and Support for Policies That Support Cessation

Programs to encourage tobacco users to quit using tobacco start with activities to increase the number of smokers who intend to quit.[1] Increasing the number of smokers who intend to quit involves (1) providing tobacco users with the tools needed to quit successfully and (2) eliminating barriers to services that will help them to quit. Evidence shows that media campaigns increase tobacco cessation rates.[1] Evidence also shows that policies that encourage people to stop using tobacco (e.g., increasing the price of cigarettes or providing insurance coverage for cessation treatment) increase rates of successful cessation.[1]

Listed below are the indicators associated with this outcome:

- 3.8.1 Level of confirmed awareness of media campaign messages on the dangers of smoking and the benefits of cessation
- 3.8.2 Level of receptivity to anti-tobacco media messages on the dangers of smoking and the benefits of cessation
- 3.8.3 Proportion of smokers who intend to quit
- 3.8.4 Proportion of smokers who intend to quit smoking by using proven cessation methods
- 3.8.5 Level of support for increasing excise tax on tobacco products
- 3.8.6 Proportion of smokers who are aware of the cessation services available to them
- 3.8.7 Proportion of smokers who are aware of their insurance coverage for cessation treatment
- 3.8.8 Level of support for increasing insurance coverage for cessation treatment
- 3.8.9[NR] Proportion of employers who are aware of the benefits of providing coverage for cessation treatment

Reference

1. Task Force on Community Preventive Services. The guide to community preventive services: tobacco use prevention and control. *American Journal of Preventive Medicine.* 2001;20(Suppl 2):1–88.

For Further Reading

Commonwealth Department of Health and Aged Care. *Australia's National Tobacco Campaign: evaluation report volume one: every cigarette is doing you damage.* Canberra, Australia: Commonwealth Department of Health and Aged Care; 1999. Available from: http://www.health.gov.au/pubhlth/publicat/document/metadata/tobccamp.htm. Accessed March 2005.

Flay BR. Mass media and smoking cessation: a critical review. *American Journal of Public Health.* 1987;77(2):153–60.

Glantz SA, Begay ME. Tobacco industry campaign contributions are affecting tobacco control policymaking in California. *Journal of the American Medical Association.* 1994; 272(15):1176–82.

Halpern M, Warner K. Motivations for smoking cessation: a comparison of successful quitters and failures. *Journal of Substance Abuse.* 1993;5(3):247–56.

Haug NA, Stitzer ML, Svikis DS. Smoking during pregnancy and intention to quit: a profile of methadone-maintained women. *Nicotine and Tobacco Research.* 2001;3(4):333–9.

Heiser PF, Begay ME. The campaign to raise the tobacco tax in Massachusetts. *American Journal of Public Health.* 1997;87(6):968–73.

Hellman R, Cummings KM, Haughey BP, Zielezny MA, O'Shea RM. Predictors of attempting and succeeding at smoking cessation. *Health Education Research.* 1991;6(1):77–86.

National Cancer Institute. Population-based smoking cessation: proceedings of a conference on What Works to Influence Cessation in the General Population. *Smoking and Tobacco Control Monograph No. 12.* Bethesda, MD: National Cancer Institute; 2000. NIH Publication No. 00-4892.

Sussman S, Dent CW, Wang E, Cruz NT, Sanford D, Johnson CA. Participants and nonparticipants of a mass media self-help smoking cessation program. *Addictive Behaviors.* 1994;19(6):643–54.

Sussman S, Dent CW, Severson H, Burton D, Flay BR. Self-initiated quitting among adolescent smokers. *Preventive Medicine.* 1998;27(5 Pt 3):A19–28.

Wakefield M, Borland R. Saved by the bell: the role of telephone helpline services in the context of mass-media anti-smoking campaigns. *Tobacco Control.* 2000;9(2):117–9.

Zhu S, Rosbrook B, Anderson CM, Gilpin E, Sadler GPJ. The demographics of help-seeking for smoking cessation in California and the role of the California Smoker's Helpline. *Tobacco Control.* 1995;4(1):9–15.

Outcome 8

Increased Awareness, Knowledge, Intention to Quit, and Support for Policies That Support Cessation

Indicator Rating
← ○ ◐ ● ● → better

Number	Indicator	Overall quality (low → high)	Resources needed	Strength of evaluation evidence	Utility	Face validity	Accepted practice
3.8.1	Level of confirmed awareness of media campaign messages on the dangers of smoking and the benefits of cessation	▬▬▬▬	$$†	●	●	●	●
3.8.2	Level of receptivity to anti-tobacco media messages on the dangers of smoking and the benefits of cessation	▬▬▬	$$†	◐	●	●	●
3.8.3	Proportion of smokers who intend to quit	▬▬▬	$$†	●	●	●	●
3.8.4	Proportion of smokers who intend to quit smoking by using proven cessation methods	▬▬▬	$$$†	○	●	◐	●
3.8.5	Level of support for increasing excise tax on tobacco products	▬▬▬	$$†	◐	●	●	●
3.8.6	Proportion of smokers who are aware of the cessation services available to them	▬▬▬	$$	●	●	●	●
3.8.7	Proportion of smokers who are aware of their insurance coverage for cessation treatment	▬▬▬	$$$	⊘	●	●	●
3.8.8	Level of support for increasing insurance coverage for cessation treatment	▬▬▬	$$$	⊘	●	●	●
3.8.9[NR]	Proportion of employers who are aware of the benefits of providing coverage for cessation treatment	▬▬▬	⊘	⊘	⊘	⊘	⊘

† Denotes low agreement among reviewers: that is, fewer than 75% of the valid ratings for this indicator were within one point of each other (see Appendix B for an explanation).
⊘ Denotes no data.
[NR] Denotes an indicator that is not rated (see Appendix B for an explanation).

Indicator 3.8.1

Level of Confirmed Awareness of Media Campaign Messages on the Dangers of Smoking and the Benefits of Cessation

Goal area 3	Promoting quitting among adults and young people
Outcome 8	Increased awareness, knowledge, intention to quit, and support for policies that support cessation
What to measure	Proportion of the target population that can accurately recall a media message about the dangers of smoking and the benefits of cessation
Why this indicator is useful	Evaluators should measure exposure to media messages to confirm awareness of these messages by asking respondents to provide specific information about the messages.[1] Evidence shows that mass media campaigns are effective in increasing tobacco-use cessation.[1,2]
Example data source(s)	Legacy Media Tracking Survey (LMTS), 2003 Information available at: http://tobacco.rti.org/data/lmts.cfm
Population group(s)	Young people less than 18 years of age
Example survey question(s)	**From LMTS** Have you recently seen an anti-smoking or anti-tobacco ad on TV that shows _____? ☐ Yes ☐ Maybe, not sure ☐ No ☐ Refused to answer What happens in this ad? (DO NOT READ RESPONSE CATEGORIES.) _____ What do you think the main message of this ad was? _____
Comments	The example questions could also be asked of adults. Evaluators may want to categorize awareness of the medium (e.g., billboard, television, or print) through which respondents learned of the message. Programs may want to evaluate confirmed awareness of an advertisement by respondents' smoking status (current, former, or never) and addiction level (e.g., light, moderate, or heavy) because awareness levels may differ significantly among groups with different levels of addiction. Evaluators should work closely with countermarketing campaign managers to (1) develop a separate series of questions for each main media message and (2) coordinate data collection with the timing of the media campaign.

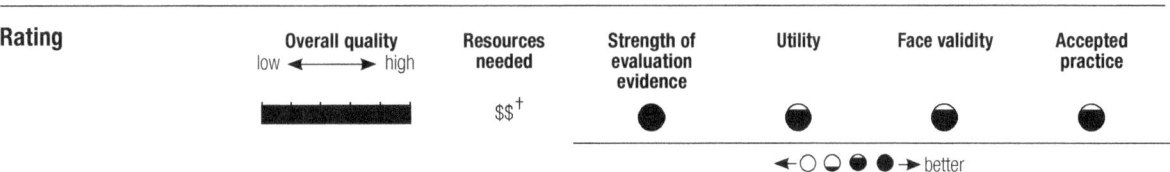

† Denotes low agreement among reviewers: that is, fewer than 75% of the valid ratings for this indicator were within one point of each other (see Appendix B for an explanation).

References
1. Sly DF, Heald GR, Ray S. The Florida "truth" anti-tobacco media evaluation: design, first year results, and implications for planning future state media evaluations. *Tobacco Control.* 2001;10(1):9–15.
2. Task Force on Community Preventive Services. The guide to community preventive services: tobacco use prevention and control. *American Journal of Preventive Medicine.* 2001;20(Suppl 2):1–88.

Indicator 3.8.2

Level of Receptivity to Anti-tobacco Media Messages on the Dangers of Smoking and the Benefits of Cessation

Goal area 3	Promoting quitting among adults and young people
Outcome 8	Increased awareness, knowledge, intention to quit, and support for policies that support cessation
What to measure	Level of receptivity to media messages by the intended audience. Receptivity is generally defined as the extent to which people are willing to listen to a persuasive message. In tobacco control evaluation, however, the definition is narrower; receptivity is the extent to which people believe that the message was convincing, made them think about their behavior, and stimulated discussion with others.[1]
Why this indicator is useful	Message awareness is necessary but not sufficient to change the knowledge, attitudes, and intentions of young people and adults. Media campaigns are effective only if their messages reach and resonate with the intended audience. A well-received message helps ensure campaign effectiveness.[2-5]
Example data source(s)	Legacy Media Tracking Survey (LMTS), 2003 Information available at: http://tobacco.rti.org/data/lmts.cfm
Population group(s)	Young people less than 18 years of age
Example survey question(s)	**From LMTS** Tell me how much you agree or disagree with the following statement: This ad is convincing. Would you say you: ☐ Strongly agree ☐ Agree ☐ Disagree ☐ Strongly disagree ☐ No opinion ☐ Don't know ☐ Refused Would you say the ad gave you good reasons not to smoke? ☐ Yes ☐ No ☐ Don't know ☐ Refused Did you talk to your friends about this ad? ☐ Yes ☐ No ☐ Don't know ☐ Refused
Comments	The example questions could also be asked of adults. Evaluators may want to assess the public's level of receptivity to anti-tobacco media campaigns that address (1) smoking during pregnancy and (2) telephone quitlines and other quitting strategies. Evaluators may want to assess media message receptivity by communication medium (e.g., television, print, or radio). Evaluators should work closely with countermarketing campaign managers to (1) develop a separate series of questions for each main media message and (2) coordinate data collection with the timing of the media campaign.

Rating

Overall quality low ⟷ high	Resources needed	Strength of evaluation evidence	Utility	Face validity	Accepted practice
▬▬▬▬▬	$$[†]	◐	◐	◐	●

◀─ ○ ◔ ◐ ● ─▶ better

† Denotes low agreement among reviewers: that is, fewer than 75% of the valid ratings for this indicator were within one point of each other (see Appendix B for an explanation).

References
1. Sly DF, Heald GR, Ray S. The Florida "truth" anti-tobacco media evaluation: design, first year results, and implications for planning future state media evaluations. *Tobacco Control.* 2001;10(1):9–15.
2. McGuire WJ. Public communication as a strategy for inducing health-promoting behavioral change. *Preventive Medicine.* 1984;13(3):299–319.
3. Kotler P, Armstrong G. *Principles of marketing,* 9th ed. Upper Saddle River, NJ: Prentice-Hall; 2001.
4. Carter WB. Health behavior as a rational process: theory of reasoned action and multiattribute utility theory. In: Glanz K, Lewis F, Rimer B, editors. *Health behavior and health education: theory, research, and practice.* San Francisco, CA: Jossey-Bass; 1990. pp. 63–91.
5. Maibach E, Parrott RL, editors. *Designing health messages: approaches from communication theory and public health practice.* Thousand Oaks, CA: Sage; 1995.

Indicator 3.8.3

Proportion of Smokers Who Intend to Quit

Goal area 3	Promoting quitting among adults and young people
Outcome 8	Increased awareness, knowledge, intention to quit, and support for policies that support cessation
What to measure	Proportion of smokers who are seriously considering stopping smoking
Why this indicator is useful	Evidence shows that intention to quit using tobacco is a strong predictor of actual quit attempts.[1,2]
Example data source(s)	▸ Adult Tobacco Survey (ATS): CDC Recommended Questions: Core, 2003 ▸ Youth Tobacco Survey (YTS): CDC Recommended Questions: Core, 2004
Population group(s)	▸ Smokers 18 years of age or older ▸ Smokers aged less than 18 years
Example survey question(s)	**From ATS** Are you seriously considering stopping smoking within the next 6 months? ☐ Yes ☐ No ☐ Don't know/Not sure ☐ Refused Are you planning to stop smoking within the next 30 days? ☐ Yes ☐ No ☐ Don't know/Not sure ☐ Refused **From YTS** Do you want to stop smoking cigarettes? ☐ I do not smoke now ☐ Yes ☐ No
Comments	None

Rating

Overall quality low ◀——▶ high	Resources needed	Strength of evaluation evidence	Utility	Face validity	Accepted practice
▬▬▬▬▬▬	$$[†]	●	●	◐	●

◀ ○ ◌ ● ● ▶ better

† Denotes low agreement among reviewers: that is, fewer than 75% of the valid ratings for this indicator were within one point of each other (see Appendix B for an explanation).

References
1. U.S. Department of Health and Human Services. *Reducing tobacco use: a report of the Surgeon General.* Atlanta, GA: Centers for Disease Control and Prevention; 2000.
2. Hellman R, Cummings KM, Haughey BP, Zielezny MA, O'Shea RM. Predictors of attempting and succeeding at smoking cessation. *Health Education Research.* 1991;6(1):77–86.

GOAL AREA 3
Outcome 8

Indicator 3.8.4

Proportion of Smokers Who Intend to Quit Smoking by Using Proven Cessation Methods

Goal area 3	Promoting quitting among adults and young people
Outcome 8	Increased awareness, knowledge, intention to quit, and support for policies that support cessation
What to measure	Proportion of smokers who report that they intend to quit smoking using proven cessation methods (FDA-approved pharmacotherapies, in-person individual counseling, counseling from telephone quitlines, or stop-smoking classes)
Why this indicator is useful	Approximately 46% of smokers attempt to quit each year in the United States, but only about 5% of those attempting to quit are still abstinent 1 year later.[1] The use of proven cessation strategies—such as FDA-approved pharmacotherapies, counseling, and telephone quitlines—improves the chances of a successful quit attempt.[1]
Example data source(s)	No commonly used data sources were found
Population group(s)	Smokers 18 years of age or older Smokers aged less than 18 years
Example survey question(s)	Do you intend to quit smoking in the next 30 days? ☐ Yes ☐ No ☐ Don't know/Not sure ☐ Refused to answer *If yes to above, then ask:* Which of the following cessation methods do you intend to use? ☐ Call a quitline ☐ See a physician ☐ Join a cessation program ☐ Use a nicotine patch, gum, nasal spray, inhaler, lozenge, or tablet ☐ Use a prescription pill, such as Zyban, Buproprion, or Wellbutrin ☐ Quit with a friend, relative, or acquaintance ☐ Other methods ☐ Quit on your own
Comments	The authors created these example questions. They are not in any commonly used data source. Evaluators may want to assess smokers' intention to quit by respondents' tobacco use (current, former, or never) and addiction level (e.g., light, moderate, or heavy) because awareness levels may differ significantly among groups with different levels of addiction. Addiction levels are often inversely related to strength of intention to quit.

Rating

Overall quality low ◄──────► high	Resources needed	Strength of evaluation evidence	Utility	Face validity	Accepted practice
■■■■■■■■■	$$$[†]	○	●	◐	●

◄ ○ ◐ ● ● → better

[†] Denotes low agreement among reviewers: that is, fewer than 75% of the valid ratings for this indicator were within one point of each other (see Appendix B for an explanation).

Reference

1. Fiore MC, Bailey WC, Cohen SJ, Dorfman SF, Goldstein MG, Gritz EG, Heyman RB, Jaén CR, Kottke TE, Lando HA, Mecklenburg RE, Mullen PD, Nett LM, Robinson L, Stitzer ML, Tommasello AC, Villejo L, Wewers ME. *Treating tobacco use and dependence: clinical practice guideline.* Rockville, MD: U.S. Department of Health and Human Services; 2000.

Indicator 3.8.5

Level of Support for Increasing Excise Tax on Tobacco Products

Goal area 3	Promoting quitting among adults and young people
Outcome 8	Increased awareness, knowledge, intention to quit, and support for policies that support cessation
What to measure	Proportion of the population that supports an increase in excise tax on cigarettes and the amount of tax increase they support
Why this indicator is useful	Public opinion is a major determinant of the feasibility of enacting an excise tax increase on tobacco products. Tobacco policies are unlikely to be adopted without support among business owners, policy makers, and the general public.[1-4] Measuring policy makers' support for a tax increase will also assess their willingness to support legislation for a tax increase.[5]
Example data source(s)	Adult Tobacco Survey (ATS): CDC Recommended Questions: Supplemental Section F: Policy Issues, 2003
Population group(s)	Adults aged 18 years or older
Example survey question(s)	**From ATS** How much additional tax on a pack of cigarettes would you be willing to support if some or all the money raised was used to support tobacco control programs? ☐ More than two dollars a pack ☐ Less than fifty cents a pack ☐ Two dollars a pack ☐ No tax increase ☐ One dollar a pack ☐ Don't know/Not sure ☐ Fifty to ninety-nine cents a pack ☐ Refused
Comments	The example question could be asked of decision makers or opinion leaders. Evaluators may want to analyze the level of support for increasing an excise tax on tobacco products according to the smoking status of the respondent. To gather more complete data on tobacco use, evaluators can also ask questions about the use of other tobacco products such as spit tobacco (smokeless), bidis, small cigars, and loose tobacco (roll-your-own).

Rating

Overall quality low ⟵⟶ high	Resources needed	Strength of evaluation evidence	Utility	Face validity	Accepted practice
▬▬▬▬▬	$$†	○	●	◐	●

⟵ ○ ◐ ● ● ⟶ better

† Denotes low agreement among reviewers: that is, fewer than 75% of the valid ratings for this indicator were within one point of each other (see Appendix B for an explanation).

References
1. U.S. Department of Health and Human Services. *Reducing tobacco use: a report of the Surgeon General.* Atlanta, GA: Centers for Disease Control and Prevention; 2000.
2. U.S. Department of Health and Human Services. *Women and smoking: a report of the Surgeon General.* Rockville, MD: U.S. Department of Health and Human Services, Public Health Service, Office of the Surgeon General; 2001.
3. Thomson GW, Wilson N. Public attitudes about tobacco smoke in workplaces: the importance of workers' rights in survey questions. *Tobacco Control.* 2004;13(2):206–7.
4. Howard KA, Rogers T, Howard-Pitney B, Flora JA, Norman GJ, Ribisl KM. Opinion leaders' support for tobacco control policies and participation in tobacco control activities. *American Journal of Public Health.* 2000;90(8):1283–7.
5. O'Connell P. Tobacco control in the land of the golden leaf: has political perception kept pace with reality? *North Carolina Medical Journal.* 2002;63(3):175–6.

GOAL AREA 3
Outcome 8

Indicator 3.8.6

Proportion of Smokers Who Are Aware of the Cessation Services Available to Them

Goal area 3	Promoting quitting among adults and young people
Outcome 8	Increased awareness, knowledge, intention to quit, and support for policies that support cessation
What to measure	Proportion of smokers who know about available cessation services, such as individual counseling (face-to-face), group counseling (face-to-face), telephone counseling, self-help programs (such as brochures, videos, and Internet support), on-site treatment, follow-up counseling, and FDA-approved pharmacotherapies[1-3]
Why this indicator is useful	An increase in the availability of cessation services will not have an effect if tobacco users do not learn about these services.[2-5]
Example data source(s)	Adult Tobacco Survey (ATS): CDC Recommended Questions: Supplemental Section C : Cessation, 2003
Population group(s)	Smokers aged 18 years or older
Example survey question(s)	**From ATS** Are you aware of assistance that might be available to help you quit smoking, such as telephone quitlines, local health clinic services? ☐ Yes ☐ No ☐ Don't know/Not sure ☐ Refused
Comments	The example survey question could be modified to include a more expansive list of cessation services. The example survey question could be asked of young people.
Rating	Overall quality: low ◄──► high — filled bar Resources needed: $$ Strength of evaluation evidence: ● Utility: ● Face validity: ● Accepted practice: ● ◄ ○ ◐ ● ● ► better

References

1. McMenamin SB, Halpin HA, Ibrahim JK, Orleans CT. Physician and enrollee knowledge of Medicaid coverage for tobacco-dependence treatments. *American Journal of Preventive Medicine.* 2004;26(2):99–104.
2. Schauffler HH, Barker DC, Orleans CT. Medicaid coverage for tobacco-dependence treatments. *Health Affairs.* 2001;20(1):298–303.
3. Centers for Disease Control and Prevention. *Coverage for tobacco use cessation treatments.* Atlanta, GA: Centers for Disease Control and Prevention; 2004.
4. Miller CL, Wakefield M, Roberts L. Uptake and effectiveness of the Australian telephone quitline service in the context of a mass media campaign. *Tobacco Control.* 2003;12(Suppl 2):ii53–8.
5. The Pacific Center on Health & Tobacco. *Linking a network: integrate quitlines with health care systems.* Portland, OR: The Pacific Center on Health & Tobacco: 2003. Available from: http://www.paccenter.org/pages/pub_reports.htm. Accessed March 2005.

Indicator 3.8.7

Proportion of Smokers Who Are Aware of Their Insurance Coverage for Cessation Treatment

Goal area 3	Promoting quitting among adults and young people
Outcome 8	Increased awareness, knowledge, intention to quit, and support for policies that support cessation
What to measure	Proportion of smokers who know whether their insurance coverage includes smoking cessation treatments. Such coverage could include individual counseling (face-to-face), group counseling (face-to-face), telephone counseling, self-help programs (such as brochures, videos, and Internet support), on-site treatment, follow-up counseling, and all types of FDA-approved pharmacotherapies.[1-3]
Why this indicator is useful	Insurance coverage lowers barriers to cessation services if tobacco users know about the coverage. Increased awareness of the cessation services that are covered by insurers may lead to greater use of these services.[3]
Example data source(s)	American Smoking and Health Survey (ASHES), 2003 Information available at: http://tobacco.rti.org/data/New/surveys.cfm
Population group(s)	Smokers aged 18 years or older
Example survey question(s)	**From ASHES** Does any of your health insurance include coverage for treatment to quit smoking cigarettes or to stop using other tobacco products? ☐ Yes ☐ No ☐ Don't know/Not sure ☐ Refused
Comments	Evaluators may want to assess awareness of the specific types of cessation treatments covered rather than awareness of cessation treatment coverage in general.

Rating

Overall quality low ⟵⟶ high	Resources needed	Strength of evaluation evidence	Utility	Face validity	Accepted practice
▬▬▬▬	$$$	⊘	●	●	●

⟵ ○ ◐ ◉ ● ⟶ better

⊘ Denotes no data.

References
1. McMenamin SB, Halpin HA, Ibrahim JK, Orleans CT. Physician and enrollee knowledge of Medicaid coverage for tobacco-dependence treatments. *American Journal of Preventive Medicine.* 2004;26(2):99–104.
2. Schauffler HH, Barker DC, Orleans CT. Medicaid coverage for tobacco-dependence treatments. *Health Affairs.* 2001;20(1):298–303.
3. Centers for Disease Control and Prevention. *Coverage for tobacco use cessation treatments.* Atlanta, GA: Centers for Disease Control and Prevention; 2004.

GOAL AREA 3
Outcome 8

Indicator 3.8.8

Level of Support for Increasing Insurance Coverage for Cessation Treatment

Goal area 3	Promoting quitting among adults and young people
Outcome 8	Increased awareness, knowledge, intention to quit, and support for policies that support cessation
What to measure	Proportion of decision makers or opinion leaders who support increasing health care coverage to include proven behavioral and pharmacologic treatments that help people stop smoking
Why this indicator is useful	Studies show that the number of managed care organizations offering even partial coverage of cessation services is still low.[1] Measuring decision maker support for increasing insurance coverage of cessation treatment may assist with efforts to improve coverage.[2]
Example data source(s)	Decision Maker or Opinion Leader Survey
Population group(s)	Decision makers
Example survey question(s)	Proven therapies for treatment of tobacco dependence should be covered by health insurance plans. Do you… ☐ Strongly agree ☐ Agree ☐ Disagree ☐ Strongly disagree
Comments	The authors created this example question. It is not in any commonly used data source. This example question could be asked of adults in the general population.

Rating

Overall quality low ⟷ high	Resources needed	Strength of evaluation evidence	Utility	Face validity	Accepted practice
▬▬▬▬	$$$	⊘	●	●	●

←○◐●●→ better

⊘ Denotes no data.

References
1. McPhillips-Tangum C. Results from the first annual survey on addressing tobacco in managed care. *Tobacco Control.* 1998;7(Suppl):S11–3.
2. Centers for Disease Control and Prevention. *Coverage for tobacco use cessation treatments.* Atlanta, GA: Centers for Disease Control and Prevention; 2004.

Indicator 3.8.9[NR]

Proportion of Employers Who Are Aware of the Benefits of Providing Coverage for Cessation Treatment

Goal area 3	Promoting quitting among adults and young people
Outcome 8	Increased awareness, knowledge, intention to quit, and support for policies that support cessation
What to measure	Proportion of employers or other group insurance purchasers (e.g., purchasing coalitions) that are aware of the benefits (e.g., improved employee health and greater employee productivity) of providing insurance coverage for proven behavioral and pharmacologic treatments that help people stop smoking
Why this indicator is useful	If purchasers of group insurance packages are aware of the direct benefits of providing coverage for tobacco dependence treatments, they may demand such coverage.[1]
Example data source(s)	No commonly used data sources were found
Population group(s)	Employers
Example survey question(s)	Health plan coverage that includes proven therapies for tobacco cessation lead to improved employee heath. Do you… ☐ Strongly agree ☐ Agree ☐ Disagree ☐ Strongly disagree Health plan coverage that includes proven therapies for tobacco cessation lead to greater employee productivity. Do you… ☐ Strongly agree ☐ Agree ☐ Disagree ☐ Strongly disagree
Comments	The authors created these example questions. They are not in any commonly used data source. This indicator was not rated by the panel of experts, and therefore no rating information is available. See Appendix B for an explanation.
Rating	Overall quality (low → high): — ; Resources needed: no data; Strength of evaluation evidence: no data; Utility: no data; Face validity: no data; Accepted practice: no data ← ○ ◐ ● ● → better ⊘ Denotes no data.

[NR] Denotes an indicator that is not rated (see Appendix B for an explanation).

Reference
1. Centers for Disease Control and Prevention. *Coverage for tobacco use cessation treatments.* Atlanta, GA: Centers for Disease Control and Prevention; 2004.

Outcome 9

Increase in the Number of Health Care Providers and Health Care Systems Following Public Health Service (PHS) Guidelines

The Clinical Practice Guideline: Treating Tobacco Use and Dependence was produced by a consortium of experts charged with "identifying effective, experimentally validated, tobacco-dependence treatment and practices."[1] To ensure that the *Guideline* would be based on the best evidence available, the experts reviewed approximately 6,000 scientific publications on how health care providers and health care systems can reduce tobacco use. Given that many tobacco users visit a primary care clinician each year, it is important that clinicians be prepared to intervene with tobacco users who are willing to quit. The five major steps (the "5 A's") to intervention include asking the patient if he or she uses tobacco, advising him or her to quit, assessing the patient's willingness to make a quit attempt, assisting him or her in making a quit attempt, and arranging for follow-up contact to prevent relapse.[1] Evidence shows that cessation counseling and FDA-approved pharmacotherapies contribute to increases in quit rates. In addition, evidence is strong that institutionalizing cessation counseling in health care settings leads to an increase in the number of patients who quit smoking.[1]

Listed below are the indicators associated with this outcome:

3.9.1   Proportion of health care providers and health care systems that have fully implemented the Public Health Service (PHS) guidelines

3.9.2   Proportion of adults who have been asked by a health care professional about smoking

3.9.3   Proportion of smokers who have been advised to quit smoking by a health care professional

3.9.4   Proportion of smokers who have been assessed regarding their willingness to make a quit attempt by a health care professional

3.9.5   Proportion of smokers who have been assisted in quitting smoking by a health care professional

3.9.6   Proportion of smokers for whom a health care professional has arranged for follow-up contact regarding a quit attempt

3.9.7   Proportion of pregnant women who report that a health care professional advised them to quit smoking during a prenatal visit

3.9.8   Proportion of health care systems that have provider-reminder systems in place

Reference

1. Fiore MC, Bailey WC, Cohen SJ, Dorfman S, Goldstein M, Gritz E, Heyman RB, Jaén CR, Kottke TE, Lando HA, Mecklenburg RE, Mullen PD, Nett LM, Robinson L, Stitzer ML, Tommasello AC, Villejo L, Wewers ME. *Treating tobacco use and dependence: clinical practice guideline.* Rockville, MD: U.S. Department of Health and Human Services; 2000.

For Further Reading

Barker DC, Robinson LA, Rosenthal AC. A survey of managed care strategies for pregnant smokers. *Tobacco Control.* 2000;9(Suppl 3):iii46–50.

Borland R, Segan CJ, Livingston PM, Owen N. The effectiveness of callback counseling for smoking cessation: a randomized trial. *Addiction.* 2001;96(6):881–9.

Campion P, Owen L, McNeill A, McGuire C. Evaluation of a mass media campaign on smoking and pregnancy. *Addiction.* 1994;89(10):1245–54.

Commonwealth Department of Health and Aged Care. *Australia's National Tobacco Campaign: evaluation report volume one: every cigarette is doing you damage.* Canberra, Australia: Commonwealth Department of Health and Aged Care; 1999. Available from: http://www.health.gov.au/pubhlth/publicat/document/metadata/tobccamp.htm. Accessed March 2005.

Glasgow RE, Hollis JF, McRae SG, Lando HA, LaChance P. Providing an integrated program of low intensity tobacco cessation services in a health maintenance organization. *Health Education Research.* 1991;6(1):87–99.

Halpin Schauffler H, Mordavsky JK, McMenamin S. Adoption of the AHCPR clinical practice guideline for smoking cessation: a survey of California's HMOs. *American Journal of Preventive Medicine.* 2001;21(3):153–61.

Lichtenstein E, Glasgow RE, Lando HA, Ossip-Klein DJ, Boles SM. Telephone counseling for smoking cessation: rationales and meta-analytic review of evidence. *Health Education Research.* 1996;11(2):243–57.

McFall SL, Michener A, Rubin D, Flay BR, Mermelstein RJ, Burton D, Jelen P, Warnecke RB. The effects and use of maintenance newsletters in a smoking cessation intervention. *Addictive Behaviors.* 1993;18(2):151–8.

McPhillips-Tangum C. Results from the first annual survey on addressing tobacco in managed care. *Tobacco Control.* 1998;7(Suppl):S11–3.

National Cancer Institute. Population-based smoking cessation: proceedings of a conference on What Works to Influence Cessation in the General Population. *Smoking and Tobacco Control Monograph No. 12.* Bethesda, MD: National Cancer Institute; 2000. NIH Publication No. 00-4892.

Oregon Health Division. *Oregon's Tobacco Prevention and Education Program.* Portland, OR: Oregon Health Division; 1999.

Owen L. Impact of a telephone helpline for smokers who called during a mass media campaign. *Tobacco Control.* 2000;9(2):148–54.

Platt S, Tannahill A, Watson J, Fraser E. Effectiveness of antismoking telephone helpline: follow up survey. *British Medical Journal.* 1997;314(7091):1371–5.

Rigotti NA, Quinn VP, Stevens VJ, Solberg LI, Hollis JF, Rosenthal AC, Zapka JG, France E, Gordon N, Smith S, Monroe M. Tobacco-control policies in 11 leading managed care organizations: progress and challenges. *Effective Clinical Practice.* 2002;5(3):130–6.

Task Force on Community Preventive Services. The guide to community preventive services: tobacco use prevention and control. *American Journal of Preventive Medicine.* 2001;20(Suppl 2):1–88.

Zhu S, Rosbrook B, Anderson CM, Gilpin E, Sadler GPJ. The demographics of help-seeking for smoking cessation in California and the role of the California Smoker's Helpline. *Tobacco Control.* 1995;4(1):9–15.

Zhu SH, Anderson CM, Johnson CE, Tedeschi G, Roeseler A. A centralised telephone service for tobacco cessation: the California experience. *Tobacco Control.* 2000;9 (Suppl 2):ii48–55.

Zhu SH, Anderson CM, Tedeschi GJ, Rosbrook B, Johnson CE, Byrd M, Gutierrez-Terrell E. Evidence of real-world effectiveness of a telephone quitline for smokers. *New England Journal of Medicine.* 2002;347(14):1087–93.

Outcome 9

Increase in the Number of Health Care Providers and Health Care Systems Following Public Health Service (PHS) Guidelines

Indicator Rating
← ○ ◔ ◑ ● → better

Number	Indicator	Overall quality (low → high)	Resources needed	Strength of evaluation evidence	Utility	Face validity	Accepted practice
3.9.1	Proportion of health care providers and health care systems that have fully implemented the Public Health Service (PHS) guidelines	▬▬▬	$$$	◑	◑	◑	●
3.9.2	Proportion of adults who have been asked by a health care professional about smoking	▬▬	$$	●	◑	◑	●
3.9.3	Proportion of smokers who have been advised to quit smoking by a health care professional	▬▬	$$	●	◑	◑	●
3.9.4	Proportion of smokers who have been assessed regarding their willingness to make a quit attempt by a health care professional	▬▬	$$$	●	◑	◑	●
3.9.5	Proportion of smokers who have been assisted in quitting smoking by a health care professional	▬▬	$$	●	◑	◑	●
3.9.6	Proportion of smokers for whom a health care professional has arranged for follow-up contact regarding a quit attempt	▬▬†	$$$†	◑	◑	◑	●
3.9.7	Proportion of pregnant women who report that a health care professional advised them to quit smoking during a prenatal visit	▬▬	$$$†	◔	●	●	●
3.9.8	Proportion of health care systems that have provider-reminder systems in place	▬▬	$$$	●	●	●	●

† Denotes low agreement among reviewers: that is, fewer than 75% of the valid ratings for this indicator were within one point of each other (see Appendix B for an explanation).

Indicator 3.9.1

Proportion of Health Care Providers and Health Care Systems That Have Fully Implemented the Public Health Service (PHS) Guidelines

Goal area 3	Promoting quitting among adults and young people
Outcome 9	Increase in the number of health care providers and health care systems following the Public Health Service (PHS) guidelines
What to measure	Proportion of health care system administrators (or managed care providers) who have fully implemented PHS recommendations. For a list of the recommendations, see "Comments" below.
Why this indicator is useful	Policies implemented by managed care administrators affect whether tobacco-dependence treatment services are offered to patients. Increases in the use of these proven services will result in increases in the number of successful quit attempts.[1,2]
Example data source(s)	Addressing Tobacco in Managed Care (ATMC), 1997–1998 Information available at: http://www.aahp.org/atmc/mainindex.cfm
Population group(s)	Managed care administrators
Example survey question(s)	**From ATMC** With regard to the AHCPR [Agency for Health Care Policy and Research] guidelines, has your plan implemented them: ☐ Fully ☐ Partially ☐ The plan has not implemented the guidelines
Comments	Note: The Agency for Health Care Policy and Research is now named the Agency for Healthcare Research and Quality (AHRQ). The AHRQ published the most recent Public Health Service (PHS) guidelines. A more thorough way to measure this indicator would be to ask managed care administrators the example question for each of the PHS guideline recommendations for health care administrators, insurers, and purchasers. The PHS guideline recommendations are: 1. Implement a tobacco-use identification system in every clinic 2. Provide education, resources, and feedback to promote provider intervention 3. Dedicate staff to provide tobacco-dependence treatment and assess the delivery of this treatment in staff performance evaluations 4. Promote hospital policies that support and provide inpatient tobacco-dependence services 5. Include tobacco-dependence treatment (both counseling and pharmacotherapy) identified as effective in this guideline as paid or covered services for all subscribers or members of health insurance packages 6. Reimburse clinicians and specialists for delivery of effective tobacco-dependence treatments, and include these interventions in the defined duties of clinicians

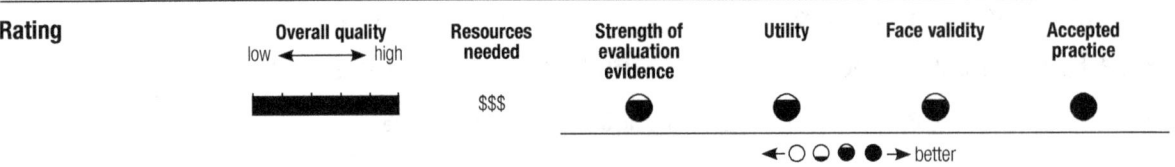

References
1. Fiore MC, Bailey WC, Cohen SJ, Dorfman SF, Goldstein MG, Gritz EG, Heyman RB, Jaén CR, Kottke TE, Lando HA, Mecklenburg RE, Mullen PD, Nett LM, Robinson L, Stitzer ML, Tommasello AC, Villejo L, Wewers ME. *Treating tobacco use and dependence: clinical practice guideline.* Rockville, MD: U.S. Department of Health and Human Services; 2000.
2. Task Force on Community Preventive Services. The guide to community preventive services: tobacco use prevention and control. *American Journal of Preventive Medicine.* 2001;20(Suppl 2):1–88.

Indicator 3.9.2

Proportion of Adults Who Have Been Asked by a Health Care Professional About Smoking

Goal area 3	Promoting quitting among adults and young people
Outcome 9	Increase in the number of health care providers and health care systems following the Public Health Service (PHS) guidelines
What to measure	Proportion of adults who had been asked about their smoking status by a health care professional during the previous 12 months
Why this indicator is useful	Evidence shows that when patients are asked about their tobacco use by a health care professional and when that response is documented, clinician interventions increase.[1]
Example data source(s)	Adult Tobacco Survey (ATS): CDC Recommended Questions: Core, 2003 Adult Tobacco Survey (ATS): CDC Recommended Questions: Supplemental Section C: Cessation, 2003
Population group(s)	Adults aged 18 years or older
Example survey question(s)	**From ATS** During the past 12 months, did any doctor, nurse, or other health professional ask if you smoke? ☐ Yes ☐ No ☐ Don't know/Not sure ☐ Refused **From ATS, Supplemental Section C** In the past 12 months, did a dentist ask if you smoked? ☐ Yes ☐ No ☐ Don't know/Not sure ☐ Refused
Comments	The example question could also be asked of young people.

Rating

Overall quality low ←→ high	Resources needed	Strength of evaluation evidence	Utility	Face validity	Accepted practice
▬▬▬▬	$$	●	◐	◐	●

←○ ◔ ◐ ● →better

Reference

1. Fiore MC, Bailey WC, Cohen SJ, Dorfman SF, Goldstein MG, Gritz EG, Heyman RB, Jaén CR, Kottke TE, Lando HA, Mecklenburg RE, Mullen PD, Nett LM, Robinson L, Stitzer ML, Tommasello AC, Villejo L, Wewers ME. *Treating tobacco use and dependence: clinical practice guideline.* Rockville, MD: U.S. Department of Health and Human Services; 2000.

Indicator 3.9.3

Proportion of Smokers Who Have Been Advised to Quit Smoking by a Health Care Professional

Goal area 3	Promoting quitting among adults and young people
Outcome 9	Increase in the number of health care providers and health care systems following the Public Health Service (PHS) guidelines
What to measure	Proportion of smokers who had been advised to quit smoking by a health care professional during the previous 12 months
Why this indicator is useful	Evidence shows that quit rates increase when health care professionals advise their patients to stop using tobacco.[1]
Example data source(s)	▸ Adult Tobacco Survey (ATS): CDC Recommended Questions: Core, 2003 ▸ Adult Tobacco Survey (ATS): CDC Recommended Questions: Supplemental Section C: Cessation, 2003
Population group(s)	Smokers aged 18 years or older
Example survey question(s)	**From ATS** During the past 12 months, did any doctor, nurse, or other health professional advise you to not smoke? ☐ Yes ☐ No ☐ Don't know/Not sure ☐ Refused **From ATS: Supplemental Section C** In the past 12 months, did a dentist advise you to quit smoking? ☐ Yes ☐ No ☐ Don't know/Not sure ☐ Refused
Comments	The example questions could also be asked of young smokers.

Rating

Overall quality low ←→ high	Resources needed	Strength of evaluation evidence	Utility	Face validity	Accepted practice
▬▬▬▬▬	$$	●	◐	◐	●

← ○ ◐ ● ● → better

Reference

1. Fiore MC, Bailey WC, Cohen SJ, Dorfman SF, Goldstein MG, Gritz EG, Heyman RB, Jaén CR, Kottke TE, Lando HA, Mecklenburg RE, Mullen PD, Nett LM, Robinson L, Stitzer ML, Tommasello AC, Villejo L, Wewers ME. *Treating tobacco use and dependence: clinical practice guideline.* Rockville, MD: U.S. Department of Health and Human Services; 2000.

GOAL AREA 3
Outcome 9

Indicator 3.9.4

Proportion of Smokers Who Have Been Assessed Regarding Their Willingness to Make a Quit Attempt by a Health Care Professional

Goal area 3	Promoting quitting among adults and young people
Outcome 9	Increase in the number of health care providers and health care systems following the Public Health Service (PHS) guidelines
What to measure	Proportion of smokers who have been evaluated by a health care professional regarding their willingness to stop smoking
Why this indicator is useful	Evidence suggests that once a tobacco-using patient is advised to quit, assessing that patient's willingness to quit can help to tailor the cessation counseling provided to the patient.[1]
Example data source(s)	No commonly used data sources were found.
Population group(s)	Smokers aged 18 years or older
Example survey question(s)	During the past 12 months, did any doctor, nurse, or other health care professional ask you if you were willing to make a quit attempt? ☐ Yes ☐ No ☐ Don't know/Not sure ☐ Refused to answer In the past 12 months, did a dentist ask you if you were willing to make a quit attempt? ☐ Yes ☐ No ☐ Don't know/Not sure ☐ Refused to answer
Comments	The authors created the example questions. They are not in any commonly used data source. The example questions could also be asked of young smokers. Evaluators might also wish to evaluate whether the physician inquired about the patient's willingness to use assistance in quitting (e.g., calling a quitline, joining a group cessation program, or using FDA-approved pharmacotherapies).
Rating	Overall quality: low ◄───► high — high Resources needed: $$$ Strength of evaluation evidence: ● Utility: ● Face validity: ● Accepted practice: ● ←○◐●●→ better

Reference
1. Fiore MC, Bailey WC, Cohen SJ, Dorfman SF, Goldstein MG, Gritz EG, Heyman RB, Jaén CR, Kottke TE, Lando HA, Mecklenburg RE, Mullen PD, Nett LM, Robinson L, Stitzer ML, Tommasello AC, Villejo L, Wewers ME. *Treating tobacco use and dependence: clinical practice guideline*. Rockville, MD: U.S. Department of Health and Human Services; 2000.

Indicator 3.9.5

Proportion of Smokers Who Have Been Assisted in Quitting Smoking by a Health Care Professional

Goal area 3	Promoting quitting among adults and young people
Outcome 9	Increase in the number of health care providers and health care systems following the Public Health Service (PHS) guidelines
What to measure	Proportion of smokers who have had a health care professional actively assist them in an attempt to quit smoking. Examples of assistance include prescribing FDA-approved cessation medications, providing educational material, providing counseling or a counseling referral, and establishing a firm quit date.
Why this indicator is useful	Evidence is strong that clinician assistance in cessation leads to improved quit rates.[1]
Example data source(s)	▸ Adult Tobacco Survey (ATS): CDC Recommended Questions: Core, 2003 ▸ American Smoking and Health Survey (ASHES), 2003 Information available at: http://tobacco.rti.org/data/New/surveys.cfm
Population group(s)	Smokers aged 18 years or older

Example survey question(s)

From ATS

In the past 12 months, when a doctor, nurse, or other health professional advised you to quit smoking, did they also do any of the following?

	Yes	No	Don't know / Not sure	Refused
1. Prescribe or recommend a patch, nicotine gum, nasal spray, an inhaler, or pills such as Zyban®	☐	☐	☐	☐
2. Suggest that you set a specific date to stop smoking	☐	☐	☐	☐
3. Suggest that you use a smoking cessation class, program, quit line, or counseling	☐	☐	☐	☐
4. Provide you with booklets, videos, or other material to help you quit smoking on your own	☐	☐	☐	☐

From ASHES

During the past 12 months, that is since [FILL IN DATE], when a doctor, dentist, nurse, or other health professional advised you to quit smoking cigarettes, did they do any of the following: suggest that you use a smoking cessation class, program, quitline, or seek counseling for stopping smoking?
☐ Yes ☐ No ☐ Don't know/Not sure ☐ Refused

Comments The example questions could also be asked of young smokers.

Rating

Overall quality low ←——→ high	Resources needed	Strength of evaluation evidence	Utility	Face validity	Accepted practice
▰▰▰▱▱	$$	●	●	◐	●

←○◔●◑→ better

Reference

1. Fiore MC, Bailey WC, Cohen SJ, Dorfman SF, Goldstein MG, Gritz EG, Heyman RB, Jaén CR, Kottke TE, Lando HA, Mecklenburg RE, Mullen PD, Nett LM, Robinson L, Stitzer ML, Tommasello AC, Villejo L, Wewers ME. *Treating tobacco use and dependence: clinical practice guideline.* Rockville, MD: U.S. Department of Health and Human Services; 2000.

GOAL AREA 3
Outcome 9

Indicator 3.9.6

Proportion of Smokers for Whom a Health Care Professional Has Arranged for Follow-up Contact Regarding a Quit Attempt

Goal area 3	Promoting quitting among adults and young people
Outcome 9	Increase in the number of health care providers and health care systems following the Public Health Service (PHS) guidelines
What to measure	Proportion of smokers who have had a health care professional schedule follow-up contact to help them quit smoking
Why this indicator is useful	Brief interventions may not be sufficient to help every patient quit successfully. Arranging for follow-up contact ensures continued cessation assistance and can increase the likelihood of a successful quit attempt.[1]
Example data source(s)	No commonly used data sources were found.
Population group(s)	Smokers aged 18 years or older Smokers aged less than 18 years
Example survey question(s)	In the past 12 months, when a doctor or other health professional advised you to quit smoking, did he or she also do any of the following? Yes No 1. Call and ask you about your quit attempt within one week ☐ ☐ 2. Ask you about your quit attempt in person (during an office visit) within one week ☐ ☐ 3. Call and ask you about your quit attempt within one month ☐ ☐ 4. Ask you about your quit attempt in person (during an office visit) within one month ☐ ☐ 5. Arrange for a cessation counselor, program, or quitline to make follow-up contact with you regarding your quit attempt ☐ ☐
Comments	The authors created these example questions. They are not in any commonly used data source.

Rating

Overall quality low ⟷ high	Resources needed	Strength of evaluation evidence	Utility	Face validity	Accepted practice
▬▬▬▬▬[†]	$$$[†]	◕	◕	◕	◕

⟵ ○ ◔ ◕ ● ⟶ better

[†] Denotes low agreement among reviewers: that is, fewer than 75% of the valid ratings for this indicator were within one point of each other (see Appendix B for an explanation).

Reference
1. Task Force on Community Preventive Services. The guide to community preventive services: tobacco use prevention and control. *American Journal of Preventive Medicine.* 2001;20(Suppl 2):1–88.

Indicator 3.9.7

Proportion of Pregnant Women Who Report That a Health Care Professional Advised Them to Quit Smoking During a Prenatal Visit

Goal area 3	Promoting quitting among adults and young people
Outcome 9	Increase in the number of health care providers and health care systems following the Public Health Service (PHS) guidelines
What to measure	Proportion of pregnant women who were advised by a health care professional during a prenatal visit of the ill effects of smoking
Why this indicator is useful	Tobacco use by pregnant women and exposure to tobacco smoke are causal factors in both maternal and child morbidity and mortality. Evidence shows that advising pregnant women to quit, coupled with intensive counseling, increases abstinence rates.[1]
Example data source(s)	CDC Pregnancy Risk Assessment Monitoring System (PRAMS), Phase 4, 2000–2003
Population group(s)	Pregnant women
Example survey question(s)	**From PRAMS** During any of your prenatal care visits, did a doctor, nurse, or other health care worker talk with you about how smoking during pregnancy could affect your baby? ☐ No ☐ Yes
Comments	Evaluators could also collect information on whether the health care professional advised the patient to quit smoking or provided assistance in quitting.

Rating

Overall quality low ←——→ high	Resources needed	Strength of evaluation evidence	Utility	Face validity	Accepted practice
▬▬▬▬▬	$$$[†]	◐	◐	◐	●

←○◐◑●→ better

[†] Denotes low agreement among reviewers: that is, fewer than 75% of the valid ratings for this indicator were within one point of each other (see Appendix B for an explanation).

Reference
1. Fiore MC, Bailey WC, Cohen SJ, Dorfman SF, Goldstein MG, Gritz EG, Heyman RB, Jaén CR, Kottke TE, Lando HA, Mecklenburg RE, Mullen PD, Nett LM, Robinson L, Stitzer ML, Tommasello AC, Villejo L, Wewers ME. *Treating tobacco use and dependence: clinical practice guideline.* Rockville, MD: U.S. Department of Health and Human Services; 2000.

Indicator 3.9.8

Proportion of Health Care Systems That Have Provider-reminder Systems in Place

Goal area 3	Promoting quitting among adults and young people
Outcome 9	Increase in the number of health care providers and health care systems following the Public Health Service (PHS) guidelines
What to measure	Proportion of health care systems that include smoking status information (e.g., stickers) in their patients' records. This information is recorded in order to prompt health care professionals to discuss smoking cessation during patients' visits.
Why this indicator is useful	Evidence shows that reminder systems for health care providers increase the rate of clinician intervention to assist patients in quitting, thereby increasing the number of patients who successfully quit.[1,2]
Example data source(s)	Addressing Tobacco in Managed Care (ATMC), Survey of Health Plans, 1997–1998
Population group(s)	Managed care administrators
Example survey question(s)	**From ATMC** *Mark all that apply* Has your plan implemented systems for any of the following? (Yes/No) 1. Documentation of patient smoking status in an administrative computer database 2. Documentation of patient smoking status in the medical record 3. Computerized clinic reminders to encourage providers to advise patients to quit 4. Provider training in effective smoking cessation interventions 5. Routine cessation advice/brief provider counseling of patients 6. Provider incentives that promote tobacco cessation assessment and intervention 7. Patient incentives for use of/adherence to recommended cessation treatment Are the providers in your plan required to carry out any of the following activities? 1. Ask new patients about their smoking status 2. Include smoking status as a vital sign (i.e., ask about and document smoking status at every visit) 3. Document smoking status in the patient's medical record 4. Strongly advise all patients who smoke to quit 5. Assess willingness of patient to make a quit attempt 6. Refer the patient who smokes to intensive treatment when the physician considers it appropriate or the patient prefers it 7. Arrange for follow-up with patients who are trying to quit smoking 8. Ensure that support staff is trained to counsel patients about smoking cessation 9. Have literature about smoking cessation and the health risks of smoking readily available in waiting rooms and exam rooms 10. Encourage parents who smoke to provide a smoke-free environment for their children at home and in day care 11. Other (please specify)_____

Comments None

Rating

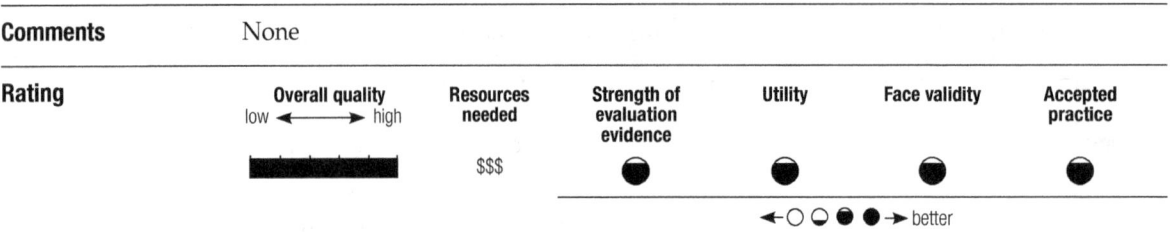

References
1. Fiore MC, Bailey WC, Cohen SJ, Dorfman SF, Goldstein MG, Gritz EG, Heyman RB, Jaén CR, Kottke TE, Lando HA, Mecklenburg RE, Mullen PD, Nett LM, Robinson L, Stitzer ML, Tommasello AC, Villejo L, Wewers ME. *Treating tobacco use and dependence: clinical practice guideline.* Rockville, MD: U.S. Department of Health and Human Services; 2000.
2. Task Force on Community Preventive Services. The guide to community preventive services: tobacco use prevention and control. *American Journal of Preventive Medicine.* 2001;20(Suppl 2):1–88.

Outcome 10

Increased Insurance Coverage for Cessation Services

The Guide to Community Preventive Services recommends that insurance carriers cover proven cessation therapies and strongly recommends reducing patients' out-of-pocket costs for cessation therapies to increase quit rates.[1] A review of five studies showed that pre-paid or discounted prescription drug benefits increased the percentage of patients who received pharmacotherapy and increased smoking abstinence rates.[1] *The Guide to Community Preventive Services* and *Treating Tobacco Use and Dependence: Clinical Practice Guideline* also recommends that smoking cessation treatment (both pharmacotherapy and counseling) be included as a covered benefit by health plans because doing so increases the use of these services and improves overall abstinence rates.[1,2] Full coverage of tobacco-dependence treatment is an effective and relatively low-cost strategy for significantly increasing the use of proven interventions and increasing quit attempts and quit rates.[3] Reviewers of tobacco-dependence treatments found that full insurance coverage of treatment services produced the highest level of use of these services.[4] In addition, full coverage produced the highest use of nicotine replacement therapy, increased the number of quit attempts, and yielded the greatest decline in overall smoking prevalence.[4]

Listed below are the indicators associated with this outcome:

- **3.10.1** Proportion of insurance purchasers and payers that reimburse for tobacco cessation services

References

1. Task Force on Community Preventive Services. The guide to community preventive services: tobacco use prevention and control. *American Journal of Preventive Medicine.* 2001;20(Suppl 2):1–88.

2. Fiore MC, Bailey WC, Cohen SJ, Dorfman S, Goldstein M, Gritz E, Heyman RB, Jaén CR, Kottke TE, Lando HA, Mecklenburg RE, Mullen PD, Nett LM, Robinson L, Stitzer ML, Tommasello AC, Villejo L, Wewers ME. *Treating tobacco use and dependence: clinical practice guideline.* Rockville, MD: U.S. Department of Health and Human Services; 2000.

3. Schauffler HH, McMenamin S, Olson K, Boyce-Smith G, Rideout JA, Kamil J. Variations in treatment benefits influence smoking cessation: results of a randomised controlled trial. *Tobacco Control.* 2001;10(2):175–80.

4. Fiore MC, Hatsukami DK, Baker TB. Effective tobacco-dependence treatment. *Journal of the American Medical Association.* 2002;288(14):1768–71.

For Further Reading

Borland R, Owen N, Hill D, Schofield P. Predicting attempts and sustained cessation of smoking after the introduction of workplace smoking bans. *Health Psychology.* 1991;10(5):336–42.

Borland R, Segan CJ, Livingston PM, Owen N. The effectiveness of callback counseling for smoking cessation: a randomized trial. *Addiction.* 2001;96(6):881–9.

Hellman R, Cummings KM, Haughey BP, Zielezny MA, O'Shea RM. Predictors of attempting and succeeding at smoking cessation. *Health Education Research.* 1991;6(1):77–86.

Hennrikus DJ, Jeffery RW, Lando HA. The smoking cessation process: longitudinal observations in a working population. *Preventive Medicine.* 1995;24(3):235–44.

Hymowitz N, Cummings KM, Hyland A, Lynn WR, Pechacek TF, Hartwell TD. Predictors of smoking cessation in a cohort of adult smokers followed for five years. *Tobacco Control.* 1997;6(Suppl 2):S57–62.

Morabia A, Costanza MC, Bernstein MS, Rielle JC. Ages at initiation of cigarette smoking and quit attempts among women: a generation effect. *American Journal of Public Health.* 2002;92(1):71–4.

National Cancer Institute. Population-based smoking cessation: proceedings of a conference on What Works to Influence Cessation in the General Population. *Smoking and Tobacco Control Monograph No. 12.* Bethesda, MD: National Cancer Institute; 2000. NIH Publication No. 00-4892.

Sargent JD, Mott LA, Stevens M. Predictors of smoking cessation in adolescents. *Archives of Pediatric and Adolescent Medicine.* 1998;152(4):388–93.

Zhu SH, Anderson CM, Tedeschi GJ, Rosbrook B, Johnson CE, Byrd M, Gutierrez-Terrell E. Evidence of real-world effectiveness of a telephone quitline for smokers. *New England Journal of Medicine.* 2002;347(14):1087–93.

Outcome 10

Increased Insurance Coverage for Cessation Services

Indicator Rating

◄ ○ ◐ ● ● ► better

Number	Indicator	Overall quality low ◄——► high	Resources needed	Strength of evaluation evidence	Utility	Face validity	Accepted practice
3.10.1	Proportion of insurance purchasers and payers that reimburse for tobacco cessation services	├──┼──┼──┤ │ │	$$$	●	●	●	●

Indicator 3.10.1

Proportion of Insurance Purchasers and Payers That Reimburse for Tobacco Cessation Services

Goal area 3	Promoting quitting among adults and young people
Outcome 10	Increased insurance coverage for cessation services
What to measure	Proportion of purchasers and payers of health insurance (public and private) who reimburse for some level of tobacco cessation services. Examples of such services are (1) medications approved by the FDA and (2) individual, group, and telephone counseling.
Why this indicator is useful	Reducing out-of-pocket costs for cessation treatment increases the use of both effective cessation therapies and cessation.[1] In addition, reimbursement of expenses increases the number of quit attempts and decreases smoking relapse rates.[2,3]
Example data source(s)	Addressing Tobacco in Managed Care (ATMC), Survey of Health Plans, 1997–1998
Population group(s)	Managed care administrators

Example survey question(s)

From ATMC

Coverage for smoking cessation intervention is:
- ☐ Available to selected members as outlined in their coverage agreement
- ☐ Available to selected members with specific co-morbidities
  Please list: _____
- ☐ Available to all members
- ☐ Not available
- ☐ Other (please specify) _____

Is there an annual or lifetime limit on coverage for smoking cessation interventions?
- ☐ Yes, annual
- ☐ Yes, lifetime
- ☐ No limit
- ☐ Other (please specify) _____

Which of the following cessation interventions are available in your plan, and which are included in your plan's formulary? (Mark all that apply.)

	Unavailable	Full coverage	Partial coverage	In Formulary
1. Nicotine replacement therapy				
Over-the-counter	☐	☐	☐	☐
Prescription	☐	☐	☐	☐
Only with enrollment in cessation program	☐	☐	☐	☐
2. Buproprion (e.g., Zyban®)	☐	☐	☐	☐
3. Telephone counseling	☐	☐	☐	☐
4. Face-to-face counseling	☐	☐	☐	☐
5. Classes or group meeting	☐	☐	☐	☐
6. Self-help materials	☐	☐	☐	☐

GOAL AREA 3
Outcome 10

Comments	Evaluators need to determine which employers and/or health insurance organizations provide coverage for that state's population in order to obtain meaningful data regarding reimbursement of tobacco cessation services.
	Evaluators may also want to measure whether tobacco cessation treatment is fully or partially reimbursed by public and private health insurance purchasers or payers.

Rating	Overall quality low ⟵⟶ high	Resources needed	Strength of evaluation evidence	Utility	Face validity	Accepted practice
	▬▬▬▬	$$$	◐	●	●	●

⟵ ○ ◔ ◐ ● ⟶ better

References
1. Task Force on Community Preventive Services. The guide to community preventive services: tobacco use prevention and control. *American Journal of Preventive Medicine.* 2001;20(Suppl 2):1–88.
2. Centers for Disease Control and Prevention. *Coverage for tobacco use cessation treatments.* Atlanta, GA: Centers for Disease Control and Prevention; 2004.
3. Centers for Disease Control and Prevention. State Medicaid coverage for tobacco-dependence treatments—United States, 1994–2002. M*orbidity and Mortality Weekly Report.* 2004;53(3):54–7.

Outcome 11

Increased Number of Quit Attempts and Quit Attempts Using Proven Cessation Methods

Quitting smoking has immediate and long-term benefits, such as reducing smokers' risk of diseases caused by smoking and improving health in general.[1] Attempting to quit is the first step in becoming tobacco-free. Although some smokers can quit without help, the probability of a quit attempt leading to sustained abstinence is increased by using behavioral and pharmaceutical interventions.[2] Effective interventions include FDA-approved pharmacotherapies and various forms of counseling (individual or group, in person or by telephone).[3]

Listed below are the indicators associated with this outcome:

- **3.11.1** Proportion of adult smokers who have made a quit attempt
- **3.11.2** Proportion of young smokers who have made a quit attempt
- **3.11.3** Proportion of adult and young smokers who have made a quit attempt using proven cessation methods

References

1. U.S. Department of Health and Human Services. *The health consequences of smoking: a report of the Surgeon General.* Atlanta, GA: Centers for Disease Control and Prevention; 2004.

2. U.S. Department of Health and Human Services. *Reducing tobacco use: a report of the Surgeon General.* Atlanta, GA: Centers for Disease Control and Prevention; 2000.

3. Task Force on Community Preventive Services. The guide to community preventive services: tobacco use prevention and control. *American Journal of Preventive Medicine.* 2001;20(Suppl 2):1–88.

For Further Reading

Doescher MP, Saver BG. Physicians' advice to quit smoking: the glass remains half empty. *Journal of Family Practice.* 2000;49(6):543–7.

Fiore MC, Bailey WC, Cohen SJ, Dorfman S, Goldstein M, Gritz E, Heyman RB, Jaén CR, Kottke TE, Lando HA, Mecklenburg RE, Mullen PD, Nett LM, Robinson L, Stitzer ML, Tommasello AC, Villejo L, Wewers ME. *Treating tobacco use and dependence: clinical practice guideline.* Rockville, MD: U.S. Department of Health and Human Services; 2000.

Fiore MC, Hatsukami DK, Baker TB. Effective tobacco-dependence treatment. *Journal of the American Medical Association.* 2002;288(14):1768–71.

Hollis JF, Bills R, Whitlock E, Stevens VJ, Mullooly J, Lichtenstein E. Implementing tobacco interventions in the real world of managed care. *Tobacco Control.* 2000;9 (Suppl 1):i18–24.

McBride PE, Plane MB, Underbakke G, Brown RL, Solberg LI. Smoking screening and management in primary care practices. *Archives of Family Medicine.* 1997;6(2):165–72.

Outcome 11

Increased Number of Quit Attempts and
Quit Attempts Using Proven Cessation Methods

Indicator Rating
←○◐●●→ better

Number	Indicator	Overall quality (low ← → high)	Resources needed	Strength of evaluation evidence	Utility	Face validity	Accepted practice
3.11.1	Proportion of adult smokers who have made a quit attempt	▬▬▬▬▬▬	$$†	●	●	●	●
3.11.2	Proportion of young smokers who have made a quit attempt	▬▬▬▬▬†	$$	○	●	●	●
3.11.3	Proportion of adult and young smokers who have made a quit attempt using proven cessation methods	▬▬▬▬▬▬	$$	●	●	●	●

† Denotes low agreement among reviewers: that is, fewer than 75% of the valid ratings for this indicator were within one point of each other (see Appendix B for an explanation).

GOAL AREA 3
Outcome 11

Indicator 3.11.1

Proportion of Adult Smokers Who Have Made a Quit Attempt

Goal area 3	Promoting quitting among adults and young people
Outcome 11	Increased number of quit attempts and quit attempts using proven cessation methods
What to measure	Proportion of adult smokers who have stopped smoking for at least 1 day during the previous 12 months in an attempt to quit smoking
Why this indicator is useful	Attempting to quit is an essential step in the process of becoming tobacco-free. Stopping tobacco use entirely is often preceded by several quit attempts.[1] Increasing the number of quit attempts may lead to increased smoking cessation rates and a lower prevalence of smoking.[1]
Example data source(s)	Adult Tobacco Survey (ATS): CDC Recommended Questions: Core, 2003 Behavioral Risk Factor Surveillance System (BRFSS), 2002 Current Population Survey: Tobacco Use Supplement (CPS TUS), 2003
Population group(s)	Smokers aged 18 years or older
Example survey question(s)	**From ATS, BRFSS, and CPS TUS** During the past 12 months, have you stopped smoking for one day or longer because you were trying to quit smoking? ☐ Yes ☐ No ☐ Don't know/Not sure ☐ Refused
Comments	Evaluators may also want to measure the number of quit attempts made by smokers over a given time period.
Rating	Overall quality: low ◄──► high Resources needed: $$[†] Strength of evaluation evidence: ◐ Utility: ● Face validity: ◐ Accepted practice: ● ◄ ○ ◔ ◐ ● ► better

† Denotes low agreement among reviewers: that is, fewer than 75% of the valid ratings for this indicator were within one point of each other (see Appendix B for an explanation).

Reference
1. Fiore MC, Bailey WC, Cohen SJ, Dorfman SF, Goldstein MG, Gritz EG, Heyman RB, Jaén CR, Kottke TE, Lando HA, Mecklenburg RE, Mullen PD, Nett LM, Robinson L, Stitzer ML, Tommasello AC, Villejo L, Wewers ME. *Treating tobacco use and dependence: clinical practice guideline.* Rockville, MD: U.S. Department of Health and Human Services; 2000.

Indicator 3.11.2

Proportion of Young Smokers Who Have Made a Quit Attempt

Goal area 3	Promoting quitting among adults and young people
Outcome 11	Increased number of quit attempts and quit attempts using proven cessation methods
What to measure	Proportion of young smokers who have stopped smoking for at least 1 day during the previous 12 months in an attempt to quit smoking
Why this indicator is useful	Attempting to quit is an essential step in the process of becoming tobacco-free. Successful cessation of tobacco use is often preceded by several quit attempts.[1] Increasing the number of quit attempts can lead to increased smoking cessation rates and a lower prevalence of smoking.[1]
Example data source(s)	▸ Youth Tobacco Survey (YTS): CDC Recommended Questions: Core, 2004 ▸ CDC Youth Risk Behavior Surveillance System (YRBSS), 2003
Population group(s)	Smokers less than 18 years of age
Example survey question(s)	**From YTS** How many times during the past 12 months have you stopped smoking for one day or longer because you were trying to quit smoking? ☐ I have not smoked in the past 12 months ☐ I have not tried to quit ☐ 1 time ☐ 2 times ☐ 3 to 5 times ☐ 6 to 9 times ☐ 10 or more times **From YTS and YRBSS** During the past 12 months, did you ever try to quit smoking cigarettes? ☐ I did not smoke during the past 12 months ☐ Yes ☐ No
Comments	None

Rating

Overall quality low ⟷ high	Resources needed	Strength of evaluation evidence	Utility	Face validity	Accepted practice
▬▬▬▬▬†	$$	○	●	●	●

← ○ ◐ ● ● → better

† Denotes low agreement among reviewers: that is, fewer than 75% of the valid ratings for this indicator were within one point of each other (see Appendix B for an explanation).

Reference
1. Fiore MC, Bailey WC, Cohen SJ, Dorfman SF, Goldstein MG, Gritz EG, Heyman RB, Jaén CR, Kottke TE, Lando HA, Mecklenburg RE, Mullen PD, Nett LM, Robinson L, Stitzer ML, Tommasello AC, Villejo L, Wewers ME. *Treating tobacco use and dependence: clinical practice guideline.* Rockville, MD: U.S. Department of Health and Human Services; 2000.

Indicator 3.11.3

Proportion of Adult and Young Smokers Who Have Made a Quit Attempt Using Proven Cessation Methods

Goal area 3	Promoting quitting among adults and young people
Outcome 11	Increased number of quit attempts and quit attempts using proven cessation methods
What to measure	The proportion of adult and young smokers who have stopped smoking for at least 1 day during the previous 12 months using proven cessation methods in an attempt to quit smoking entirely. Examples of proven cessation strategies are (1) FDA-approved pharmacotherapies, (2) in-person individual counseling, (3) counseling from telephone quitlines, and (4) stop-smoking classes.
Why this indicator is useful	Evidence shows that among adult tobacco users, the use of effective cessation strategies such as counseling or FDA-approved pharmaceuticals can double quit rates compared to unassisted quit attempts.[1] Less evidence is available concerning young tobacco users, but preliminary studies suggest that cognitive-behavioral interventions are a promising approach.[2]
Example data source(s)	Adult Tobacco Survey (ATS): CDC Recommended Questions: Core, 2003 Youth Tobacco Survey (YTS): Supplemental Questions, 2004
Population group(s)	Smokers aged 18 years or older Smokers aged less than 18 years
Example survey question(s)	**From ATS** During the past 12 months, have you stopped smoking for one day or longer because you were trying to quit smoking? ☐ Yes ☐ No ☐ Don't know/Not sure ☐ Refused The last time you tried to quit smoking, did you use any other assistance such as classes or counseling? ☐ Yes ☐ No *If yes, ask* Did you use? *(Check all that apply)* Yes No 1. A stop-smoking clinic or class ☐ ☐ 2. A telephone quitline ☐ ☐ 3. One-on-one counseling from a doctor or nurse ☐ ☐ 4. Self-help material, books or videos ☐ ☐ 5. Acupuncture ☐ ☐ 6. Hypnosis ☐ ☐ 7. Other, specify_____ The last time you tried to quit smoking, did you use the nicotine patch, gum, or any other medication to help you quit? ☐ ☐ Did you use? 1. Nicotine gum ☐ ☐ 2. A patch ☐ ☐ 3. A nasal spray ☐ ☐ 4. An inhaler ☐ ☐ 5. Buproprion, Zyban,® Wellbutrin® ☐ ☐ 5. Other, specify_____

Example survey question(s) (cont.)	**From YTS Supplemental Questions** Have you ever participated in a program at school to help you quit using tobacco? ☐ I have never used tobacco ☐ Yes ☐ No
Comments	This example YTS Supplemental question could be expanded to include multiple types of cessation methods, as well as the number of quit attempts in the previous year (see ATS questions).

Rating

Overall quality low ←——→ high	Resources needed	Strength of evaluation evidence	Utility	Face validity	Accepted practice
▬▬▬▬	$$	●	◐	◐	●

←○ ◔ ◑ ● → better

References
1. Fiore MC, Bailey WC, Cohen SJ, Dorfman SF, Goldstein MG, Gritz EG, Heyman RB, Jaén CR, Kottke TE, Lando HA, Mecklenburg RE, Mullen PD, Nett LM, Robinson L, Stitzer ML, Tommasello AC, Villejo L, Wewers ME. *Treating tobacco use and dependence: clinical practice guideline.* Rockville, MD: U.S. Department of Health and Human Services; 2000.
2. Milton MH, Maule CO, Yee SL, Backinger C, Malarcher AM, Husten CG. *Youth tobacco cessation: a guide for making informed decisions.* Atlanta, GA: Centers for Disease Control and Prevention; 2004.

Outcome 12

Increased Price of Tobacco Products

Evidence is strong that raising the price of cigarettes encourages smokers to quit and reduces smoking prevalence and tobacco use.[1] A comprehensive review of studies of the effect of tobacco price increases shows that a 10% increase in price yields a 4% decrease in tobacco consumption (approximately 2% of which is due to reduced consumption and the remaining 2% is due to quitting smoking).[1] Certain populations—such as adolescents, young adults, and low-income smokers—are particularly price sensitive and are more likely to quit or cut back in response to cigarette price increases than other populations.[2] Even the tobacco industry recognizes the effect of price increases, as revealed by an internal Philip Morris document stating, "A high cigarette price, more than any other cigarette attribute, has the most direct impact on the share of the quitting population. Price, not tar level, is the main driving force for quitting."[3]

Listed below is the indicator associated with this outcome:

3.12.1 Amount of tobacco product excise tax

References

1. Task Force on Community Preventive Services. The guide to community preventive services: tobacco use prevention and control. *American Journal of Preventive Medicine.* 2001;20(Suppl 2):1–88.

2. Centers for Disease Control and Prevention. Responses to cigarette prices by race/ethnicity, income, and age groups—United States, 1976–1993. *Morbidity and Mortality Weekly Report.* 1998;47(29):605–9.

3. Schwab C. Cigarette attributes and quitting. Philip Morris Doc. 2045447810, March 4, 1993. Available from: http://www.pmdocs.com. Accessed December 2004.

For Further Reading

Fiore MC, Bailey WC, Cohen SJ, Dorfman S, Goldstein M, Gritz E, Heyman RB, Jaén CR, Kottke TE, Lando HA, Mecklenburg RE, Mullen PD, Nett LM, Robinson L, Stitzer ML, Tommasello AC, Villejo L, Wewers ME. *Treating tobacco use and dependence: clinical practice guideline.* Rockville, MD: U.S. Department of Health and Human Services; 2000.

Fiore MC, Hatsukami DK, Baker TB. Effective tobacco dependence treatment. *Journal of the American Medical Association.* 2002;288(14):1768–71.

Sciamanna CN, Hoch JS, Duke GC, Fogle MN, Ford DE. Comparison of five measures of motivation to quit smoking among a sample of hospitalized smokers. *Journal of General Internal Medicine.* 2000;15(1):16–23.

U.S. Department of Health and Human Services. *Reducing tobacco use: a report of the Surgeon General.* Atlanta, GA: Centers for Disease Control and Prevention; 2000.

Outcome 12

Increased Price of Tobacco Products

Indicator Rating

←○◐●●→ better

Number	Indicator	Overall quality low ←——→ high	Resources needed	Strength of evaluation evidence	Utility	Face validity	Accepted practice
3.12.1	Amount of tobacco product excise tax	▬▬▬▬▬	$	●	●	◐	●

Indicator 3.12.1

Amount of Tobacco Product Excise Tax

Goal area 3	Promoting quitting among adults and young people
Outcome 12	Increased price of tobacco products
What to measure	(1) The state excise tax per pack of cigarettes and (2) the percentage of the total price of a pack of cigarettes that is attributable to tax
Why this indicator is useful	Increasing the tax on tobacco products reduces tobacco consumption and prevalence, especially among the most price-sensitive populations (e.g., young people).[1,2] Increasing cigarette excise tax is an effective method of increasing the real price of cigarettes, although maintaining high prices requires further tax increases to offset the effects of inflation.[1,2]
Example data source(s)	• CDC State Tobacco Activities Tracking and Evaluation (STATE) system Data available at: http://www.cdc.gov/tobacco/STATEsystem • Campaign For Tobacco-Free Kids (CTFK) Information available at: http://tobaccofreekids.org/research/factsheets • State departments of revenue
Population group(s)	Not applicable. This indicator is best measured by tracking and monitoring state excise tax on tobacco products.
Example survey question(s)	Not applicable
Comments	States can also independently track the price of tobacco products by collecting "scanner data" (data obtained from product bar codes), which provide information on product price, brand, and promotions. However, this type of data collection can be cost prohibitive. To gather more complete data on tobacco use, evaluators can also ask questions about the use of other tobacco products such as spit tobacco (smokeless), bidis, small cigars, and loose tobacco (roll-your-own).

Rating

Overall quality low ◄——► high	Resources needed	Strength of evaluation evidence	Utility	Face validity	Accepted practice
▬▬▬▬	$	●	●	◐	●

◄ ○ ◔ ◉ ● ► better

References
1. U.S. Department of Health and Human Services. *Preventing tobacco use among young people: a report of the Surgeon General.* Atlanta, GA: Centers for Disease Control and Prevention; 1994.
2. Task Force on Community Preventive Services. The guide to community preventive services: tobacco use prevention and control. *American Journal of Preventive Medicine.* 2001;20(Suppl 2):1–88.

Outcome 13

Increased Cessation Among Adults and Young People

Scientific evidence shows that stopping smoking yields major and immediate health benefits. Former smokers live longer than smokers and they have a decreased risk of lung cancer, other cancers, heart attack, stroke, and chronic lung disease.[1] In addition, newborns of women who stop smoking before pregnancy or during the first 3 months of pregnancy have birth weights that are the same as those of nonsmokers.[1] Quitting even later than 3 months in pregnancy confers some benefit. Regardless of the age at which they stop smoking, former smokers live longer and frequently healthier lives than smokers. The excess risk of death from smoking begins to decrease shortly after cessation and continues to decrease for at least 10–15 years.[1]

Listed below are the indicators associated with this outcome:

- **3.13.1** Proportion of smokers who have sustained abstinence from tobacco use
- **3.13.2**[NR] Proportion of recent successful quit attempts

Reference

1. U.S. Department of Health and Human Services. *The health benefits of smoking cessation: a report of the Surgeon General.* Atlanta, GA: Centers for Disease Control and Prevention; 1990. CDC Publication No. 90-8416.

For Further Reading

Fiore MC, Bailey WC, Cohen SJ, Dorfman S, Goldstein M, Gritz E, Heyman RB, Jaén CR, Kottke TE, Lando HA, Mecklenburg RE, Mullen PD, Nett LM, Robinson L, Stitzer ML, Tommasello AC, Villejo L, Wewers ME. *Treating tobacco use and dependence: clinical practice guideline.* Rockville, MD: U.S. Department of Health and Human Services; 2000.

Fiore MC, Hatsukami DK, Baker TB. Effective tobacco dependence treatment. *Journal of the American Medical Association.* 2002;288(14):1768–71.

Haug NA, Stitzer ML, Svikis DS. Smoking during pregnancy and intention to quit: a profile of methadone-maintained women. *Nicotine and Tobacco Research.* 2001;3(4): 333–9.

Nicholson J, Hennrikus D, Lando H, McCarty M, Vessey J. Patient recall versus physician documentation in report of smoking cessation counseling performed in the inpatient setting. *Tobacco Control.* 2000;9(4):382–8.

Task Force on Community Preventive Services. The guide to community preventive services: tobacco use prevention and control. *American Journal of Preventive Medicine.* 2001;20(Suppl 2):1–88.

U.S. Department of Health and Human Services. *Reducing tobacco use: a report of the Surgeon General.* Atlanta, GA: Centers for Disease Control and Prevention; 2000.

Windsor RA, Warner KE, Cutter GR. A cost-effectiveness analysis of self-help smoking cessation methods for pregnant women. *Public Health Reports.* 1988;103(1):83–8.

Windsor RA, Woodby LL, Miller TM, Hardin JM, Crawford MA, DiClemente CC. Effectiveness of Agency for Health Care Policy and Research clinical practice guideline and patient education methods for pregnant smokers in Medicaid maternity care. *American Journal of Obstetrics and Gynecology.* 2000;182(Pt 1):68–75.

Outcome 13

Increased Cessation Among Adults and Young People

Indicator Rating

←○ ◔ ● ●→ better

Number	Indicator	Overall quality low ←——→ high	Resources needed	Strength of evaluation evidence	Utility	Face validity	Accepted practice
3.13.1	Proportion of smokers who have sustained abstinence from tobacco use	├─┼─┼─┤ │	$$	●	●	●	●
3.13.2^{NR}	Proportion of recent successful quit attempts	▬▬▬▬▬	⊘	⊘	⊘	⊘	⊘

⊘ Denotes no data.
^{NR} Denotes an indicator that is not rated (see Appendix B for an explanation).

Indicator 3.13.1

Proportion of Smokers Who Have Sustained Abstinence from Tobacco Use

Goal area 3	Promoting quitting among adults and young people
Outcome 13	Increased cessation among adults and young people
What to measure	Proportion of former smokers who have sustained abstinence from tobacco use for 6 months or longer[1]
Why this indicator is useful	The longer the time since a person smoked, the more likely that person will continue not smoking.[2]
Example data source(s)	Adult Tobacco Survey (ATS): CDC Recommended Questions: Core, 2003 Behavioral Risk Factor Surveillance System (BRFSS): Tobacco Use Prevention Module, 2002 Youth Tobacco Survey (YTS): CDC Recommended Questions: Core, 2004
Population group(s)	Former smokers aged 18 years or older Former smokers aged less than 18 years
Example survey question(s)	**From ATS and BRFSS** About how long has it been since you last smoked cigarettes regularly? ☐ Within the past month (0 to 1 month ago) ☐ Within the past 3 months (1 to 3 months ago) ☐ Within the past 6 months (3 to 6 months ago) ☐ Within the past year (6 to 12 months ago) ☐ Within the past 5 years (1 to 5 years ago) ☐ Within the past 15 years (5 to 15 years ago) ☐ 15 or more years ago ☐ Don't know/Not sure ☐ Refused **From YTS** When was the last time you smoked a cigarette, even one or two puffs? ☐ I have never smoked even one or two puffs ☐ Earlier today ☐ Not today but sometime during the past 7 days ☐ Not during the past 7 days but sometime during the past 30 days ☐ Not during the past 30 days but sometime during the past 6 months ☐ Not during the past 6 months but sometime during the past year ☐ 1 to 4 years ago ☐ 5 or more years ago When you last tried to quit, how long did you stay off cigarettes? ☐ I have never smoked cigarettes ☐ I have never tried to quit ☐ Less then a day ☐ 1 to 7 days ☐ More than 7 days but less than 30 days ☐ 30 days or more but less than 6 months ☐ 6 months or more but less than a year ☐ 1 year or more

Comments	Evaluators could also ask the example questions of current smokers regarding their last quit attempt or longest quit attempt, since an increase in the duration of a quit attempt (even if the smoker begins smoking again) could indicate progress toward cessation.
	This indicator can be used as a proxy for smokers who have "permanently quit."
	Evaluators can determine a proxy for "former smokers" using YTS data by combining the variable of lifetime smoking (≥ 100 cigarettes) and current cigarette smoking (smoked zero cigarettes during the past 30 days).
	Evaluators could also modify the example questions to measure sustained abstinence from all tobacco products.

Rating	Overall quality low ◄——► high	Resources needed	Strength of evaluation evidence	Utility	Face validity	Accepted practice
	▬▬▬▬▬	$$	●	●	●	●

◄─○ ◐ ● ●─► better

References
1. Schwartz JL. *Review and evaluation of smoking cessation methods: the United States and Canada, 1978–1985.* Bethesda, MD: National Cancer Institute; 1987.
2. Hughes JR, Keely JP, Niaura RS, Ossip-Klein DJ, Richmond RL, Swan GE. Measures of abstinence in clinical trials: issues and recommendations. *Nicotine and Tobacco Research.* 2003;5(1):13–25. Erratum in: *Nicotine and Tobacco Research.* 2003;5(4):603.

GOAL AREA 3
Outcome 13

Indicator 3.13.2[NR]

Proportion of Recent Successful Quit Attempts

Goal area 3	Promoting quitting among adults and young people
Outcome 13	Increased cessation among adults and young people
What to measure	Proportion of smokers who made a quit attempt in the previous 12 months and are still not smoking
Why this indicator is useful	It is important to measure the proportion of recent successful quit attempts to document progress toward increased cessation.[1]
Example data source(s)	• Adult Tobacco Survey (ATS): CDC Recommended Questions: Core, 2003 • Behavioral Risk Factor Surveillance System (BRFSS), 2002 • Youth Tobacco Survey (YTS): CDC Recommended Questions: Core, 2004
Population group(s)	• Smokers aged 18 years or older • Smokers aged less than 18 years
Example survey question(s)	**From ATS and BRFSS** Have you smoked at least 100 cigarettes in your entire life? ☐ Yes ☐ No ☐ Don't know/Not sure ☐ Refused Do you now smoke cigarettes every day, some days, or not at all? ☐ Everyday ☐ Some days ☐ Not at all ☐ Refused During the past 12 months, have you stopped smoking for one day or longer because you were trying to quit smoking? ☐ Yes ☐ No ☐ Don't know/Not sure ☐ Refused **From YTS** During the past 30 days, on how many days did you smoke cigarettes? ☐ 0 days ☐ 1 or 2 days ☐ 3 to 5 days ☐ 6 to 9 days ☐ 10 to 19 days ☐ 20 to 29 days ☐ All 30 days How many times during the past 12 months have you stopped smoking for one day or longer because you were trying to quit smoking? ☐ I have not smoked in the past 12 months ☐ I have not tried to quit ☐ 1 time ☐ 2 times ☐ 3 to 5 times ☐ 6 to 9 times ☐ 10 or more times

Example survey question(s) (cont.)	When you last tried to quit, how long did you stay off cigarettes? ☐ I have never smoked cigarettes ☐ I have never tried to quit ☐ Less than a day ☐ 1 to 7 days ☐ More than 7 days but less than 30 days ☐ 30 days or more but less than 6 months ☐ 6 months or more but less than a year ☐ 1 year or more
Comments	Evaluators should ask all three example questions of respondents in the target population to obtain the information necessary to measure this indicator. Evaluators may also want to report the percentage of *ever-smokers* that have quit. This percentage is calculated by dividing the number of *former smokers* by the number of *ever-smokers*. This indicator was not rated by the panel of experts, and therefore no rating information is provided. See Appendix B for an explanation.
Rating	Overall quality / Resources needed / Strength of evaluation evidence / Utility / Face validity / Accepted practice — no data

⊘ Denotes no data.

NR Denotes an indicator that is not rated (see Appendix B for an explanation).

Reference
1. Task Force on Community Preventive Services. The guide to community preventive services: tobacco use prevention and control. *American Journal of Preventive Medicine*. 2001;20(Suppl 2):1–88.

Outcome 14

Reduced Tobacco-use Prevalence and Consumption

Evidence is strong that tobacco use, particularly cigarette smoking, is the leading cause of preventable illness and death in the United States. Cigarette smoking is responsible for more than 440,000 deaths each year, or one of every five deaths.[1] In the United States, nearly one in four adults and about one in four teenagers smoke.[1,2] If current trends continue, 25 million people (including 5 million of today's children) will die prematurely of a smoking-related disease.[3] Paralleling this enormous health and personal toll is the economic burden of tobacco use: more than $75 billion in medical expenditures and another $80 billion in indirect costs resulting from lost productivity.[1] Reducing the number of smokers is the best strategy for decreasing preventable disease and death.[4-6]

Listed below are the indicators associated with this outcome:

- **3.14.1** Smoking prevalence
- **3.14.2** Prevalence of tobacco use during pregnancy
- **3.14.3** Prevalence of postpartum tobacco use
- **3.14.4** Per capita consumption of tobacco products

References

1. Centers for Disease Control and Prevention. *Targeting tobacco use: the nation's leading cause of death, 2004* [At a Glance]. Atlanta, GA: Centers for Disease Control and Prevention, National Center for Chronic Disease Prevention and Health Promotion; 2004. Available from: http://www.cdc.gov/nccdphp/aag/aag_osh.htm. Accessed March 2005.

2. Centers for Disease Control and Prevention. Youth risk behavior surveillance–United States, 2003. *Morbidity and Mortality Weekly Report CDC Surveillance Summaries.* 2004;53(SS-2):1–29.

3. Centers for Disease Control and Prevention. Projected smoking-related deaths among youth—United States. *Morbidity and Mortality Weekly Report.* 1996;45(44):971–4.

4. U.S. Department of Health and Human Services. *Women and smoking: a report of the Surgeon General.* Rockville, MD: U.S. Department of Health and Human Services, Public Health Service, Office of the Surgeon General; 2001.

5. U.S. Department of Health and Human Services. *The health consequences of smoking: cardiovascular disease. A report of the Surgeon General.* Atlanta, GA: Centers for Disease Control; 1983. PHS Publication No. 84-50204.

6. U.S. Department of Health and Human Services. *The health consequences of smoking: cancer. A report of the Surgeon General.* Atlanta, GA: Centers for Disease Control; 1982. PHS Publication No. 82-50179.

For Further Reading

U.S. Department of Health and Human Services. *Reducing tobacco use: a report of the Surgeon General.* Atlanta, GA: Centers for Disease Control and Prevention; 2000.

U.S. Department of Health and Human Services. *Preventing tobacco use among young people: a report of the Surgeon General.* Atlanta, GA: Centers for Disease Control and Prevention; 1994.

U.S. Department of Health and Human Services. *The health benefits of smoking cessation: a report of the Surgeon General.* Atlanta, GA: Centers for Disease Control and Prevention; 1990. CDC Publication No. 90-8416.

National Cancer Institute. Population based smoking cessation: proceedings of a conference on What Works to Influence Cessation in the General Population. *Smoking and Tobacco Control Monograph No. 12.* Bethesda, MD: U.S. Department of Health and Human Services, National Institutes of Health, National Cancer Institute; 2000. NIH Publication No. 00-4892.

Outcome 14

Reduced Tobacco-use Prevalence and Consumption

Indicator Rating

← ○ ◐ ● ● → better

Number	Indicator	Overall quality low ←→ high	Resources needed	Strength of evaluation evidence	Utility	Face validity	Accepted practice
3.14.1	Smoking prevalence	▬▬▬	$$†	●	●	●	●
3.14.2	Prevalence of tobacco use during pregnancy	▬▬▬	$$	●	●	●	●
3.14.3	Prevalence of postpartum tobacco use	▬▬▬	$$$	●	◐	◐	●
3.14.4	Per capita consumption of tobacco products	▬▬▬	$	●	●	●	●

† Denotes low agreement among reviewers: that is, fewer than 75% of the valid ratings for this indicator were within one point of each other (see Appendix B for an explanation).

Indicator 3.14.1

Smoking Prevalence

Goal area 3	Promoting quitting among adults and young people
Outcome 14	Reduced tobacco-use prevalence and consumption
What to measure	Proportion of adults who have ever smoked at least 100 cigarettes in their lives and who smoke every day or some days[1] Proportion of young people who have smoked on at least 1 day during the previous 30 days[2]
Why this indicator is useful	Tobacco use remains the leading preventable cause of death and disease in the United States, resulting in more than 440,000 deaths each year.[3] Although smoking prevalence continues to decline, nearly one in four adults and about one in four teenagers smoke.[4] Reducing the number of smokers is the best strategy for decreasing preventable disease and death.[6-8]
Example data source(s)	▸ Adult Tobacco Survey (ATS): CDC Recommended Questions: Core, 2003 ▸ Behavioral Risk Factor Surveillance System (BRFSS), 2003 ▸ Youth Tobacco Survey (YTS): CDC Recommended Questions: Core, 2004 ▸ CDC Youth Risk Behavior Surveillance System (YRBSS), 2003
Population group(s)	▸ Adult smokers aged 18 years or older ▸ Young smokers aged less than 18 years
Example survey question(s)	**From ATS and BRFSS** Have you smoked at least 100 cigarettes in your entire life? ☐ Yes ☐ No ☐ Don't know/Not sure ☐ Refused Do you now smoke cigarettes everyday, some days, or not at all? ☐ Everyday ☐ Some days ☐ Not at all ☐ Refused **From YTS and YRBSS** During the past 30 days, on how many days did you smoke cigarettes? ☐ 0 days ☐ 1 or 2 days ☐ 3 to 5 days ☐ 6 to 9 days ☐ 10 to 19 days ☐ 20 to 29 days ☐ All 30 days
Comments	To gather more complete data on tobacco use, evaluators can also ask questions about the use of other tobacco products such as spit tobacco (smokeless), bidis, small cigars, and loose tobacco (roll-your-own).

GOAL AREA 3
Outcome 14

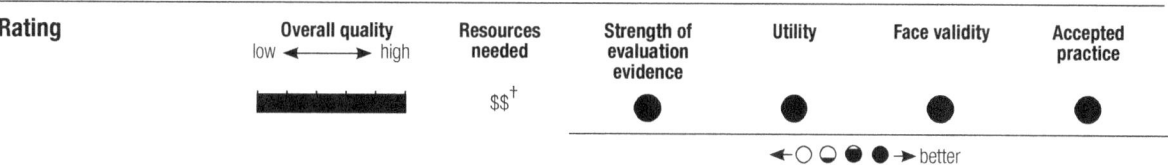

† Denotes low agreement among reviewers: that is, fewer than 75% of the valid ratings for this indicator were within one point of each other (see Appendix B for an explanation).

References
1. Centers for Disease Control and Prevention. Prevalence of current cigarette smoking among adults and changes in prevalence of current and some-day smoking—United States, 1996–2001. *Morbidity and Mortality Weekly Report.* 2003;52(14):303–7.
2. Centers for Disease Control and Prevention. Cigarette use among high school students—United States, 1991–2003. *Morbidity and Mortality Weekly Report.* 2004;53(23);499–502.
3. Centers for Disease Control and Prevention. *Targeting tobacco use: the nation's leading cause of death, 2004* [At a Glance]. Atlanta, GA: Centers for Disease Control and Prevention; 2004. Available from: http://www.cdc.gov/nccdphp/aag/aag_osh.htm. Accessed March 2005.
4. Centers for Disease Control and Prevention. State laws on tobacco control—United States, 1998. *Morbidity and Mortality Weekly Report CDC Surveillance Summaries.* 1999;48(SS-3):21–40.
5. Centers for Disease Control and Prevention. Projected smoking-related deaths among youth—United States. *Morbidity and Mortality Weekly Report.* 1996;45(44):971–4.
6. U.S. Department of Health and Human Services. *Women and smoking: a report of the Surgeon General.* Rockville, MD: U.S. Department of Health and Human Services, Public Health Service, Office of the Surgeon General; 2001.
7. U.S. Department of Health and Human Services. *The health consequences of smoking: cardiovascular disease. A report of the Surgeon General.* Atlanta, GA: Centers for Disease Control; 1983. PHS Publication No. 84-50204.
8. U.S. Department of Health and Human Services. *The health consequences of smoking: cancer. A report of the Surgeon General.* Atlanta, GA: Centers for Disease Control; 1982. PHS Publication No. 82-50179.

Indicator 3.14.2

Prevalence of Tobacco Use During Pregnancy

Goal area 3	Promoting quitting among adults and young people
Outcome 14	Reduced tobacco-use prevalence and consumption
What to measure	Proportion of pregnant women who smoked during pregnancy
Why this indicator is useful	Smoking is associated with a variety of complications before, during, and after pregnancy, including ectopic pregnancy, premature membrane rupture, placental complications, preterm delivery, stillbirth, neonatal and perinatal mortality, increased rates of hospital care, and low birth weight.[1] Reducing maternal smoking prevalence can lead to a reduced probability of these complications.
Example data source(s)	▸ Birth certificate data ▸ CDC Pregnancy Risk Assessment Monitoring System (PRAMS), Phase 4, 2000–2003
Population group(s)	▸ Not applicable. This indicator is best measured by examining birth certificate data from vital statistic records. ▸ Pregnant women
Example survey question(s)	**Birth certificate data are available from states' vital statistics data.** **From PRAMS** In the *last 3 months* of your pregnancy, how many cigarettes or packs of cigarettes did you smoke on an average day? ☐ _____cigarettes OR _____ packs ☐ Less than 1 cigarette a day ☐ I didn't smoke ☐ I don't smoke
Comments	Using birth certificate data may lead to underestimates of smoking rates during pregnancy due to underreporting.[1] Surveys such as PRAMS might yield more accurate data regarding smoking behaviors. To gather more complete data on tobacco use, evaluators can also ask questions about the use of other tobacco products such as cigars, chewing tobacco, and loose tobacco.

Rating

Overall quality low ◄──► high	Resources needed	Strength of evaluation evidence	Utility	Face validity	Accepted practice
███████░░	$$	●	●	●	●

◄ ○ ◐ ● ● ► better

Reference
1. U.S. Department of Health and Human Services. *Women and smoking: a report of the Surgeon General.* Rockville, MD: U.S. Department of Health and Human Services, Public Health Service, Office of the Surgeon General; 2001.

GOAL AREA 3
Outcome 14

Indicator 3.14.3

Prevalence of Postpartum Tobacco Use

Goal area 3	Promoting quitting among adults and young people
Outcome 14	Reduced tobacco-use prevalence and consumption
What to measure	Proportion of women who use tobacco in the postpartum period (6 months after giving birth)
Why this indicator is useful	Although smoking prevalence among women decreases significantly during pregnancy, most mothers resume smoking within a year of delivery.[1,2] In such cases, not only is the health of the mother affected, but also that of her child; exposure to secondhand smoke is a major cause of lower respiratory infections, asthma, and chronic middle inner ear infections among infants and children.[2,3]
Example data source(s)	CDC Pregnancy Risk Assessment Monitoring System (PRAMS), Phase 4, 2000–2003
Population group(s)	Pregnant women
Example survey question(s)	Are you currently pregnant? ☐ Yes ☐ No ☐ Don't know/Not sure ☐ Refused to answer Have you given birth in the past 6 months? ☐ Yes ☐ No ☐ Don't know/Not sure ☐ Refused to answer **From PRAMS** How many cigarettes or packs of cigarettes do you smoke on an average day now? ☐ _____cigarettes OR _____packs ☐ Less than 1 cigarette a day ☐ I didn't smoke ☐ I don't smoke
Comments	The authors created the first two example questions to screen survey respondents for pregnancy status. The questions are not found in any commonly used data source. Evaluators may want to differentiate between women who continued smoking throughout pregnancy into the postpartum period and women who relapsed during the postpartum period.

Rating

Overall quality low ←→ high	Resources needed	Strength of evaluation evidence	Utility	Face validity	Accepted practice
▆▆▆▆	$$$	●	◐	●	●

←○◔●●→ better

References
1. U.S. Department of Health and Human Services. *The health benefits of smoking cessation.* Atlanta, GA: Centers for Disease Control; 1990. CDC Publication No. 90-8416.
2. U.S. Department of Health and Human Services. *Women and smoking: a report of the Surgeon General.* Rockville, MD: U.S. Department of Health and Human Services, Public Health Service, Office of the Surgeon General; 2001.
3. National Cancer Institute. Health effects of exposure to environmental tobacco smoke: the report of the California Environmental Protection Agency. *Smoking and Tobacco Control Monograph No. 10.* Bethesda, MD: National Cancer Institute; 1999. NIH Publication No. 99-4645.

Indicator 3.14.4

Per Capita Consumption of Tobacco Products

Goal area 3	Promoting quitting among adults and young people
Outcome 14	Reduced tobacco-use prevalence and consumption
What to measure	The number of cigarette packs sold per adult aged 18 years or older in the state
Why this indicator is useful	Decreases in overall tobacco consumption indicate the success of a comprehensive tobacco control program.[1,2]
Example data source(s)	‣ CDC State Tobacco Activities Tracking and Evaluation (STATE) system Data available at: http://www.cdc.gov/tobacco/STATEsystem ‣ State departments of revenue
Population group(s)	Not applicable. This indicator is best measured by examining tax records to assess the states' sales of cigarettes.
Example survey question(s)	Not applicable
Comments	Evaluators need to measure statewide consumption of cigarettes, smokeless tobacco, and other tobacco products separately.

Rating

Overall quality low ⟵⟶ high	Resources needed	Strength of evaluation evidence	Utility	Face validity	Accepted practice
▬▬▬▬▬	$	●	●	●	●

⟵ ○ ◐ ● ● ⟶ better

References
1. Farrelly MC, Pechacek TF, Chaloupka FJ. The impact of tobacco control expenditures on aggregate cigarette sales: 1981–2000. *Journal of Health Economics.* 2003;22(5):843–59. Erratum in: *Journal of Health Economics.* 2004;23(2):419.
2. Orzechowski W, Walker RC. *The tax burden on tobacco: historical compilation.* Volume 38. Arlington, VA: Orzechowski and Walker; 2003.

Future Directions

In this publication, we discuss key outcome indicators to evaluate comprehensive state tobacco control programs. Outcome indicators are important for program planning, monitoring, and evaluation. In addition, increasing demands for timelier program performance measures and the need to synthesize existing evidence for evaluation of tobacco control programs contributed to the need for this publication.

The Centers for Disease Control and Prevention's (CDC's) future plans include (1) developing process indicators for evaluating comprehensive tobacco control programs, (2) developing process and outcome indicators for evaluating activities that address tobacco-related disparities (National Tobacco Control Program [NTCP] goal area 4), and (3) conducting research and building scientific evidence for indicators and theories related to tobacco control.

Process Indicators

Process indicators are used to measure success in program planning and implementation. Indicators in this area help to answer questions about the planning, infrastructure, and implementation of a program's activities and the extent to which these activities are reaching the target population. Process indicators are also used to understand why outcomes were or were not achieved as planned. For example, program managers can learn whether implementation of a program component could be improved or whether a new strategy is needed to overcome an unexpected obstacle (e.g., political opposition).

In the NTCP logic models, the emphasis is on environmental, behavioral, and health outcomes; it is assumed that the capacity and infrastructure needed for goal-specific activities are, for the most part, in place. However, for fully informed program planning and evaluation, the program's capacity, infrastructure, and processes must also be assessed. To do so, well-defined indicators of these aspects of the program are needed. Although considerable work has been completed on defining indicators that can be used by program planners and evaluators for measuring program capacity, working with CDC partners to define these indicators in a meaningful and systematic way is necessary.

Indicators for NTCP Goal Area 4: Eliminating Tobacco-related Disparities

Unlike activities to prevent initiation of tobacco use by young people, eliminate nonsmokers' exposure to secondhand smoke, and promote quitting among adults and young people, activities to identify and eliminate tobacco-related disparities lack a definitive evidence base for implementing a program and identifying target outcomes. Sufficient public health knowledge and experience exists, however, to provide a well-founded framework for approaching tasks associated with improving the public health infrastructure and related capacities so that tobacco control programs can address tobacco-related disparities among specific populations.

Building on successful capacity-building and infrastructure activities during the past 10 years, CDC began the Disparities Pilot Training Project, an initiative to improve the state and territorial public health capacity and infrastructure needed to address tobacco-related disparities. To assist health departments and their partners with planning and implementing strategic activities to identify and eliminate tobacco-related disparities, CDC prepared a draft logic model that is based on state practices, published scientific findings, and input from external partners (see draft logic model, page 271). Instead of focusing on traditional health outcomes, this logic model focuses on the minimum capacity needed by state and territorial health departments to pursue strategic activities that would identify and eliminate tobacco-related disparities.

In cooperation with its partners, CDC will continue the task of developing an approach to identifying, evaluating, and eliminating tobacco-related disparities. The draft logic model is a window to the work that is being done now and that needs to continue.

Research Opportunities

We encourage researchers outside CDC who read this publication to identify research opportunities. For example, where the strength of the evidence for using certain indicators is low, expanding that evidence base would be beneficial. Researchers might also consider developing new evaluation designs that could (1) further refine theories related to tobacco control or (2) identify other outcome indicators, especially indicators for program components that need additional research or scientific evidence to support them. In addition, researchers might work on developing methods for measuring indicators for which no well-established methods are currently available.

Goal Area 4

Identifying and Eliminating Tobacco-Related Disparities

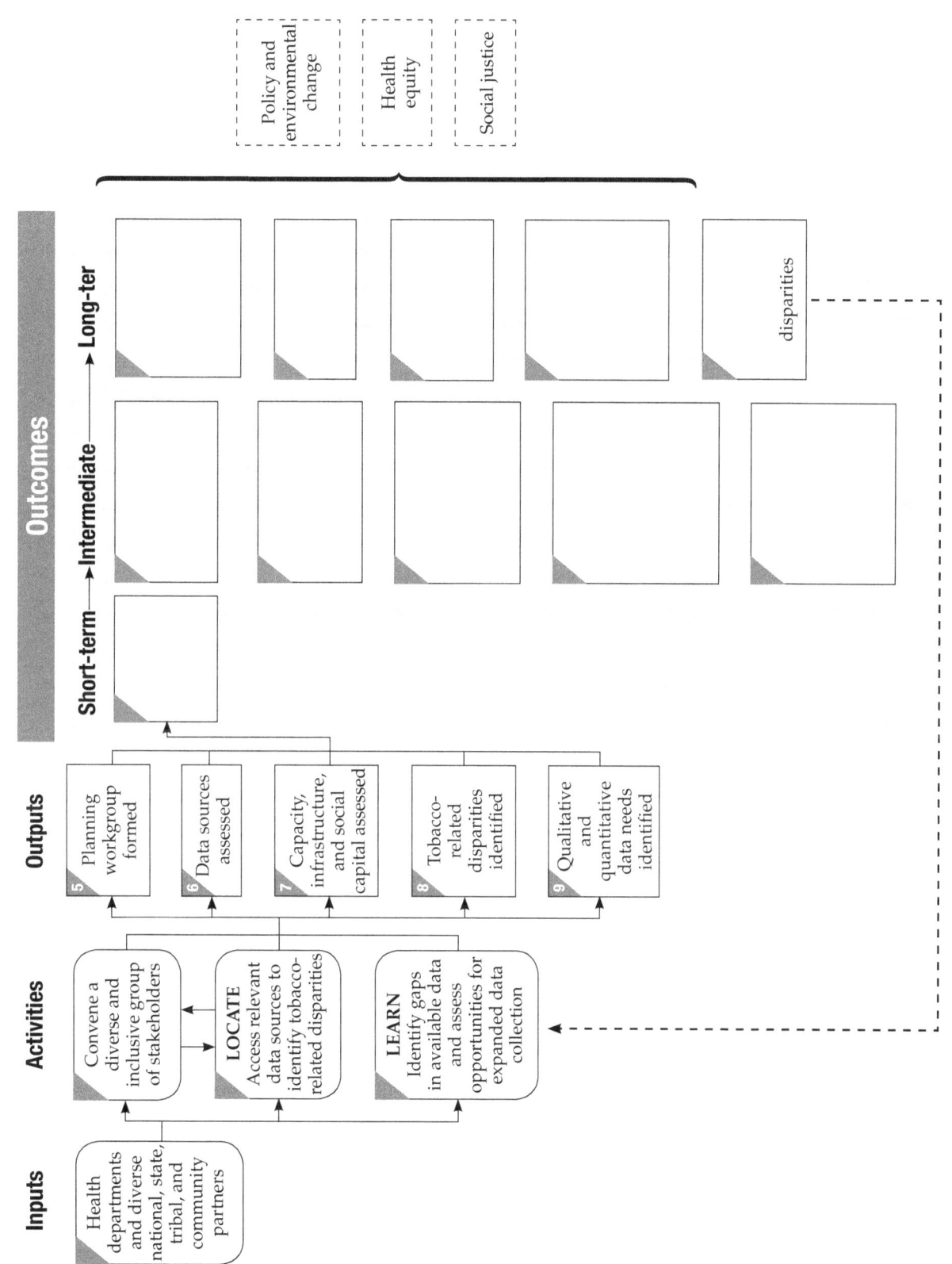

CHAPTER 5 — *Future Directions*

Appendices and Glossary

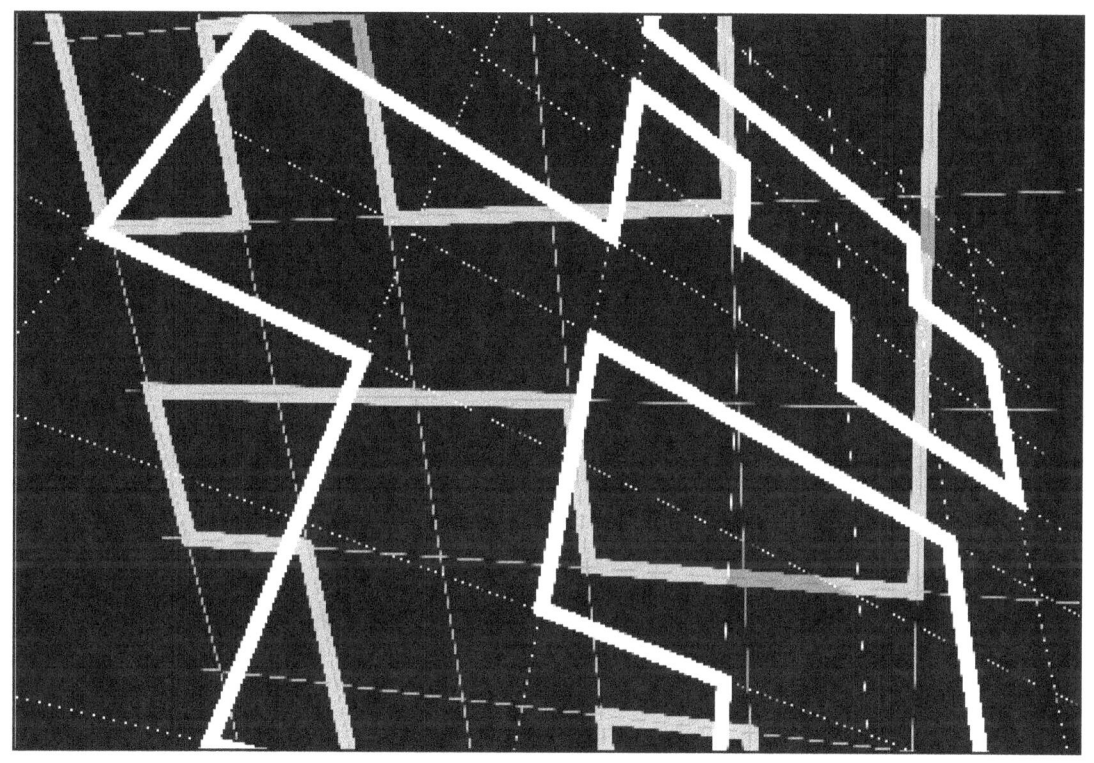

APPENDIX A

National Tobacco Control Program

An Overview

The Centers for Disease Control and Prevention (CDC) is the lead federal agency for comprehensive tobacco prevention and control. CDC develops, conducts, and supports strategic activities to protect the public's health from the harmful effects of tobacco use.

To carry out its mission, CDC:

- Expands the science base for effective tobacco control.

- Builds sustainable capacity and infrastructure for comprehensive tobacco control programs and policies.

- Communicates information about tobacco issues to policy makers, health professionals, and the public.

- Provides technical assistance on developing, implementing, and evaluating tobacco control policies, strategies, and initiatives.

- Builds strategic partnerships with national and international organizations.

Through its Office on Smoking and Health, CDC manages the National Tobacco Control Program (NTCP), which funds comprehensive tobacco control programs in state health departments and territories. NTCP-funded programs work to implement the strategies described in the following publications:

- *Best Practices for Comprehensive Tobacco Control Programs*[1]

- *Reducing Tobacco Use: A Report of the Surgeon General*[2]

- *The Guide to Community Preventive Services: Tobacco Use Prevention and Control*[3]

- *Treating Tobacco Use and Dependence: Clinical Practice Guideline*[4]

- *The Health Consequences of Smoking: A Report of the Surgeon General*[5]

- *Preventing Tobacco Use Among Young People: A Report of the Surgeon General*[6]

- *Women and Smoking: A Report of the Surgeon General*[7]

- *Tobacco Use Among U.S. Racial/Ethnic Minority Groups—African Americans, American Indians and Alaska Natives, Asian Americans and Pacific Islanders, and Hispanics: A Report of the Surgeon General*[8]

CDC created NTCP to encourage coordinated, nationwide activities to reduce tobacco-related disease and death. NTCP provides funds and technical support to all 50 states, the District of Columbia, seven U.S. territories, and eight national networks of Indian tribes, Alaskan Natives, and other minority ethnic groups.

NTCP's Goals

The overall goal of NTCP's comprehensive tobacco control programs is to reduce tobacco-related disease, disability, and death. This goal is subdivided into four goal areas:

- Preventing initiation of tobacco use among young people.
- Eliminating nonsmokers' exposure to secondhand smoke.
- Promoting quitting among adults and young people.
- Identifying and eliminating tobacco-related disparities.

The Four Strategies of the NTCP

- Population-based community interventions.
- Countermarketing.
- Public policies and regulations to reduce tobacco use.
- Surveillance and evaluation.

For more information on the NTCP go to http://www.cdc.gov/tobacco.

References

1. Centers for Disease Control and Prevention. *Best practices for comprehensive tobacco control programs*. Atlanta, GA: Centers for Disease Control and Prevention; 1999.

2. U.S. Department of Health and Human Services. *Reducing tobacco use: a report of the Surgeon General*. Atlanta, GA: Centers for Disease Control and Prevention; 2000.

3. Task Force on Community Preventive Services. The guide to community preventive services: tobacco use prevention and control. *American Journal of Preventive Medicine*. 2001;20(Suppl 2):1–88.

4. Fiore MC, Bailey WC, Cohen SJ, Dorfman SF, Goldstein MG, Gritz EG, Heyman RB, Jaén CR, Kottke TE, Lando HA, Mecklenburg RE, Mullen PD, Nett LM, Robinson L, Stitzer ML, Tommasello AC, Villejo L, Wewers ME. *Treating tobacco use and dependence: clinical practice guideline*. Rockville, MD: U.S. Department of Health and Human Services. Public Health Service; 2000.

5. U.S. Department of Health and Human Services. *The health consequences of smoking: a report of the Surgeon General*. Atlanta, GA: Centers for Disease Control and Prevention; 2004.

6. U.S. Department of Health and Human Services. *Preventing tobacco use among young people: a report of the Surgeon General*. Atlanta, GA: Centers for Disease Control and Prevention; 1994.

7. U.S. Department of Health and Human Services. *Women and smoking: a report of the Surgeon General*. Rockville, MD: U.S. Department of Health and Human Services, Public Health Service, Office of the Surgeon General; 2001.

8. U.S. Department of Health and Human Services. *Tobacco Use Among U.S. Racial/Ethnic Minority Groups—African Americans, American Indians and Alaska Natives, Asian Americans and Pacific Islanders, and Hispanics: a report of the Surgeon General.* Atlanta, GA: U.S. Department of Health and Human Services, Centers for Disease Control and Prevention, National Center for Chronic Disease Prevention and Health Promotion, Office on Smoking and Health; 1998.

APPENDIX B

Selecting and Rating the Indicators

The Centers for Disease Control and Prevention (CDC) began producing this publication by appraising the logic models for three of the four goal areas of the National Tobacco Control Program (NTCP):

- Preventing initiation of tobacco use among young people.
- Eliminating nonsmokers' exposure to secondhand smoke.
- Promoting quitting among adults and young people.

As a result of the appraisal, our previously published logic models were updated, and the new versions are published here.[1]

Selecting the Indicators and Data Sources

After an extensive review of published and fugitive literature, we selected candidate indicators for the outcome components of each NTCP goal area's logic model. Then we reviewed the scientific evidence for an association between the candidate indicators and the outcome components in the NTCP logic models. For example, we looked for evidence that an increase in levels of support for policies, and enforcement of policies, to decrease young people's access to tobacco (indicator 1.6.4) is associated with a reduction in the percentage of teenagers who experiment with tobacco (outcome 10 in goal area 1).

Next, we selected example data sources and survey questions for each indicator. One important criterion used to select example data sources was their easy availability to state tobacco control programs. Such data sources include the Behavioral Risk Factor Surveillance System; Adult Tobacco Survey: CDC-Recommended Questions; Youth Tobacco Survey: CDC-Recommended Questions; Current Population Survey: Tobacco Use Supplement; CDC Pregnancy Risk Assessment Monitoring System; and the CDC Youth Risk Behavior Surveillance System.

The selected survey questions come primarily from these survey or surveillance systems. However, if these sources had no appropriate questions to measure the indicator, we developed example questions or chose questions from national or state surveys and evaluation protocols (e.g., Legacy Media Tracking Survey) that are not widely used by state tobacco control programs, although they are available to them.

Rating the Indicators

We assembled a panel of experts (whose names are listed in Appendix C) to rate the final set of candidate indicators. The principal reason for having experts rate the indicators was to have them advise CDC on which indicators were key for evaluation of comprehensive state tobacco control programs. The experts also assessed the indicators on the basis of several criteria and advised us about which data sources are most useful for tracking these indicators. In developing the rating process, we first did a pilot test. As a result of that test, we refined the indicator rating process, instructions to raters, and supportive materials (see page 284).

The panelists were asked to rate each of the 136 candidate indicators separately according to the following criteria:

- **Strength of the evaluation evidence.** The extent to which the literature supports use of the indicator for the evaluation of comprehensive, statewide tobacco control programs, as characterized by the logic models.

  Reference citations on each indicator rating form were intended to provide guidance for reviewer ratings.

- **Resources needed for data collection and analysis.** The amount of funds, time, and effort needed to collect reliable and precise data on the indicator and to analyze primary or secondary data.

  In making their judgments, reviewers were instructed to consider the availability of existing data (e.g., archival records or other secondary data) and the difficulties related to sampling and data collection methods. We reminded reviewers that many state health departments do not have extensive data collection systems for use in comprehensive evaluations of their tobacco control programs. However, all states have access to data on adults from the Behavioral Risk Factor Surveillance System, as well as periodic data on attitudes and policies through the Tobacco Use Supplements of the Current Population Survey. In addition, CDC synthesizes behavioral and policy data on the State Tobacco Activities Tracking and Evaluation (STATE) system. The resources needed for data collection and analysis are less when data are already available than when new data must be collected and analyzed.

- **Utility.** The extent to which the indicator would help to answer key evaluation questions for a state comprehensive tobacco control program.

  Although many indicators are also appropriate and useful for evaluating local tobacco control programs, reviewers were asked to consider the utility of each indicator for evaluating state tobacco control programs.

- **Face validity.** The extent to which judgments about and measurements of the indicator would appear valid and relevant to policy makers and other decision makers who use the results of an evaluation to justify their continued support.

- **Uniqueness.** Whether the indicator contributes distinctive information for the evaluation of tobacco control efforts.

  Reviewers who believed that an indicator was not unique were instructed to identify the redundant indicator.

- **Conformity with accepted practice.** The degree to which use of the indicator as a measure of a tobacco control program's progress is consistent with accepted, real-world tobacco control practice.

- **Overall quality.** A global rating that reflects the reviewer's opinion of the overall quality of the indicator.

- **Summary rating.** The reviewer's opinion of how essential a particular indicator is for the evaluation of comprehensive, statewide tobacco control programs.

After the rating process, 31 indicators were merged, 4 eliminated, and 7 added, leaving a total of 120 indicators for which we provide information in this publication.

In addition, we asked the expert raters to:

- Comment on the data sources and survey questions that CDC had selected for each proposed indicator.
- Suggest alternative data sources and questions.
- Suggest additional indicators that would be useful for evaluation of comprehensive state tobacco control programs.

Each expert used a separate rating form for each indicator (see end of this appendix for a reprint of the rating form and rater instructions).

The form has three sections:

- A summary of information on CDC's proposed indicator and logic model component to which it relates, suggested data sources and survey questions, and (when available) a reference to the scientific evidence supporting the use of the indicator.
- A rating scale for each criterion.
- Space for reviewer comments.

We also encouraged the experts to write notes on the rating forms and to provide additional information, references, or other documentation.

Analysis and Synthesis of Data from the Expert Reviews

After CDC received the completed rating forms from the experts, all data (including written comments) were entered into an electronic file. We adjusted for multiple responses, skipped items, and coding errors. If, for example, a rater circled more than one response for a criterion, we averaged the responses unless the rater had noted a preference for one response over another. Skipped items and "don't know" responses were combined into a "no answer" category. All data were analyzed using the Statistical Analysis System (SAS v.8.02).[2]

For each type of rating, numerical data were analyzed in various ways. Frequency distributions of numerical data were analyzed to help us understand the raters' perceptions about the indicators. Narrative comments included on the raters' rating sheets were also reviewed to help us understand why raters gave an indicator a particularly high or low rating. To limit the effect of outliers, we used the median scores for each indicator.

After reviewing the experts' ratings, we decided to combine indicators that were originally divided by population group (e.g., young people, adults). The experts' numeric ratings for the 31 merged indicators are not provided in this publication but are noted with NR. In addition, after reviewing the rating data and comments carefully, we eliminated four indicators that were rated "not essential" by most panel members.

CDC also reviewed the expert panelists' "resources needed" scores (their estimate of the intensity of resources required to collect and analyze data on each indicator). CDC substituted scores for six indicators that were rated by the experts. For example, the experts rated the "resources needed" criterion for indicator 1.9.12 (amount of tobacco industry campaign contributions to local and state politicians) as 2.5 out of 4. We know, however, that data about this indicator are readily available from archival sources, so we lowered the score to 1 out of 4.

The indicator rating tables include seven indicators that were not rated by the experts. Most of those were suggested by the experts themselves, and CDC used its best judgment to select which expert-proposed indicators to include. These indicators are not rated (and noted by an NR), but some information about them is provided in the indicator profiles.

Two criteria used by expert panelists were not included in the final rating tables: "uniqueness" and the "summary rating." "Uniqueness" was only used to determine redundant indicators, and we found that the "summary rating" was highly correlated with "quality."

After extensive analysis and consideration, we also decided not to use the expert panelists' assessment for the "strength of evaluation evidence" criterion because, among other reasons, several panelists were concerned that their knowledge of the scientific literature on certain areas of tobacco control was limited. Instead, ratings for this criterion are based on the findings from an independent literature review conducted by the Battelle Centers for Public Health Research and Evaluation under contract to CDC. Battelle staff reviewed 847 articles to assess the evidence supporting the use of each indicator to measure a downstream outcome of a tobacco control program.

We evaluated and scored each relevant article or report on the following factors:

Type of Article
One designation per article as follows:

- **Research article.** Article with new data, generally from a single study.
- **Review article.** Article with summaries of multiple published studies and no original data.
- **Background article.** Article with information relevant to the indicator but no evidence of a relationship between the indicator and outcomes.

   Score:
   Research article = 0.5
   Review article = 1.0
   Background article = 0.0

Linkage

The extent of evidence provided in the article for a link between the indicator and the expected downstream outcomes in the NTCP goal area logic models.

Score:
Article shows *any* evidence of link between the indicator and an expected outcome = 1.0

Article shows only evidence *against* a link between the indicator and expected outcome = –1.0

Relevance

The degree to which the article specifically focuses on the indicator.

Score:
Article focuses directly on the indicator = 1.0
Article does not focus directly on the indicator = 0.0

Study Strength

How well the study was designed and how well it showed a link between the indicator and outcomes in the NTCP goal area logic models.

Score:
Article shows *strong* links between the indicator and an expected outcome = 1.0
Article shows a *weak* link = 0.5*

These data were used to calculate the Strength of Evaluation Evidence (SEE) criterion, as follows:

$$SEE = \sum(T*L*R*S)$$

where, for each article,

T = article type
L = linkage
R = relevance
S = study strength

The product of T*L*R*S for each article was summed across all articles for each indicator. The result was translated into the relative score in the indicator rating tables, symbolized as follows:

- No data (⊘): Indicators for which no studies tested an association between the indicator and a downstream outcome in one of NTCP's goal area logic models.

- No support (○): Indicators for which most studies that tested an association between the indicator and outcomes in the logic models found that the association was not significant (SEE score = – 0.5–0.0).

---

*An article that showed a weak link was given a value of 0.5 rather than 0 (zero) because a weak link is stronger than no link.

- Minimal support (◐): Indicators for which roughly an equal amount of research showed a significant association as showed no association between the indicator and downstream logic model outcomes. This category also includes indicators for which studies with weak designs supported an association between the indicator and an outcome (SEE score: 0.01–0.5).

- Moderate support (◉): Indicators for which more research showed a significant association between the indicator and a logic model outcome than research showing a non-significant association. This category also includes indicators for which studies supported an association between the indicator and a downstream outcome in the logic models, but the study designs were not strong (SEE score = 0.51–2.5).

- Strong support (●): Indicators for which research showed a strong relationship between the indicator and a logic model outcome. Included in this category are all long-term indicators because the research supporting these indicators as predictive of beneficial health effects is well established (SEE score > 2.5).

We also footnoted indicators that had low reviewer response, low agreement among reviewers, or a modified "resources needed" criterion with the following symbols:

- An asterisk (*) indicates low reviewer response: if less than 75% of experts rated the indicator or if more than 75% of experts gave a certain criterion an invalid rating (e.g., "don't know"), we considered the indicator to have low reviewer response. A low response suggests a high degree of uncertainty among raters. An example of such an indicator is 2.3.2: Level of receptivity to media messages about secondhand smoke.

- A dagger (†) indicates a low level of agreement among reviewers: if less than 75% of the valid ratings were within one point of each other, we considered the rating to have a low level of agreement. An example of an indicator with a low level of agreement is 1.6.3: Proportion of students who would ever wear or use something with a tobacco company name or picture. This low level of agreement represents a relatively high degree of variability in the raters' responses for the criterion.

- A diamond (◊) indicates that the "resources needed" rating for this indicator was modified by CDC after the experts provided their ratings for this criterion. An example of such an indicator is 1.9.1: Extent and type of retail tobacco advertising and promotions.

Review of this Publication

This publication was peer reviewed internally at CDC and externally by program managers of state tobacco control programs and by other experts in the field of tobacco control.

CDC/OSH Key Indicators Report: Instructions for Expert Panel Reviewers

Purpose

CDC's Office on Smoking and Health (OSH) is developing a report intended to assist state and territorial tobacco control program evaluation efforts under the National Tobacco Control Program (NTCP). State Program Managers, State Evaluators, OSH staff, and national partners will be the primary audiences for the report. The report will aim to accomplish the following functions:

- Serve as a companion to OSH's Best Practices for *Comprehensive Tobacco Control Programs* and *Introduction to Program Evaluation for Comprehensive Tobacco Control Programs*.

- Describe key outcome indicators for evaluation of statewide, comprehensive tobacco control programs, and suggest appropriate data sources and measures for these indicators.

- Encourage states to use consistent evaluation measures and comparable data sources.

- Help OSH determine evaluation criteria for the NTCP, assess Best Practices recommendations, and provide consistent surveillance and evaluation technical assistance to states.

Methods

Report development began with a critical appraisal of OSH logic models for three of the four NTCP goal areas: (1) preventing initiation of tobacco use among youth; (2) eliminating nonsmokers' exposure to secondhand smoke; and (3) promoting quitting among youth and adults. The logic models (figures 1, 2, and 3) graphically display the links among input, activity, output, and short, intermediate, and long-term outcome components.

The fourth NTCP goal area—identify and eliminate disparities among population groups—will be incorporated through guidance on population-specific data collection methods and measures.

Almost every identified outcome indicator may be tracked for various population groups, including groups with high tobacco use prevalence rates or excess tobacco-related disease morbidity and mortality. In addition, OSH is currently developing a logic model specific to this disparities goal. The primary focus is currently on identifying appropriate program activities and process measures.

The indicators are organized by CDC/OSH goal area and logic model component. Extensive review of published and fugitive literature identified candidate indicators for the outcome components of each logic model. Selection decisions were guided by a need to highlight key indicators for evaluation of statewide, comprehensive tobacco control programs. Linkages connecting antecedent and consequent indicators were reviewed for evidence of association; for example, what is the evidence that implementation of tobacco-free policies in schools is associated with "downstream" outcomes? Each goal indicator list (tables 1, 2, and 3) shows the proposed indicators and references to supportive evaluation research. However, the references provided are not intended to be a comprehensive bibliography.

Next, optimal data sources and measures were selected for each indicator. The primary criterion used to select measures was whether the data sources are readily available to state tobacco control programs. These include the Behavioral Risk Factor Surveillance System (BRFSS), CDC Adult and Youth Tobacco Surveys, and other similar surveys and surveillance data sources. Where necessary, measures were drawn from other national and state-specific surveys and evaluation protocols that are not widely used at present but are accessible to state tobacco control programs.

Finally, a pilot study was conducted to test the rating process. Refinements in the instructions, rating forms, and supportive materials were made in response to feedback from pilot study participants.

Rating Process

The principal purpose of this expert review process is to advise CDC/OSH on which of the proposed indicators are considered key for the evaluation of comprehensive state tobacco control programs, and what data sources and measures would be most useful for tracking these indicators. Reviewers are asked to do the following:

- Rate each indicator on a set of criteria.
- Comment on the data sources and measures that have been identified for each proposed indicator.
- Suggest alternative data sources and measures.
- Offer additional indicators that may be useful for state tobacco control program evaluation.

Rating Form

Each indicator is presented on a separate rating form in the same order as the indicators are listed in tables 1, 2, and 3. The rating forms have three sections:

- Summary information on the proposed indicator, including the goal area, logic model component, suggested data sources and measures, other relevant information, and a reference regarding the evidence supporting use of the indicator, where available.
- Eight rating criteria scales for reviewer response.
- Space for open-ended reviewer comments on the proposed indicator and data sources/measures.

In the summary information section on the rating forms, the data sources/measures suggested are intended only to help operationalize the indicators and do not represent a comprehensive list of all possible measures for the indicators. In several instances where existing data sources or measures have not been identified, they have been labeled generically (e.g., "State Adult Tobacco Survey") and the measure noted as "No question identified." This suggests that a measure could be added to a state-specific survey. For measures involving data collection at levels other than for an individual respondent, only the data source is identified (e.g., "Environmental scan of tobacco advertising and promotional practices in retail outlets" or "Local level policy tracking system"). Finally, to conserve space, response options for the suggested measures have been abbreviated.

Rating Criteria

The following criteria are to be used to rate each indicator:

1. **Strength of the evaluation evidence**—extent to which you believe that the literature supports use of the indicator for the evaluation of comprehensive, statewide tobacco control programs, as characterized by the logic models. The reference citations included in tables 1, 2, and 3 and on each indicator rating form are intended to provide guidance in your ratings on this criterion, but your knowledge about other citations should also be used.

2. **Data collection and analysis resource needs**—your rating of the intensity of resource use (cost, time, and effort) required to collect reliable and precise measures, and to analyze appropriately primary or secondary data on the indicator. In making your judgments, please consider availability of existing data (e.g., archival records or other secondary data) and methodology and sampling frame issues. Please recognize that, with few exceptions (e.g., California, Massachusetts, Florida, Oregon, Texas, and a few others), most state health departments currently do not implement comprehensive, statewide evaluations of their tobacco control programs.

   All states have access to basic prevalence data for adults from the BRFSS, periodic data on attitudes and policies through the Current Population Survey (CPS) tobacco use supplements, and School Health Education Profile (SHEP). CDC synthesizes the available state-level data on many behavioral and policy areas in the State Tobacco Activities Tracking and Evaluation System (STATE). Beyond these "common denominator" data sources, some states collect additional data through youth or adult surveys, policy tracking systems, media tracking systems, or other specific data collection methods. The intensity of resource use for data collection and analysis will obviously be less for those "common denominator" data sources than for other sources.

3. **Utility**—extent to which you believe that the indicator would help to answer key statewide comprehensive tobacco control program evaluation questions. Although these indicators may also be appropriate and useful for community-level evaluation, the utility criterion refers primarily to state efforts.

4. **Face validity**—your estimation of how valid the indicator would appear to be in the eyes of policy makers and decision makers who may be users of tobacco control program evaluation results.

5. **Uniqueness**—your opinion of whether the indicator contributes distinct information for the evaluation of tobacco control efforts. If you believe that the indicator is not unique, please note the redundant indicator in the space provided. [Note: Pilot study reviewers suggested that the best way to rate indicators on their uniqueness was to review all indicators in a given area once through, and then adjust ratings on this criterion as necessary.]

6. **Conformity with accepted practice**—your opinion of the degree to which use of the indicator is consistent with currently accepted, "real-world" tobacco control practice.

7. **Overall quality**—a summary rating that reflects your opinion of the overall quality of the indicator.
8. **Priority rating**—your opinion of how essential this indicator is for the evaluation of comprehensive, statewide tobacco control programs. [Note: Pilot study participants suggested that this criterion be reviewed again and adjusted once all indicators in an area have been rated.]

Reviewer Comments

In addition to providing comments and suggestions regarding the proposed indicator, data sources, and measures in the spaces provided, reviewers are encouraged to write notes anywhere on the rating forms or provide additional information, references, or other documentation, as necessary.

Product

Expert ratings of the indicators will be taken into account when determining the final list of key indicators. The report will also present information on each indicator, as in Box 1.

Box 1: Indicator Summary (Sample)	
Proposed Indicator:	Proportion of youth who report never having tried a cigarette
Goal Area:	Preventing Initiation of Tobacco Use Among Youth
Logic Model Component:	Long-term—Reduced initiation among youth
Definition:	Proportion of respondents under 18 years of age who report that they have never tried even one puff of a cigarette.
Purpose:	By employing periodic cross-sectional surveys of youth sampled from school or communitywide frames, this indicator may be used to track the rate of initiation of cigarette smoking among youth in a given population. With sufficient sampling, initiation may be measured with good precision in various subpopulation groups to look at gender, age, geographic, and ethnic/racial group disparities.
Rationale:	Reduced initiation of tobacco use by youth will lower the youth smoking prevalence rate in the population. And, if youth reach adulthood without any tobacco use, chances are they will not initiate use as an adult.
Demographic Group:	Youth, under the age of 18 years.
Data Sources/Measures:	CDC Youth Tobacco Survey Have you ever tried cigarette smoking, even one or two puffs? Yes No
Additional Data Needs:	Age, gender, race, ethnicity, city/county of residence.
Limitations:	None
Other Information:	This indicator may also encompass measurement of other forms of tobacco use, such as smokeless tobacco.

References

1. MacDonald G, Starr G, Schooley M, Yee SL, Klimowski K, Turner K. *Introduction to program evaluation for comprehensive tobacco control programs.* Atlanta, GA: Centers for Disease Control and Prevention; 2001.

2. SAS Institute, Inc. *SAS Language reference: dictionary.* Version 8. Cary, NC: SAS Institute Inc.; 1999.

CDC/OSH Tobacco Control Indicator Rating Form

Proposed Indicator: Proportion of schools/districts with policies that regulate display of tobacco industry promotional items (01.06.XX)

Goal Area: Preventing Initiation of Tobacco Use Among Youth (01)

Logic Model Component: Short-term—Changes in school curricula and policies (06)

Data Sources/Measures: CDC SHPPS, State School Policy and Environment (2000)

Has your [school/district] adopted a policy that prohibits students from wearing tobacco name-brand apparel or carrying merchandise with tobacco company names, logos, or cartoon characters in it?

Other Information: Question modified for use with school and/or district samples

Reference: _____

Indicator Ratings

a. Please circle the response number that reflects the extent to which evaluation evidence supports use of the indicator for the associated construct:

No Support	Minimal Support	Moderate Support	Strong Support	Don't Know
1	2	3	4	0

b. Please circle the response number that reflects your estimate of the intensity of resource utilization required to collect and analyze indicator data adequately:

Low Intensity	Moderate Intensity	High Intensity	Very High Intensity	Don't Know
1	2	3	4	0

c. Please circle the response number that reflects your rating of the utility of the indicator to answer important questions on program effectiveness and impact:

No Utility	Low Utility	Moderate Utility	High Utility	Don't Know
1	2	3	4	0

d. Please circle the response number that reflects your estimation of how face valid the indicator would appear to be in the eyes of policy- and decision-makers:

Not at All Valid	A Little Valid	Somewhat Valid	Highly Valid	Don't Know
1	2	3	4	0

e. Please circle the response number that reflects your opinion of whether the indicator contributes unique information for tobacco control evaluation efforts:

Unique	Not Unique	If "Not Unique" write the number(s) of the redundant indicator(s):	Don't Know
1	2		0

f. Please circle the response number that reflects your opinion of the degree to which use of the indicator is consistent with currently accepted, "real-world" tobacco control practice:

Not at all Consistent	A Little Consistent	Somewhat Consistent	Highly Consistent	Don't Know
1	2	3	4	0

g. Please circle the response number that reflects your view of the overall quality of the indicator:

Low				High
1	2	3	4	5

h. Please circle the response number that reflects your summary rating of how essential this indicator is for the evaluation of comprehensive state tobacco control programs:

Not Essential	Optional	Essential
1	2	3

Reviewer Comments

a. Please provide any additional comments on your ratings of this indicator:

b. If you feel there is a better indicator of this logic model construct, please specify here:

c. Please provide comments on the proposed data sources/measures for this indicator:

d. If you feel there are better data sources/measures, please specify here:

APPENDIX C

Expert Panel Members

We thank the following panel of experts members (in alphabetical order) who rated the indicators. Without their generosity in sharing their expertise and donating their time, this publication would not have been possible.

Ursula Bauer, Ph.D., M.P.H.
Director
Tobacco Control Program
New York State Department of Health

Carolyn Celebucki, Ph.D.
Associate Professor
Department of Psychology
University of Rhode Island, Providence Campus

Thomas Chapel, M.A., M.B.A.
Senior Health Scientist
Office of Program Planning & Evaluation
Centers for Disease Control and Prevention

K. Michael Cummings, M.P.H., Ph.D.
Chairman
Department of Behavioral Epidemiology
Division of Cancer Prevention and Population Sciences
Roswell Park Cancer Institute

Cristine Delnevo, Ph.D., M.P.H.
Associate Professor
School of Public Health
University of Medicine and Dentistry of New Jersey

Matthew Farrelly, Ph.D.
Senior Program Director
Tobacco Use Research Program
Research Triangle Institute

Ellen Feighery, R.N., M.S.
Program Director
Public Health Institute

Gary Giovino, Ph.D., M.S.
Senior Research Scientist
Tobacco Control Research Program
Department of Health Behavior
Division of Cancer Prevention and Population Sciences
Roswell Park Cancer Institute

Stanton Glantz, Ph.D.
Professor of Medicine (Cardiology)
University of California at San Francisco

Nell Gottlieb, Ph.D.
Professor
Department of Kinesiology and Health Education
University of Texas at Austin

Douglas Luke, Ph.D.
Associate Professor of Community Health
School of Public Health
Saint Louis University

Danny McGoldrick, Ph.D.
Director of Research
Campaign for Tobacco-Free Kids

Jesse Nodora, Dr.P.H.
Evaluation Administrator
Tobacco Education and Prevention
Arizona Department of Health Services

John Pierce, Ph.D.
Sam M. Walton Professor for Cancer Research
Department of Family and Preventive Medicine
Associate Director, Cancer Prevention and Control Program
University of California at San Diego

April Roeseler, M.S.P.H.
Chief
Local Programs and Evaluation
Tobacco Control Section
California Department of Health Services

Mike Stark, Ph.D.
Evaluation Manager
Office of Disease Prevention and Epidemiology
Oregon Department of Human Services and Multnomah County Health Department

Data Source Indicator Table

The following table cross-references example data sources and indicators in this publication. The example data sources do not represent all data sources available. When possible, Web addresses are provided. For additional information on tobacco-related data sources and data collection methods, refer to *The Introduction to Program Evaluation for Comprehensive Tobacco Control Programs* or *Surveillance and Evaluation Data Resources for Comprehensive Tobacco Control Programs*.[1,2]

Data source	Indicator numbers	For more information
Addressing Tobacco in Managed Care (ATMC), Survey of Health Plans, 1997–1998	3.7.5; 3.9.1; 3.9.8; 3.10.1	http://www.aahp.org/atmc/mainindex.cfm
Adult Tobacco Survey (ATS): CDC Recommended Questions: Core, 2003	2.3.5; 2.3.6; 2.3.7; 2.4.2; 2.4.3; 2.4.4; 2.6.1; 2.6.4; 2.7.3; 2.8.2; 2.8.3; 3.8.3; 3.9.2; 3.9.3; 3.9.5; 3.11.1; 3.11.3; 3.13.1; 3.13.2[NR]; 3.14.1	State health departments Office on Smoking and Health, Centers for Disease Control and Prevention, (770) 488–5703
Adult Tobacco Survey (ATS): CDC Recommended Questions: Supplemental Section C: Cessation, 2003	3.7.4; 3.8.6; 3.9.2; 3.9.3	State health departments Office on Smoking and Health, Centers for Disease Control and Prevention, (770) 488–5703
Adult Tobacco Survey (ATS): CDC Recommended Questions: Supplemental Section D: Environmental Tobacco Smoke, 2003	2.3.4; 2.3.7	State health departments Office on Smoking and Health, Centers for Disease Control and Prevention, (770) 488–5703
Adult Tobacco Survey (ATS): CDC Recommended Questions: Supplemental Section F: Policy Issues, 2003	1.6.4; 1.6.5; 1.6.7[NR]; 2.3.10[NR]; 3.8.5	State health departments Office on Smoking and Health, Centers for Disease Control and Prevention, (770) 488–5703
Adult Tobacco Survey (ATS): CDC Recommended Questions: Supplemental Section G: Parental Involvement, 2003	1.10.4	State health departments Office on Smoking and Health, Centers for Disease Control and Prevention, (770) 488–5703
American Lung Association's State Legislated Actions on Tobacco Issues (SLATI)	1.8.1	http://slati.lungusa.org See "Policy tracking"

Data source	Indicator numbers	For more information
American Smoking and Health Survey (ASHES), 2003	3.8.7; 3.9.5	▷ http://tobacco.rti.org/data/New/surveys.cfm
Americans for Nonsmokers' Rights (ANR)	1.8.1; 1.8.2; 1.8.3; 1.8.4; 2.4.1	▷ http://www.no-smoke.org ▷ See "Policy tracking"
Arizona Workplace Survey	2.4.2	▷ http://www.tepp.org/evaluation ▷ See "Worksite survey"
Behavioral Risk Factor Surveillance System (BRFSS), 2002	3.11.1; 3.13.2[NR]	▷ http://www.cdc.gov/brfss
Behavioral Risk Factor Surveillance System (BRFSS), 2003	2.8.3; 3.14.1	▷ http://www.cdc.gov/brfss
Behavioral Risk Factor Surveillance System (BRFSS): Tobacco Use Prevention Module, 2000	1.6.7[NR]; 2.3.7; 2.3.10[NR]	▷ http://www.cdc.gov/brfss
Behavioral Risk Factor Surveillance System (BRFSS): Tobacco Use Prevention Module, 2002	3.13.1	▷ http://www.cdc.gov/brfss
Birth certificate data	3.14.2	▷ State vital statistics and records
California Adult Tobacco Survey (CATS), 1999	2.3.4; 2.7.1; 2.7.2	▷ http://www.dhs.ca.gov/ps/cdic/ccb/TCS/html/Evaluation_Resources.htm
California Independent Evaluation: Adult Survey, 1997	2.3.9	▷ http://www.dhs.ca.gov/ps/cdic/ccb/TCS/html/Evaluation_Resources.htm
California Independent Evaluation: Adult Survey, 2000	2.7.5	▷ http://www.dhs.ca.gov/ps/cdic/ccb/TCS/html/Evaluation_Resources.htm
California Independent Evaluation: Policy Enforcement Survey: Exposure to Environmental Tobacco Smoke, 2000	2.5.1; 2.5.2; 2.5.3	▷ http://www.dhs.ca.gov/ps/cdic/ccb/TCS/html/Evaluation_Resources.htm
California Independent Evaluation: Policy Enforcement Survey: Youth Access to Tobacco, 2000	1.8.5; 1.8.6	▷ http://www.dhs.ca.gov/ps/cdic/ccb/TCS/html/Evaluation_Resources.htm
California Independent Evaluation: Youth Survey, 2000	1.6.8[NR]; 1.7.9; 1.7.10; 2.6.5	▷ http://www.dhs.ca.gov/ps/cdic/ccb/TCS/html/Evaluation_Resources.htm
California Tobacco Industry Monitoring Evaluation: Project SMART Money	1.9.5; 1.9.10	▷ http://www.ttac.org/enews/mailer09-30-03full.html ▷ See "Event sponsorship tracking system" and "Tobacco industry monitoring system"

Data source	Indicator numbers	For more information
California Tobacco Use Prevention Education Evaluation: District Coordinator Survey, 2003	1.7.4	http://www.dhs.ca.gov/ps/cdic/ccb/TCS/html/Evaluation_Resources.htm
California Tobacco Use Prevention Education Evaluation: Teacher Survey, 2003	1.7.2; 1.7.4; 1.7.5	http://www.dhs.ca.gov/ps/cdic/ccb/TCS/html/Evaluation_Resources.htm
California Youth Tobacco Survey (CA YTS), 1999	1.11.6[NR]	http://www.dhs.ca.gov/ps/cdic/ccb/TCS/html/Evaluation_Resources.htm
California's BREATH (Smoke-Free Bars, Workplaces, and Communities Program)	2.6.3	http://www.breath-ala.org
Campaign for Tobacco-Free Kids (CTFK)	1.12.1; 3.12.1	http://www.tobaccofreekids.org
CDC Pregnancy Risk Assessment Monitoring System (PRAMS), Phase 4, 2000–2003	3.9.7; 3.14.2; 3.14.3	http://www.cdc.gov/reproductivehealth
CDC School Health Profiles: Lead Health Education Teacher Questionnaire (Profiles), 2002	1.7.2; 1.7.3; 1.7.4; 1.7.5	Division of Adolescent and School Health, Centers for Disease Control and Prevention, (888) 231–6405 http://www.cdc.gov/HealthyYouth/index.htm State health departments
CDC School Health Profiles: School Principal Questionnaire (Profiles), 2002	1.7.1; 1.7.6; 1.7.11; 1.9.7; 2.4.5	Division of Adolescent and School Health, Centers for Disease Control and Prevention, (888) 231–6405 http://www.cdc.gov/HealthyYouth/index.htm State health departments
CDC State Tobacco Activities Tracking and Evaluation (STATE) system	1.8.7; 1.12.1; 2.4.6; 2.8.1; 2.8.2; 3.12.1; 3.14.4	http://www.cdc.gov/tobacco/STATESystem
CDC Youth Risk Behavior Surveillance System (YRBSS), 2003	1.7.10; 1.11.2; 1.11.4; 1.11.5; 1.13.1; 1.13.2; 1.14.1; 1.14.2; 2.6.5; 2.8.2; 2.8.3; 3.11.2; 3.14.1	http://www.cdc.gov/nccdphp/dash/yrbs/index.htm
Center for Responsive Politics (CRP)	1.9.11; 1.9.12	http://www.opensecrets.org
Current Population Survey: Tobacco Use Supplement (CPS TUS), 2003	2.4.2; 2.4.3; 3.11.1	http://www.riskfactor.cancer.gov/studies/tus-cps http://www.census.gov/apsd/techdoc/cps/cps-main.html

Data source	Indicator numbers	For more information
Decision Maker or Opinion Leader Survey	3.8.8	▸ State Decision Maker Tobacco Survey (California Independent Evaluation, Opinion Leader Survey), 1997 http://www.dhs.ca.gov/ps/cdic/ccb/TCS/html/Evaluation_Resources.htm
Direct observation of employees' and patrons' behavior	2.6.3	▸ http://www.breath-ala.org ▸ See "California's BREATH (Smoke-Free Bars, Workplaces, and Communities Program)"
Enforcement Agency Survey	1.8.5; 1.8.6; 2.5.1; 2.5.2; 2.5.3	▸ California Independent Evaluation: Policy Enforcement Survey, Youth Access to Tobacco, 2000
Environmental scan of tobacco advertising and promotional practices in retail outlets	1.9.1; 1.9.3; 1.9.7	▸ Operation Storefront: Youth Against Tobacco Advertising and Promotion Initiative http://www.dhs.ca.gov/ps/cdic/ccb/TCS/html/Evaluation_Resources.htm
Event sponsorship tracking system	1.9.5	▸ Project SMART Money http://www.ttac.org/enews/mailer09-30-03full.html#LinkF ▸ Rosenberg NJ, Siegel M. Use of corporate sponsorship as a tobacco marketing tool: a review of tobacco industry sponsorship in the USA, 1995–99. *Tob Control.* 2001; 10(3):239–46
Federal Election Commission (FEC)	1.9.12	▸ http://www.fec.gov ▸ See "Public records of political contributions"
Legacy Media Tracking Survey (LMTS), 2003	1.6.1; 1.6.2; 2.3.1; 2.3.2; 3.8.1; 3.8.2	▸ http://tobacco.rti.org/data/lmts.cfm
Media Tracking Service	1.9.8; 1.9.9	▸ See "TNS Media Intelligence Competitive Media Reporting (CMR)" ▸ Stillman FA, Cronin KA, Evans WD, Ulasevich A. Can media advocacy influence newspaper coverage of tobacco: measuring the effectiveness of the American Stop Smoking Intervention Study's (ASSIST) media advocacy strategies. *Tob Control.* 2001;10(2):137–44.
National Social Climate Survey of Tobacco Control, 2001	2.3.3	▸ http://www.ssrc.msstate.edu/socialclimate
Operation Storefront: Youth Against Tobacco Advertising and Promotion Initiative	1.9.1; 1.9.3; 1.9.7	▸ http://www.dhs.ca.gov/ps/cdic/ccb/TCS/html/Evaluation_Resources.htm ▸ See "Environmental scan"

Data source	Indicator numbers	For more information
Partnership for Prevention, Tobacco Survey: National Survey of Employer-sponsored Health Plans, 2002	3.7.6	http://www.mercerhr.com
Policy tracking system	1.8.1; 1.8.2; 1.8.3; 1.8.4; 1.9.2; 1.9.4; 1.9.6; 2.4.1	Americans for Nonsmokers' Rights http://www.no-smoke.org State Legislated Actions on Tobacco Issues (SLATI) online database http://slati.lungusa.org
Public records of political contributions	1.9.11; 1.9.12	Collected by the Office of State Secretary or equivalent at local level in each state See "Federal Election Commission (FEC)" Givel MS, Glantz SA. Tobacco lobby political influence on US state legislatures in the 1990s. *Tob Control.* 2001; 10 (2):124–34.
Quitline call monitoring	3.7.1; 3.7.2[NR]; 3.7.3	Miller CL, Wakefield M, Roberts L. Uptake and effectiveness of the Australian telephone quitline service in the context of a mass media campaign. *Tob Control.* 2003; 12 (Suppl 2): ii53–8.
State departments of revenue	1.12.1; 2.8.1; 3.12.1; 3.14.4	State tax sales data, tobacco product excise taxes
Substance Abuse and Mental Health Services Administration (SAMHSA) Compliance Checks	1.11.1	http://prevention.samhsa.gov/tobacco/guidance.asp
TNS Media Intelligence Competitive Media Reporting (CMR)	1.9.8	http://www.tnsmi-cmr.com/products/index.html See "Media Tracking Service"
Tobacco industry fiscal reports	1.9.11	http://www.altria.com/investors/02_01_annualreport.asp http://www.reynoldsamerican.com/Investors/sharedocs_cover.asp
Tobacco industry monitoring system	1.9.10	See "California Tobacco Industry Monitoring Evaluation: Project SMART Money"
University of California at San Diego, California Tobacco Survey (CTS): Adult Attitudes and Practices, 1996	1.6.7[NR]; 2.3.8; 2.3.10[NR]	http://ssdc.ucsd.edu/tobacco http://www.dhs.ca.gov/ps/cdic/ccb/TCS/html/Evaluation_Resources.htm
Worksite Survey	2.4.2	See "Arizona Workplace Survey"

Data source	Indicator numbers	For more information
Youth Tobacco Survey (YTS): CDC Recommended Questions: Core, 2004	1.6.3; 1.7.8; 1.7.9; 1.7.10; 1.10.1; 1.10.2; 1.10.3; 1.10.5; 1.11.2; 1.11.3; 1.11.4; 1.11.5; 1.13.1; 1.13.2; 1.14.1; 1.14.2; 2.3.5; 2.6.5; 2.7.3; 2.7.5; 2.8.2; 2.8.3; 3.8.3; 3.11.2; 3.13.1; 3.13.2^{NR}; 3.14.1	▸ State health departments ▸ Office on Smoking and Health, Centers for Disease Control and Prevention, (770) 488–5703
Youth Tobacco Survey (YTS): Supplemental Questions, 2004	3.11.3	▸ Office on Smoking and Health, Centers for Disease Control and Prevention, (770) 488–5703

References

1. MacDonald G, Starr G, Schooley M, Yee SL, Klimowski K, Turner K. *Introduction to program evaluation for comprehensive tobacco control programs.* Atlanta, GA: Centers for Disease Control and Prevention; 2001.

2. Yee SL, Schooley M. *Surveillance and evaluation data resources for comprehensive tobacco control programs.* Atlanta, GA: Centers for Disease Control and Prevention; 2001.

Glossary

Activities
The events or actions that are part of a tobacco control program.

Attitudes
Biases, inclinations, or tendencies that influence a person's response to situations, activities, other people, or program goals.

Awareness
The extent to which people in the target population know about an event, activity, or campaign.

Capacity
The resources (e.g., staff, data-collection systems, funds) needed to conduct a tobacco control program or to evaluate such a program.

CDC
Centers for Disease Control and Prevention.

Cognitive-behavioral interventions
Activities based on the premise that people can learn new behaviors to use in response to stimuli and that the thought processes that serve as intermediate steps between stimuli and behaviors can be altered, thereby influencing behavior. Basic applications of this theory for tobacco-use cessation are:

  Establishing self-awareness of tobacco use.

  Providing the motivation to quit.

  Preparing to quit.

  Providing strategies to maintain abstinence.

Consumption
The number of tax-paid cigarettes (pack of 20) purchased by consumers in a particular calendar year.

Data
Documented information or evidence.

Data sources
Surveys or surveillance systems used to gather data.

Evaluation
The process of determining whether programs—or certain aspects of programs—are appropriate, adequate, effective, or efficient and, if not, how to make them so.

Ever-smoker
A person who gives a positive answer to the question "Have you tried cigarette smoking, even one or two puffs?"

Example data source
Surveys or surveillance systems used to measure an indicator and the population on which the data are needed.

Face validity
The degree to which data on an indicator appear reliable to stakeholders and policy makers.

FDA
U.S. Food and Drug Administration.

Goal area
One of the four components of the overall goal of CDC's National Tobacco Control Program.

HHS
U.S. Department of Health and Human Services.

Implementation
Carrying out or putting into effect a plan or program.

Indicator
An observable and measurable characteristic or change that shows the progress a program is making toward achieving a specified outcome.

Indicator profile
The term used in this manual for a table with detailed information on one indicator listed in this publication (see page 29 for an example).

Indicator rating table
The term used in this publication for the list of the indicators associated with one outcome in one NTCP logic model. The experts' rating for each indicator is also included (see page 28 for an example).

Inputs
Resources used to plan and set up a tobacco control program.

Intervention
The method, device, or process used to prevent an undesirable outcome or create a desirable outcome.

Logic model
A graphic depiction of the presumed causal pathways that connect program inputs, activities, outputs, and outcomes.

Media messages
Anti-tobacco information provided to the public through various media (e.g., television, radio, billboards).

Minors
Persons younger than 18 years of age.

Morbidity
Disease or disease rate.

NCI
National Cancer Institute.

Never-smoker
A person who gives a negative answer to the question "Have you tried cigarette smoking, even one or two puffs?"

NIH
National Institutes of Health.

NTCP
National Tobacco Control Program.

Observation
A method of collecting data that does not involve any communication with the subjects being studied. The investigators merely watch for particular behaviors and record what they see.

Opinion leader survey
Collection of information (data) from leaders in the community.

Outcome
The results of an activity such as a countermarketing campaign or an effort to reduce nonsmokers' exposure to smoke. Outcomes can be short-term, intermediate, or long-term.

Outcome components
The term used in this publication for the short-term, intermediate, and long-term results described in the NTCP logic models for the first three goal areas. These are the results expected if tobacco control programs provide the needed inputs and engage in the recommended activities also described in the logic models.

Outcome evaluation
The systematic collection of information to assess the effect of a program or an activity within such a program to reduce the adverse health effects of tobacco use. Good evaluation allows evaluators to draw conclusions about the merit of a program and make recommendations about the program's direction.

Outcome overview
The term used in this publication for the summary of the scientific evidence in support of the assumption that achieving an outcome on an NTCP logic model affects all concurrent and later activities and outcomes (see page 25 for an example).

Outputs
The direct products of a program (e.g., the materials needed for a media campaign).

Payers
Health insurance organizations that reimburse providers for services when coverage is purchased by companies, government agencies, or other consortia. Also self-insured companies, government agencies, or other consortia that purchase health care benefits for a group of individuals and use an insurer as a fiscal intermediary to process claims and reimburse for services.

Population group
Individuals from which data about a given indicator can most commonly be collected.

Preemption
Federal or state legislation that prevents states or local jurisdictions from enacting tobacco control laws more stringent than or otherwise different from the federal or state law.

Prevalence
The amount of a factor of interest (e.g., tobacco use, awareness of a media campaign) present in a specified population at a specified time.

Process evaluation
Systematic collection of information to determine how well a program is set up and operating.

Program evaluation
Systematic collection of information about activities, characteristics, and outcomes of programs, used to make judgments about a program, improve its effectiveness, or inform decisions about future program activities.

Purchaser
Purchasers include companies, government agencies, or other consortia that purchase health care benefits for a group of individuals.

Rate
A measurement of how frequently an event occurs in a certain population at one point in time or during a particular period of time.

Reach
The number of people or households that receive a program's message or intervention.

Recent successful quit attempts
Proportion of former smokers who have quit in the previous 12 months.

Resources
Assets available or expected to be available for program operations. Resources include people, equipment, facilities, and other items used to plan, implement, and evaluate public health programs whether or not they are paid for directly with public funds.

Self service tobacco sales
Sales that allow customers to handle tobacco products before purchasing them.

Social source
A person or location from which tobacco products are obtained other than a tobacco product retailer.

Some-day smoker
A current smoker who gives a "smoked on some days" response.

Surveillance
The ongoing, systematic collection, analysis, and interpretation of data about a hazard, risk factor, exposure, or health event.

Survey
A quantitative method of collecting information on a target population at one point in time. Surveys can be conducted by interview (in person or by telephone) or by questionnaire.

Susceptibility
The intention to smoke or the absence of a strong intention not to smoke.

Sustained abstinence
Complete cessation of tobacco use for 6 months or longer.

Theory of change
Intellectual framework for understanding the process of behavior change.

Utility
The extent to which evaluation produces reports that are disseminated to relevant audiences, that inform program decisions, and that have a beneficial effect.

How to Use the Rating Tables

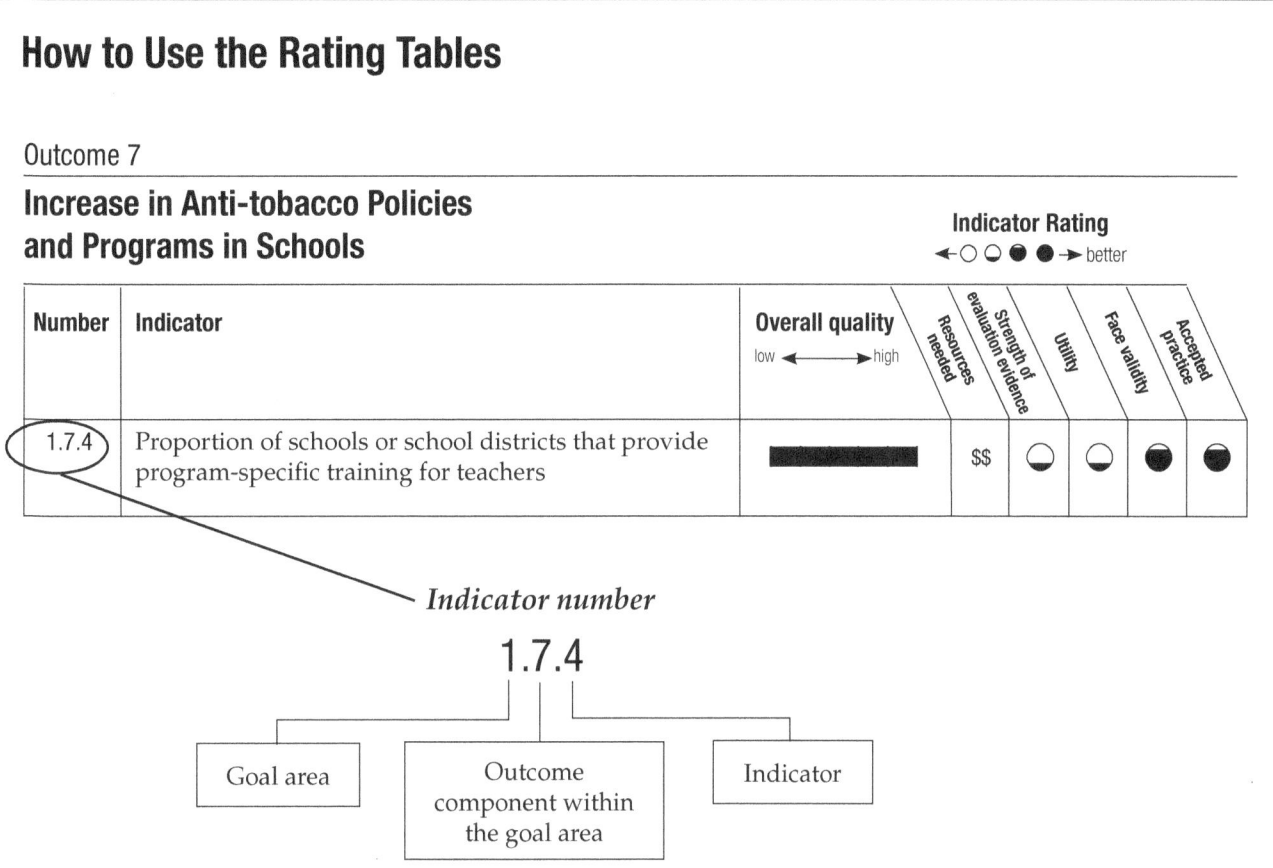

Overall quality: The general worth of the indicator as it relates to evaluating tobacco control programs.

Resources needed: Dollar signs show the amount of resources (funds, time, and effort) needed to collect and analyze data on the indicator using the most commonly available data source: the more dollar signs (maximum four), the more resources needed. The dollar signs do not represent specific amounts because the actual cost of measuring and analyzing an indicator varies according to the existing capacity of a state health department or organization to evaluate its programs.

Strength of evaluation evidence: The degree to which scientific evidence supports that implementing interventions to affect change in a given indicator (e.g., proportion of schools or school districts that provide program-specific training for teachers) will lead to a measurable downstream outcome (e.g., reduced susceptibility to experimentation with tobacco products).

Utility: The extent to which the indicator is useful for answering evaluation questions for comprehensive state tobacco control programs.

Face validity: The degree to which data on the indicator would appear valid to tobacco program stakeholders, such as policy makers.

Accepted practice: The degree to which using the indicator to measure a tobacco control program's progress is consistent with accepted practice.

www.ingramcontent.com/pod-product-compliance
Lightning Source LLC
Chambersburg PA
CBHW081719170526
45167CB00009B/3628